Physical and Occupational Therapy: Drug Implications for Practice

Physical and Occupational Therapy: Drug Implications for Practice

Edited by
Terry Malone, Ed.D., P.T., A.T.C.

Associate Professor of Physical Therapy
Assistant Professor of Surgery
Executive Director of Sports Medicine
Duke University
Durham, North Carolina
Formerly Dean of the Krannert Graduate School of Physical Therapy
University of Indianapolis
Indianapolis, Indiana

16 Contributors

J.B. Lippincott
Philadelphia
London, Mexico City, New York,
St. Louis, São Paulo, Sydney

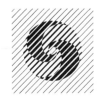

A Lippincott Physical Therapy Title

Acquisitions Editor: *Lisa Biello*
Manuscript Editor: *Marguerite Hague*
Indexer: *Ann Blum*
Design Coordinator: *Michelle Gerdes*
Cover Designer: *Joe Netherwood*
Production Manager: *Carol A. Florence*
Production Coordinator: *Kathryn Rule*
Compositor: *McFarland Graphics and Design*
Text Printer/Binder: *R. R. Donnelly and Sons*
Cover Printer: *Phoenix Color Corp.*

    3 5 6 4 2

Physical and Occupational Therapy:
Drug Implications for Practice
edited by Terry Malone with 16 contributors.
    p. cm.
    Bibliography
    Includes index.
    ISBN 0-397-50757-7
    1. Pharmacology.   2. Physical therapists.
3. Occupational therapists.   I. Malone, Terry, 1950–
RM301.P49 1989
615.8′2—dc19   88-9236
                                          CIP

The authors and publisher have exerted every effort to ensure that drug selection and dosage set forth in this text are in accord with current recommendations and practice at the time of publication. However, in view of ongoing research, changes in government regulations, and the constant flow of information relating to drug therapy and drug reactions, the reader is urged to check the package insert for each drug for any change in indications and dosage and for added warnings and precautions. This is particularly important when the recommended agent is a new or infrequently employed drug.

Contributors

Marlene A. Aldo-Benson, M.D.
Professor of Medicine, Microbiology, and Immunology
Rheumatology Division
Indiana University School of Medicine
Indianapolis, Indiana

Claudia K. Allen, M.A., O.T.R., F.A.O.T.A.
Clinical Associate Professor in Occupational Therapy and Psychiatry
    and the Behavioral Sciences
University of Southern California
Downie, California;
Chief of Occupational Therapy, Psychiatry
Los Angeles County
University of Southern California Medical Center

George R. Aronoff, M.S., M.D.
Professor of Medicine and Pharmacology
Director of Kidney Disease Program
University of Louisville Hospital
Louisville, Kentucky

Rebecca Barton, M.S., O.T.R.
Assistant Supervisor
Adult Physical Disabilities Occupational Therapy Department
Indiana University Hospitals
Indianapolis, Indiana

Lawrence P. Cahalin, B.S., P.T.
Director
Cardiovascular Assessment and Rehabilitation
CIGNA Health Plans
Pomona, California;
Blessey Cardiovascular Assessment and Treatment Services, Inc.
Manhattan Beach, California

Barbara H. Connolly, Ed.D., P.T.
Associate Professor and Chairman
Department of Rehabilitation Sciences
University of Tennessee
Memphis, Tennessee

Judy Feinberg, M.S., O.T.R., F.A.O.T.A.
Assistant Professor
Occupational Therapy Program
Indiana University School of Medicine
Indianapolis, Indiana

Anne L. Harrison, M.S., P.T.
Physical Therapist
Lexington Physical Therapy
Lexington, Kentucky

Clyde B. Killian, M.S., P.T.; Ph.D. candidate, Ohio University
Assistant Professor and Clinical Coordinator
Ohio University School of Physical Therapy
Athens, Ohio

Carole Bernstein Lewis, P.T., M.S.G., M.P.A., Ph.D.
Associate Professor of Clinical Medicine
George Washington University School of Medicine
Washington, D.C.;
Adjunct Associate Professor
Massachusetts General Hospital Institute of Health Professions
Boston, Massachusetts;
Co-Director
Physical Therapy Services of Washington, D.C., Inc.
Washington, D.C.

Terry Malone, Ed.D., P.T., A.T.C.
Associate Professor of Physical Therapy
Assistant Professor of Surgery
Executive Director of Sports Medicine
Duke University
Durham, North Carolina;
Formerly Dean of the Krannert Graduate School of Physical Therapy
University of Indianapolis
Indianapolis, Indiana

Trinda F. Metzger, M.S., P.T.
Clinical Adjunct Faculty
Krannert Graduate School of Physical Therapy
University of Indianapolis
Indianapolis, Indiana;
Outpatient Coordinator of Back Rehabilitation
Community Hospitals
Indianapolis, Indiana

Timothy E. Poe, Pharm.D.
Associate Professor of Family and Community Medicine (Clinical Pharmacy)
The Bowman Gray School of Medicine of Wake Forest University
Winston-Salem, North Carolina;
Clinical Associate Professor
University of North Carolina
School of Pharmacy
Chapel Hill, North Carolina

William E. Prentice, Ph.D., P.T., A.T.C.
Associate Professor of Physical Education
Associate Professor of Physical Therapy
Coordinator of the Sports Medicine Program
University of North Carolina
Chapel Hill, North Carolina

Christina M. Sokolek, B.S., B.A., P.T.
Senior Physical Therapist, Adult Staff
University Hospital
Indiana University
Indianapolis, Indiana

Diane M. White, B.S., P.D.
Pharmacy Doctor
University of Maryland School of Pharmacy

Cynthia Coffin Zadai, M.S., P.T.
Assistant Professor
Massachusetts General Hospital Institute of Health Professions;
Director
Chest Physical Therapy
Beth Israel Hospital
Boston, Massachusetts

Preface

Pharmacology has not been an integral part of most therapy curricula. The typical therapist has received "bits and pieces" of pharmacologic management training. The concept for this text arose from attempts to present pharmacology to students in entry level curricula and to therapists in advanced clinical programs.

Rehabilitation therapists assume a much greater role in patient management with the advent of diagnostic related groups (DRG), direct patient access to therapy services, specialization of therapy services, and ambulatory surgery. Patients that previously were hospitalized are now cared for at home and in outpatient settings. Therapists must increase their knowledge of pharmacology if they are to provide adequate patient care in these changing environments.

Physical and Occupational Therapy: Drug Implications for Practice is designed for both the student and the practicing clinician. The student will be exposed to basic pharmacology with an emphasis on "how to find the answers," while the clinician will gain perspective on how pharmacology impacts specialty areas. Generic names for drugs are used throughout the text, with trade names appearing in parentheses.

I would like to thank all the dedicated clinicians who shared their expertise in these pages. Without their efforts this text would not have been possible. I would also like to thank their "significant others" who allowed their contributions!

Terry Malone, Ed.D., P.T., A.T.C.

Contents

Physical and Occupational Therapy: Drug Implications for Practice

Pharmacology 1

Timothy E. Poe

In this chapter an attempt will be made to acquaint the student/practitioner with the general principles of pharmacology and the general classes of drugs used in the treatment of many diseases. Pharmacology may be difficult for some, primarily because of the vast numbers of agents used in the practice of medicine today. For the most part, this chapter will not concentrate on specific agents but, rather, on principles and examples to illustrate them. Also in this chapter sources of drug information are given so that the reader may obtain pertinent drug information when needed.

The word *pharmacology* was derived from the Greek *pharmakon*, which meant *drug, medicine,* or *poison,* and *logos,* meaning *reason,* and *-logy* meaning the *study of.* Thus, one may define pharmacology as the study of the interaction of chemicals with living organisms. Of course, this is usually in the context of using drugs in patients to bring about some desired effect. Drugs may be defined as chemical compounds used in the treatment, prevention, or diagnosis of disease. For example, antibiotics are chemical compounds used to treat various infections; vaccines are considered drugs because they help prevent diseases; and radiocontrast media are considered drugs because they aid in diagnosis of disease.

Pharmacology is often divided into pharmacokinetics and pharmacodynamics. *Pharmacokinetics* deals with the fate of drugs in the body, including absorption, distribution, metabolism, and excretion. One might think of this as what the body does to the drug. *Pharmacodynamics* deals with the actions and effects of the drug on tissues and organs of the body. In other words, pharmacodynamics is what the drug does to the body. These topics will be dealt with in more detail later in this chapter.

Pharmacotherapeutics is the study of the use of drugs in the treatment, prevention, or diagnosis of disease. This aspect of pharmacology correlates pharmacodynamics with the pathophysiology, microbiology, or biochemistry of the disease.

Pharmacy means the *art* of preparing, compounding, and dispensing medicines. It also is the place where such medicines are prepared, stored, and dispensed. In today's society the pharmacist may rarely compound medicines because most medications are prepared by a pharmaceutical manufacturer. However, emphasis is shifting toward the pharmacist as a provider of drug information and counselor to patients about their medications.

Toxicology is the study of the harmful effects of drugs and chemicals. Most drugs are screened in animals before studied in humans to determine their toxicologic properties.

DRUG NAMES

Sometimes the names of drugs become confusing becasue there are at least three names for every drug. The *chemical name* is usually referred to only in the product circular or original reference materials. It is the chemical description of the drug. For example, the chemical name for acetaminophen is *N*-acetyl-*p*-aminophenol. The *generic*, or *nonproprietary*, name is the name assigned to the drug when it is found to have potential therapeutic usefulness. The nonproprietary name for *N*-acetyl-*p*-aminophenol is acetaminophen. The proprietary name (trade or brand name) is the name given to the drug by the manufacturer and is usually shorter and easier to remember than the nonproprietary or chemical name. Tylenol is an example of a proprietary name for acetaminophen.

PHARMACOKINETICS

To be effective, drugs must get to their site of action, thus, a discussion of pharmacokinetics would be in order. Remember, pharmacokinetics is the absorption, distribution, metabolism, and excretion of the drug (Fig. 1-1).

Drugs usually must reach the systemic circulation to reach their site of action (except for topical or many inhaled drugs). Drugs may be administered by mouth (*p.o.*) or parenterally. Parenteral administration includes intravenous, intramuscular, subcutaneous, and intradermal administration.

The rate and extent of absorption after oral administration are dependent on several factors, including the chemical characteristics of the drug, the oral dosage form (tablet, capsule, solution, etc.), the gastric-emptying time, and sometimes, the *p*H of the stomach and intestine. There are several oral dosage forms available, some of which are discussed in the following paragraph.

Solutions are liquid preparations that contain one or more dissolved drugs, usually in water. Liquid preparations that contain alcohol are either *elixers* or *tinctures*. *Suspensions* are liquid preparations that are composed of finely divided drug particles that will not dissolve into solution. These preparations must be shaken well to obtain a uniform mixture before administration. *Solid dosage* forms include

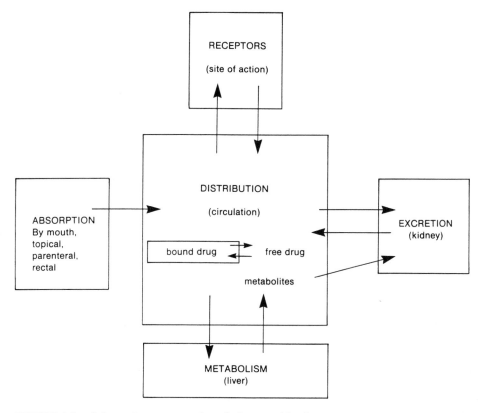

FIGURE 1-1. Schematic representation of pharmacokinetics.

capsules, which contain medication enclosed in a gelatin shell. The shell dissolves in the stomach or intestine releasing the medication for absorption. *Tablets* are solid dosage forms that contain other ingredients (in addition to the medication) to hold them together until they are taken. Tablets are sometimes coated with sugar or other coatings to prevent the patient from tasting the drug and other times are simply compressed tablets (such as most aspirin). One particular type of tablet is made such that it will not dissolve until the drug is in the small intestine. These are referred to as *enteric-coated* tablets. *Sustained-release* preparations are usually capsules or tablets and are made such that not all of the drug is released for absorption at one time. These preparations may enhance compliance because the drug does not have to be administered as often.

Only dissolved drugs can be absorbed from the intestine. Drugs are absorbed most quickly from solutions because these preparations are already in a liquid form and do not have to be dissolved. Slowest absorption would be from a sustained-release product, whereas tablets and capsules have intermediate absorption. *Bioavailability* is the study of the completeness of absorption. It is usually related to the amount of drug absorbed by mouth to the amount administered intravenously. Although the dosage form may make a difference in the bioavailability of a drug, it is usually the characteristics of the drug, itself, that determine the completeness of absorption. The rate of absorption, however, is more likely to be affected by the dosage form.

Drugs are usually absorbed by simple diffusion. Lipid- or fat- soluble drugs are absorbed more readily than drugs that are more water-soluble. Drugs that have an ionic charge do not pass readily through membranes. Hence, some drugs are affected by *p*H changes in the gastrointestinal tract and may not be absorbed as well. An example of this is a drug that is a weak acid. Aspirin is a weak acid that in the acidic environment of the stomach is relatively un-ionized. This aids absorption in the stomach and upper portion of the small intestine. If aspirin is administered with an antacid, more will be ionized and, as a result, it will not be absorbed as readily in the stomach.

Gastric-emptying time may also be important in drug absorption. As one might imagine, if a patient has a fast gastrointestinal-transit time, the drug is in contact with the intestinal mucosa for a shorter period and may not be as completely absorbed.

Drugs may also be administered *sublingually* (under the tongue) or *bucally* (between the cheek and gum) for rapid absorption. The drug usually administered in this manner is nitroglycerin, given for angina pectoris.

Parenteral administration of a drug is required usually when a patient needs a more immediate effect, the patient cannot take the drug by mouth, or the drug is not absorbed when taken orally. The quickest way to get the drug into the circulation is to inject the drug directly into the venous circulation, hence, intravenous injection. Drugs are rapidly distributed and, generally, quickly reach their site of action. The disadvantages of this method are that sterility of the drug and a sterile technique must be preserved, and caution must be taken not to administer too much drug because it would be particularly easy to produce dangerously high drug levels. *Intramuscular injection* (into a muscle mass) also requires sterile procedures. Relatively rapid absorption is obtained because of good blood supplies in muscle, but this absorption is not as rapid as with intravenous injection. This form of administration is useful when suspensions of drugs must be given, such as with procaine penicillin given for an infection. *Subcutaneous injection* is giving the drug under the skin between the skin and the muscle mass. Absorption is slower from subcutaneous tissue than from muscle. Drugs such as insulin are usually administered subcutaneously. As with other injections, sterility must be maintained. Drugs that are suspensions may be given either subcutaneously or (usually) intramuscularly to produce a sustained-release effect (Table 1-1).

After absorption, the drug is carried in the blood to its site of action. This is known as the *distribution phase*. Not only is the drug taken to its site of action, but it may also be distributed into other areas of the body, such as the central nervous system and adipose tissue. Generally, the smaller the molecular makeup and the more lipid-soluble it is, the better the drug is able to penetrate tissues and the more widely distributed it becomes. Drugs such as anesthetics (very lipid-soluble) are widely distributed and penetrate the central nervous system quite rapidly.

Transportation in the blood is facilitated by binding of the drug to serum protein, usually albumin. This is occasionally a problem with two or more drugs that compete for the same binding site, causing higher "free" levels of one of the drugs and more drug effect. *Free drug* is that portion of the total drug in the plasma that is not bound to plasma protein, whereas *bound drug* is the portion that is bound to the protein. Only free drug can penetrate capillary walls to reach its site of action. Once

TABLE 1-1
Routes of Administration

Route	Speed of Absorption*	Comments
Oral	+	Usually most convenient; nonsterile
Sublingual	++	Convenient; nonsterile; bypass liver, direct to circulation
Buccal	++	As for sublingual
Rectal	+ to ++	Bypass liver; not convenient; may irritate rectal mucosa
Subcutaneous	++ to +++	Sterility necessary; painful; may be used in unconscious patient; may be used for soluble and insoluble forms
Intramuscular	+++	More rapid absorption (blood supply good); sterility necessary; may be used in unconscious patient; may be used for soluble and insoluble forms
Intravenous	++++	Directly into circulation; most rapid absorption; sterility necessary; must use soluble forms

*Author's opinion. Speed of absorption is variable, depending on dosage form used. This is a rough comparison to give the student an overall idea of differences in absorption from various sites.

a drug is in the plasma, an equilibrium is set up such that as a drug is eliminated or reaches its site of action, more drug is released from albumin.

The magnitude of distribution is measured in terms of volume of distribution, which is a hypothetical volume that shows the relationship between the available drug and the serum concentration. The *volume of distribution* is that volume, or apparent volume, of fluid through which the drug would have to be distributed to produce the existing serum concentration.

Drugs are eliminated from the body by two primary mechanisms, metabolism and excretion. *Metabolism* is the process of transforming drugs into more water-soluble compounds so that they may be excreted by the kidneys. Metabolism takes place chiefly in the liver, although other organs may sometimes be involved, such as the kidneys and circulatory system. Although metabolism of drugs by the liver usually changes active drugs into inactive compounds, a few drugs are not active until transformed by the liver. In fact, most drugs are *detoxified* in the liver; however, in some rare instances, metabolites may be more toxic than the parent compound. Many drugs are both metabolized by the liver and excreted unchanged by the kidney. The most common drug biotransformation reactions include oxidation, reduction, hydrolysis, and conjugation. Many drugs are metabolized by the microsomal mixed-function oxidase enzyme system in the liver. This is important because these enzymes are inducible and some drugs may stimulate the metabolism of other drugs. The opposite is also true, some drugs may decrease the metabolism of the other, resulting in higher-than-normal levels. Some drug interactions occur by this mechanism.

Excretion of drugs or their metabolites is carried out by the kidney by two processes, *glomerular filtration* and *tubular secretion*. Drugs that are simply filtered through the glomerulus may be carried through the tubule into the urine or, to some extent, reabsorbed, depending on the drug's lipid solubility and *p*H of the urine. Other drugs are eliminated by active secretion by the tubule into the urine. In any event, it should be obvious that patients with decreased kidney function (for example, renal disease or elderly patients) may have problems eliminating certain drugs that are primarily excreted unchanged in the urine. Drugs may also be excreted in other body fluids, such as milk, saliva, and sweat, as well as in feces.

Although the major processes of pharmacokinetics have already been discussed, several other terms and principles need to be appreciated. The rate of disappearance of a drug from the body, whether by metabolism, excretion, or a combination, is known as a drug half-life. The *half-life* of the drug may be defined as the time it takes for half the drug in the body to be eliminated. Most of the time it is measured in hours; however, for some drugs the half-life is measured in days and, for others, in minutes. The half-life of a drug is useful information to determine how long the drug "hangs around" in the body. Not only would it tell us something about how long the drug remains in the body, but it also gives us some indication on how often to administer some drugs. The dosage interval for many drugs (mostly those that are not sustained-release) is equal to the half-life.

Drugs tend to accumulate in the body if given on a regular schedule until the amount eliminated is equal to the amount administered. This is called the *steady state* and is usually reached after five half-lives of the drug have passed, assuming the drug has been administered regularly. It is important to realize that drugs with long half-lives may take several days to weeks to reach steady state. For example, digoxin, a medication used to treat congestive heart failure, has a half-life of approximately 44 hr in an individual with normal kidney function. If the patient is not given a loading dose, he may not reach the final serum concentration equilibrium (steady state) for 10 days.

PHARMACODYNAMICS

The study of pharmacodynamics provides information on how drugs bring about their effects on the body. In general, drugs act by forming a bond, usually reversible, with some cellular constituent (receptor). Most drugs act on a specific receptor. Drugs that react with a receptor and elicit a response are called *agonists*, whereas drugs that act on a receptor and prevent the action of agonists are called *antagonists*. The typical example of this action is the histamine–antihistamine interaction. Antihistamines block the action of histamine (to produce all those symptoms of hay fever) by attaching to the histamine receptor and blocking the binding of histamine. *Partial agonists* also exist and are drugs that bind with a receptor but cannot produce maximal response compared with an agonist.

Two confusing terms are potency and efficacy. *Efficacy* is the capacity to stimulate or produce an effect for a given receptor occupancy. In other words, how well the drug works. *Potency* refers to the dose required to produce a given effect relative to a standard. Many times the use of the word *potency* misleads one into believing that because a drug is more potent, it is more effective. For example, morphine, 10 mg, is often compared with meperidine (Demerol), 75 mg. Morphine is the more potent compound because it takes less to produce the same effect as the meperidine, 75 mg.

Drugs may produce their effects in various sites throughout the body. For example, antibiotics produce their effects on the bacteria, wherever it may be, providing the antibiotic can penetrate that particular tissue. Drugs that are diuretics produce an effect because they act directly on the kidney. Some drugs may have an indirect effect, acting on one part of the body but causing an effect elsewhere. Morphine causes constriction of the pupil, not because of a direct effect on the pupil, but because of an effect on the brain. Atropine, on the other hand, acts directly on the muscle of the iris to cause dilation of the pupil.

Drugs may act *extracellularly*, at the surface of the cell, or *intracellularly* to exert their effect. Examples of drugs that act extracellularly are antacids, which neutralize excessive gastric acid; and heparin, which decreases the ability of the blood to clot. Drugs such as antihistamines act at the cellular level by interacting with a receptor to block the effects of histamine. Some drugs, such as anesthetics, act at the cellular level by nonspecifically interacting with cell membranes. Other drugs, such as antibiotics that interfere with normal growth and reproduction of the bacteria, act intracellularly (inside the bacteria).

The interaction of the drug with the body (site of action) produces some effect. When increasing amounts of drug are required to produce the same effect, *tolerance* has developed. This occurs with some drugs but not with others. Narcotics, alcohol, and barbiturates are well-known examples of drugs that produce tolerance. Rapidly developing tolerance is called *tachyphylaxis*.

Although one would like to have a drug that does only one thing, that is not possible. In addition to the desired action of a drug, there are also undesired effects called *side-effects*. Side-effects can be divided into two categories: predictable reactions and unpredictable reactions. *Predictable* reactions comprise 70% to 80% of all drug reactions and are usually extensions of the pharmacologic effects of the drug. These side-effects are usually dose related, so that as the dose increases so does the number and severity of side effects. These adverse reactions can be repeatedly demonstrated in experimental animals or in human trials. *Unpredictable* reactions may be subdivided into idiosyncratic reactions and allergic reactions. *Idiosyncratic* reactions are unusual or unexpected reactions that do not fit the usual pharmacologic actions of the drug. An example of this type of reaction is hyperactivity from phenobarbital, when the action that is expected is sedation. *Allergic* reactions comprise 6% to 10% of all drug reactions, are not related to the pharmacologic effects of the drug, are unlikely to be related at all to dose, and are not reproducible in studies (except for that individual who had the reaction). Most allergic reactions are manifested by skin reactions and, although uncomfortable (itching, burning, and the like), are not life-threatening. However, *anaphylactic* reactions may occur that result in bronchospasm, hypotension, shock, and death, if not treated quickly.

Drug interaction is a term usually used to describe an adverse event involving the interplay between two or more drugs. Although, by strict definition, an interaction does not have to be adverse, the common usage of this term implies an adverse event. Drugs may interact through pharmacokinetic mechanisms and pharmacodynamic mechanisms. A drug may interfere with the absorption of another (antacids interfere with the absorption of tetracycline), the distribution of another (displace another agent from albumin-binding sites), decrease or increase metabolism of another agent (cimetidine decreases the metabolism of drugs such as warfarin), or excretion of the other agent (probenecid blocks the excretion of penicillin, usually, a good interaction). Pharmacodynamic interactions involve the effects of the drug, rather than serum levels. For example, certain tricyclic antidepressants block the uptake into the cell of some antihypertensives, rendering the antihypertensive ineffective.

DRUG SAFETY AND EFFECTIVENESS

Before a drug can be given to a human, it must be undergo extensive toxicity testing in animals. Both acute and chronic toxicity studies are conducted in two or more species of animals. *Acute* studies attempt to identify organs or tissues affected by the drug and to determine the lethal dose. *Chronic* toxicity studies over long periods look at the likelihood that the drug may cause problems when used over an extended period, particularly the drug's carcinogenic potential. Drugs are also tested for teratogenic potential (ability to cause birth defects) in animals.

After a drug is thoroughly studied in animals, human studies are conducted. Unfortunately, there is a lack of total correlation between toxicity data in animal studies and adverse effects in humans. However, because of some similarities and because it is the "best we have" animal studies are a necessity. Human studies are conducted to determine the efficacy as well as the safety of the drug. New drugs are usually compared with drugs already in use to determine their comparative efficacy in addition to comparing them with placebo. Double-blind studies are usually necessary to eliminate patient and investigator bias. Adverse events are reported to the company conducting the investigation and, providing the drug is safe and efficacious, appear in the product package circular.

When drugs are marketed, they fall into one of two classes; *prescription* (legend) drugs or *nonprescription* (over-the-counter, or OTC) products. Prescription drugs are those that require a prescription from an authorized practitioner for their use. The term *legend* refers to the required label on the package stating: "Caution: Federal law prohibits dispensing without prescription." Drugs that are considered prescription drugs generally belong to one or more of the following categories: (1) drugs that are habit-forming and certain hypnotics; (2) drugs that are not considered safe enough for self-medication by the lay public; and (3) drugs that may not be considered safe for indiscriminate use. The OTC drugs are those determined to be safe enough for self-medication.

Drugs that have a high likelihood of being abused are not only prescription drugs, but also more rigidly controlled. These drugs are regulated under the Controlled Substances Act and termed controlled substances. Examples of controlled substances are narcotics (morphine, codeine, meperidine), barbiturates (pentobarbital, secobarbital, phenobarbital), amphetamines, and other substances that are likely to be abused. Controlled substances are divided into five classifications (Schedule I–Schedule V) and penalties for illegal use differ among them (Table 1-2).

SOURCES OF DRUG INFORMATION

With the vast amount of information available on drugs and their use, it is important to realize that even the most knowledgeable person must consult the literature frequently. Many different information sources are available. Some of the more frequently consulted sources, as well as some less well known but valuable resources, are discussed in the following paragraphs.

TABLE 1-2
Examples of Controlled Substances

Classification	Drugs (Examples)	Comments
I	Heroin, LSD, methaqualone	Not used medically; prohibited from use, except under investigation
II	Narcotics, pentobarbital, amphetamines	Abuse potential high, accepted for medical use
III	Codeine-containing drugs, paregoric, butabarbital	Medical use; less potential for abuse
IV	Phenobarbital, diazepam, propoxyphene	Less likely to cause dependence and abuse
V	Mixtures with small amounts of codeine or paregoric, others	Some available from pharmacist without prescription

The source of information most frequently consulted is probably the *Physician's Desk Reference* (PDR). This reference provides product information provided by the manufacturer of the drug. This is the same information provided in the product package circular, approved by the FDA. Although useful and a "must," this information does not satisfy some of the health provider's needs. One problem with this resource is the selectivity with which drugs are included in the PDR. Older drugs and many (if not most) generic products are not included.

One most useful source of information is *Facts and Comparisons*. This is a compendium of information similar in layout to the PDR, but much more exhaustive than the PDR. In addition, this loose-leaf book is organized by subject, rather than by manufacturer, as in the PDR. In addition to information about each drug, "Facts" gives other useful information about treatment with the various therapeutic categories of drugs. This resource has the advantage of being updated monthly instead of yearly as is the PDR (although the PDR does publish occasional supplements). Facts also contains some comparisons of many drugs by generic as well as trade name manufacturers. Dosages, side-effects, dosage forms and strengths, as well as indications and contraindications are given.

The aforementioned references are good general resources for drug information. However, it may at times be necessary to look for references for specific drug information questions. One may wish to know specifics about side-effects, drug interactions, or pharmacology of a drug. The bibliography at the end of this chapter lists sources by topic. Although more sources exist, the bibliography presents those most commonly used. In general, it is good practice to use the common references just mentioned first and supplement with the pertinent sources listed in the bibliography.

CLASSES OF DRUGS

The following discussion of drugs is divided into the different classes according to the Pharmacologic-Therapeutic Classification System developed by the American Hospital Formulary Service (AHFS). A very brief overview of these classes is provided. For more information the reader is referred to specific discussions in other chapters in this text, one of the resources mentioned in the chapter Bibliography; or specific sources cited within each class.

Antihistamines

Histamine is a naturally occurring amine that is involved in allergic reactions such as, anaphylaxis, angioedema, asthma, urticaria, and rhinitis. Antihistamines are drugs that block some of the actions of histamine by competing for binding sites. Histamine receptors are classified into two types, H_1 receptors are involved in the reactions just mentioned. The H_2 receptors are involved with acid secretion in the stomach. Antihistamines have been developed for both types of receptors. Those that are taken for allergic symptoms, such as chlorpheniramine (Chlor-Trimeton) or diphenhydramine, block H_1 receptors. Drugs that block H_2 receptors will be discussed later. There are several groups of these antihistamines based on their chemical structure (Table 1-3). Side effects of most of these agents include sedation, dry mouth, and dizziness. Patients who are troubled with drowsiness when taking cold or allergy medication are usually complaining of the side-effect of the antihistamine. Some products actually contain a combination of a decongestant and an antihistamine. Decongestants usually cause a stimulant effect rather than sedation. Uses for the antihistamines include treatment of hay fever and other allergic reactions, anxiety (because of the sedative action of some of these agents), motion sickness and nausea (some specific antihistamines).

Anti-Infective Agents

The anti-infective agents include drugs used to treat bacterial, fungal, and viral infections. These drugs are toxic to the invading organism but relatively safe for the patient. Because the most commonly used anti-infective agents are antibiotics, most of the discussion will center on antibiotics (Table 1-4).

TABLE 1-3
Examples of Antihistamines

Chemical Class	Drug	Trade Name
Ethanolamines	Diphenhydramine	Benadryl
	Dimenhydrinate	Dramamine
Ethylenediamines	Tripelennamine	Pyribenzamine
Alkylamines	Chlorpheniramine	Chlor-Trimeton
	Brompheniramine	Dimetane
Piperazines	Cyclizine	Marezine
	Meclizine	Bonine
Phenothiazines	Promethazine	Phenergan
Others	Terfenadine	Seldane

TABLE 1-4
Examples of Commonly Used Antibiotics

Class	Drug	Trade Name(s)	Comments
PENICILLINS			
	Penicillin G	Pentids	Gram +
	Penicillin V	Pen-Vee K	
	Nafcillin	Unipen	Gram +, penicillinase-
	Cloxicillin	Tegopen	resistant
	Dicloxacillin	Dynapen	
	Ampicillin	Amcill	Gram + and −
	Amoxicillin	Amoxil	
CEPHALOSPORINS			
	Cephalexin	Keflex	Gram + and −
	Cefazolin	Ancef	
	Cefaclor	Ceclor	
MACROLIDES			
	Erythromycin	E-Mycin	Gram + and −
		EES	*Mycoplasma* sp.
		Eryc	*Legionella* sp.
TETRACYCLINES			
	Tetracycline	Achromycin	Gram + and −
	Doxycycline	Vibramycin	*Chlamydia* sp.
AMINOGLYCOSIDES			
	Gentamicin	Garamycin	Gram + and −,
	Tobramycin	Nebcin	especially good against
	Amikacin	Amikin	*Pseudomona* sp.
SULFONAMIDES			
	Sulfamethoxazole	Gantanol	Gram + and −
	Sulfasoxizole	Gantrisin	
	Sulfamethoxazole/		
	trimethoprim		
	Septra		
OTHERS			
	Chloramphenicol	Chloromycetin	Gram + and −
	Clindamycin	Cleocin	Gram +, anaerobes

Antibiotics act on bacteria by inhibition of cell wall synthesis, inhibition of protein synthesis, and prevention of folic acid synthesis. Each of these mechanisms is selective for the bacteria because human cells do not contain cell walls and do not have the same mechanisms for replication of protein. In addition, humans do not synthesize folic acid, it must be obtained in the diet. Antibiotics that inhibit cell wall synthesis include penicillins and cephalosporins. Drugs that inhibit protein synthesis include erythromycin, tetracycline, chloramphenicol, streptomycin, and neomycin. Sulfonamides prevent folic acid synthesis.

Antibiotics do not kill all bacteria. Each antibiotic (or group of antibiotics) has a particular "spectrum of activity," which is the particular bacteria that it kills. For example, penicillin G is effective against many gram-positive bacteria but ineffective against gram-negative bacteria. It is usually the drug of choice for treating gram-positive infections such as streptococcal sore throat. Ampicillin, another antibiotic in the penicillin family, covers many gram-positive and gram-negative bacteria. There are many other penicillin antibiotics commonly used today. Nafcillin is an example of a group of penicillin antibiotics that are used for staphylococcal infections (gram-positive bacteria), but it has little or no effect on gram-negative bacteria.

Cephalosporin antibiotics include agents such as cephalexin (Keflex), cefazolin (Ancef or Kefzol), cefaclor (Ceclor), and many, many more. These antibiotics cover a broad spectrum of bacteria including gram-positives such as *Streptococcus* and *Staphylococcus* sp., and gram-negatives such as *Escherichia coli, Klebsiella*, and some *Proteus* sp. Penicillins and cephalosporins are available for oral and parenteral administration, although particular drugs may be better suited for one route than the other. Side-effects of the penicillins and cephalosporins are not common. Allergic reactions may occur, including anaphylaxis. The broad-spectrum agents tend to cause diarrhea.

Erythromycin is an antibiotic with a spectrum similar to penicillin, but it is also active against *Mycoplasma pneumoniae* and *Legionella*. It is commonly used in patients who are allergic to penicillin and when coverage of infections with *M. pneumoniae* or *Legionella* is needed. Like other antibiotics discussed so far, erythromycin has few side-effects. It may cause nausea, vomiting, and diarrhea in some patients. A rare but important side-effect is hepatotoxicity.

The tetracyclines are broad-spectrum antibiotics used for a variety of infectious diseases. Although these agents are effective for many gram-positive infections, they are particularly useful for those caused by gonococci, chlamydiae, and rickettsiae (Rocky Mountain spotted fever) infections. Doxycycline is a member of the tetracycline family with a similar spectrum but with a long half-life, thus it can be administered less frequently. Side-effects are primarily gastrointestinal irritation—heartburn, nausea, vomiting, and diarrhea.

Clindamycin is an antibiotic used for treating anaerobic infections. Although it is effective for many other bacteria, it is seldom used because it has been associated with a condition called pseudomembranous colitis. However, other antibiotics also cause this condition. This drug is sometimes used in treating osteomyelitis.

The aminoglycosides (gentamicin, tobramycin, others) are used to treat serious gram-negative infections. These drugs are useful only when administered parenterally and have potentially serious side-effects, i.e., nephrotoxicity and ototoxicity.

Sulfonamides (sometimes referred to as "sulfa" drugs) are useful in urinary tract infections. There are many such agents available; sulfamethoxazole is one of the commonly used drugs. The combination of sulfamethoxazole with trimethoprim (co-trimoxazole) extends the spectrum of activity and is used for urinary tract infections and otitis media. Side-effects to the sulfonamides and trimethoprim include allergic reactions, nausea, and vomiting.

Autonomic Drugs (Neuropharmacology)

The nervous system may be divided into two major categories: the *central* nervous system (CNS) and the *peripheral* nervous system (PNS). The peripheral nervous system is divided into the *voluntary* and *involuntary* systems. The voluntary system is that which is under voluntary control (somatic nervous system), i.e., the skeletal muscle. The neurotransmitter involved with the somatic system is acetylcholine.

The autonomic nervous system has two different divisions called the *parasympathetic* and *sympathetic* nervous systems. These two divisions control many internal body functions such as heart rate, vascular tone, bladder control, and gastrointestinal function. The sympathetic and parasympathetic have opposite effects on organs. For example, the parasympathetic division decreases heart rate, whereas the sympathetic system increases heart rate. Many of the drugs that will be discussed in the following sections may have some effect to accentuate or oppose each of these systems.

Acetylcholine is the neurotransmitter of the parasympathetic system (cholinergic) at both pre- and postganglionic neurons. The parasympathetic postganglionic receptors are also known as *muscarinic* receptors. Examples of agents that have muscarinic activity are bethanechol, which stimulates the bladder and intestines, and pilocarpine used to constrict the pupil (particularly in patients with glaucoma). These agents act directly on the muscarinic receptor to produce their effect.

The receptors located in the skeletel muscle and ganglia are called *nicotinic* receptors (because nicotine was found to mimic acetylcholine in the laboratory). Most drugs that are useful clinically act indirectly on these receptors by inhibiting the enzyme responsible for the breakdown of acetylcholine, acetylcholinesterase. Drugs such as neostigmine are used to restore muscle strength in patients with myasthenia gravis.

In addition to drugs that act as agonists on cholinergic receptors, some agents are used because they are antagonists to acetylcholine at the cholinergic receptor. The belladonna alkaloids (atropine, scopolamine, hyoscyamine) are used to block acetylcholine at muscarinic receptors. Clinically, atropine is used to decrease salivary secretions, depress gastrointestinal tract motility, dilate the eye, increase heart rate, and treat toxicity of cholinergic agents. Unfortunately, drugs with anticholinergic activity similar to atropine are likely to express these effects as unwanted side-effects.

The synonym for the sympathetic nervous system is the *adrenergic* nervous system. Adrenergic comes from the word *adrenaline (epinephrine)* which is one of several neurotransmitters that affect the sympathetic nervous system. Actually, *norepinephrine* (also known as noradrenaline) is the sympathetic neurotransmitter; epinephrine should be referred to as a neurohormone (released from the adrenal gland). The sympathetic nervous system produces effects opposite those of the cholinergic system mentioned earlier. Heart rate increases, bronchioles dilate, and smooth muscle of the gastrointestinal tract relaxes when the sympathetic system is stimulated (Table 1-5). It may be useful to remember that norepinephrine is important for maintenance of normal sympathetic tone and adjustment of circulatory dynamics. Epinephrine may be remembered as the emergency hormone or "fight-or-flight" hormone.

Dopamine is another neurotransmitter whose role is not completely understood. It is, however, involved as a neurotransmitter in the CNS as well as having effects on the kidney and the heart. Dopamine, norepinephrine, and epinephrine are also referred to as *catecholamines* (referring to their chemical structure). All three of these agents are important to transmitters in the CNS. Isoproterenol is a synthetic (man-made) catecholamine used in clinical practice. To understand the pharmaco-

TABLE 1-5
Examples of Organ Response (Autonomic Nervous System)

Organ	Adrenergic	Cholinergic
Eye	Mydriasis	Miosis
Heart	Increased rate	Decreased rate
Blood vessels	Constriction/dilatation	Dilatation
Bronchial muscle	Relaxation	Contraction
GI motility	Decreased	Increased
Urinary bladder (detrusor)	Relaxation	Contraction

logic effects of these agents, it is important to understand the physiology of their receptors.

Adrenergic receptors may be divided into alpha (α) and beta (β) receptors. α-Receptors regulate vasoconstriction, mydriasis, intestinal relaxation, and inhibit insulin release. β-Receptors are subdivided into β_1- and β_2-receptors. β_1-Receptors are important for increasing heart rate and increasing force of cardiac contraction. β_2-Receptors are important for bronchial relaxation and dilation of the blood vessels of the skeletal muscle, brain, and heart. Norepinephrine has both α- and β-activity (more α than β), epinephrine also has α- and β-activity but slightly more β than α, and isoproterenol has almost pure β-activity.

Drugs that have adrenergic activity may be *direct acting* or *indirect acting*. Indirect-acting adrenergic agents cause the sympathetic postganglionic neurons to release norepinephrine. Drugs such as amphetamine and ephedrine are indirect-acting agents that also have a stimulant effect on the central nervous system. Just as the cholinergics have antagonists, so do the adrenergic agents have antagonists. Drugs may be used to block α as well as β-adrenergic receptors. The uses of these agents will be discussed later in this chapter.

α-Adrenergic agents are used as decongestants. Drugs such as pseudoephedrine and phenylpropanolamine are given orally. Some patients may experience some CNS stimulation, especially from phenylpropanolamine. This drug is also used in OTC diet pills to suppress appetite. Phenylephrine (and many others) may be used topically in nasal sprays and drops.

β-adrenergic agents are used as bronchodilators in the treatment of asthma. Drugs such as metaproterenol and albuterol are given by inhalation as well as by mouth. Isoproterenol may be used for cardiac standstill and shock, as well as for bronchospasm.

Epinephrine is useful in the treatment of anaphylaxis. Dopamine is useful in shock and some cases of heart failure and kidney failure.

β-Adrenergic blockers may be divided by the type of β-receptor that is blocked. Some drugs such as propranolol are nonspecific blockers and block both β_1- and β_2-receptors. Atenolol is an example of a β-blocker that specifically blocks β_1-receptors. There are a number of β-blockers available, and they find many uses, including treatment of angina, hypertension, migraine headache, cardiac arrythmias, and others.

Anticoagulants and Coagulants

Anticoagulants are drugs used to prevent the blood from clotting. Most of the time these agents are used in patients with a recent thrombus, such as deep vein thrombosis and pulmonary embolus. Although used in acute situations, these agents do nothing to dissolve the clot but rather prevent further clotting. The anticoagulants may be divided into two groups—heparin, which has to be given parenterally, and the coumarins, which are used orally.

Heparin activates a plasma protein, antithrombin III, that affects clotting at several steps in the clotting cascade. The onset of action of heparin is immediate. It is usually administered intravenously by continuous infusion, although for some indications, it may be administered subcutaneously. Even though the onset is immediate, the dosage must be titrated for each patient to achieve optimal anticoagulation. Heparin is monitored by the activated partial thromboplastin time, a test that is sensitive to most of the plasma coagulation factors. The dosage of heparin is given in *units* as opposed to most drugs which are measured in terms of *milligrams* (mg). Side-effects of heparin are usually limited to excessive anticoagulation; however, thrombocytopenia may occur, and osteoporosis has been reported with long-term therapy.

Warfarin sodium is the most commonly used agent of the coumarin drugs. Although it is available for parenteral use, it is almost always used orally. Warfarin prevents the synthesis of the vitamin K-dependent clotting factors, II, VII, IX, and X. The onset of action of this agent occurs as the clotting factors disappear from the blood. Therefore, this agent is not useful in the acute situation as is heparin. It usually requires 5 to 7 days to become fully effective. Side-effects are usually due to excessive anticoagulation (hemorrhage), but necrosis of the skin and a condition called purple-toe syndrome occur rarely. One of the major problems with warfarin is the possibility of numerous drug interactions. Only a slight change in serum levels of warfarin can mean a dramatic change in prothrombin time. Drugs such as aspirin must be avoided in patients taking warfarin. In fact, it is wise to be aware of warfarin interactions whenever a patient needs to be taking other drugs in addition to warfarin.

Heparin is usually given to treat thrombotic events such as pulmonary embolus and deep vein thrombosis. It is also used in situations in which the physician wants to prevent clotting, such as after certain surgical procedures. Warfarin is usually given to prevent reclotting after treatment with heparin or to prevent thrombi from forming in patients with artificial valves.

Although the anticoagulants are effective in preventing venous thrombosis, they have less effect in preventing arterial thrombi. Because the platelet plays a more important role in arterial thrombi, *antiplatelet drugs* are given to prevent these thrombi. Several agents have been shown to have antiplatelet activity, including aspirin, sulfinpyrazone, dipyridamole, and the nonsteroidal anti-inflammatory drugs. Studies documenting the efficacy in the treatment of transient ischemic effects and myocardial infarction have, thus far shown that aspirin may be the agent of choice. The antiplatelet effects of aspirin last the life time of the platelet, in contrast to other agents that are effective only during the time the drug is in the plasma. The effective dosage of aspirin appears to be from 90 mg/day to 1300 mg/day (one baby aspirin to one adult tablet four times daily).

Other drugs that are used in the treatment of thrombotic disorders are the *thrombolytics.* These agents promote digestion of fibrin, dissolving the clot. Streptokinase and urokinase are enzymes used for this purpose. However, these drugs are not uniformly used for every patient because of expense and the greater likelihood for bleeding. Streptokinase is currently receiving more use in treating acute myocardial infarction.

In addition to having drugs that prevent clotting, certain agents are available to decrease bleeding (*hemostatic agents*). One such agent is aminocaproic acid which inhibits (indirectly) the dissolution of clots. Side-effects include nausea, cramps, dizziness, and headache. Other agents used as hemostatic agents are vitamin K (particularly useful to reverse the effects of warfarin) and local agents such as absorbable gelatin sponge, absorbable gelatin film, oxidized cellulose, microfibrillar collagen, and thrombin. Protamine is occasionally used to reverse the effects of heparin. Fresh-frozen plasma may be used to reverse the effects of heparin or warfarin.

Cardiovascular Drugs

ANTIANGINAL AGENTS

When the oxygen consumption of the heart becomes greater than supply, angina results. The aim of treatment is to increase oxygen to the heart or to decrease oxygen consumption or to serve both functions. Nitroglycerin and other nitrates, such as isosorbide, act as *vasodilators*. Although the nitrates were originally thought to dilate coronary arteries, the coronary vessels are probably maximally dilated from hypoxia. The nitrates may actually decrease the work load on the heart by decreasing blood pressure resulting from peripheral vasodilation.

A new class of agents used to treat angina are the *calcium channel blockers*. These agents block the slow calcium channel in smooth muscle, which decreases vessel spasm. Nifedipine, diltiazem, and verapamil are the calcium channel blockers marketed in the United States.

β-Adrenergic blockers are also used for the treatment of angina. These drugs decrease myocardial oxygen consumption, probably by decreasing heart rate and cardiac contractility.

ANTIARRHYTHMIC DRUGS

Drugs that are used to treat abnormal rhythms of the heart are known as *antiarrhythmic* drugs. These drugs modify electrical activity of the heart and work by several different mechanisms. The common action of all is to decrease automaticity. There are a number of drugs used for this purpose, and they are divided into several classes. The more commonly used drugs are quinidine, procainamide, lidocaine, propranolol, and verapamil. Although useful and lifesaving in many situations, these drugs can cause arrhythmias (proarrhythmic effect) in some situations.

CARDIAC GLYCOSIDES

One of the most common drugs used in the treatment of congestive heart failure is digitalis. Digitalis is derived from a plant called foxglove and is actually a group of drugs. Digoxin is the most common of the digitalis glycosides in use today. Digoxin increases the force of contraction of the heart and generally slows the heart. Although useful in many patients, the difference between the therapeutic dose and toxic dose is very small. The dosage must be carefully adjusted, with particular attention to the patient's age and kidney function. Digoxin is not only useful for congestive heart failure, but may be used to treat atrial fibrillation and paroxysmal supraventricular tachyarrhythmias.

ANTILIPEMIC AGENTS

Patients with elevated cholesterol and serum triglyceride levels are often treated with drugs if diet and exercise fail to control the elevated lipid levels. Cholestyramine and colestipol bind bile acids in the gastrointestinal tract, preventing their reabsorption and, thereby, decreasing serum cholesterol concentrations. Other drugs, such as gemfibrozil, nicotinic acid (niacin), and probucol, decrease triglycerides and cholesterol levels by inhibiting synthesis in the liver. Other newer agents are currently under investigation for the treatment of hyperlipidemias.

ANTIHYPERTENSIVE AGENTS

Drugs that are used to treat high blood pressure may act by several mechanisms and are actually from several different classes of drugs. The classes are diuretics, sympatholytics, vasodilators, and angiotensin-converting enzyme inhibitors (Table 1-6).

Treatment is often initiated with *diuretics* and additional drugs added as needed to control blood pressure. The thiazide diuretics, such as hydrochlorothiazide, are inexpensive and can be taken once daily. These drugs work not only because they decrease fluid volume but also because of a direct effect on the arterioles. Side-effects include hypokalemia, hyponatremia, and occasionally, impotence.

The *sympatholytics* (adrenergic-blocking agents) actually comprise several different mechanisms of action. β-Blockers, such as propranolol, are also useful in hypertension. Although one would suspect that these agents act by decreasing heart rate and, therefore, cardiac output, the β-blockers may have other less-defined effects on blood pressure. Reserpine is an older agent that depletes stores of norepinephrine. Although useful in some patients, it may cause depression in high doses and is less commonly used. Methyldopa is an agent that acts centrally to decrease sympathetic tone. This agent may cause somnolence, depression, and impotence (as do most other antihypertensives). In addition, methyldopa (and other sympatholytics) may cause orthostatic hypotension. Clonidine and guanabenz also act in the central nervous system to decrease sympathetic tone. Side-effects are similar to methyldopa, with less orthostatic hypotension, but clonidine may cause rebound hypertension if discontinued abruptly. Prazosin is an α–adrenergic-blocking agent that produces both arterial and venous dilatation. Prazosin causes an unusual side effect known as first-dose syncope. Hence, this drug is initiated with small doses of prazosin at bedtime for the first 1 to 2 days of treatment.

Vasodilators, such as hydralazine and minoxidil, lower blood pressure by directly causing vasodilatation. These drugs can cause reflex tachycardia, thus patients with angina should also receive an adrenergic-blocking drug, such as a β-blocker, before initiating therapy. Although both of these drugs can cause sodium

TABLE 1-6
Examples of Antihypertensives

Class	Drug	Trade Name(s)
DIURETICS		
Thiazide	Hydrocholorthiazide	Esidrix
(Related)	Chlorthalidone	Hygroton
LOOP DIURETICS	Furosemide	Lasix
	Bumetanide	Bumex
POTASSIUM-SPARING DIURETICS	Triamterene	Dyrenium
	Spironolactone	Aldactone
SYMPATHOLYTICS		
β-Blockers	Propranolol	Inderal
	Metoprolol	Lopressor
	Atenolol	Tenormin
	Nadolol	Corgard
Others	Reserpine	Various names
	Methyldopa	Aldomet
	Clonidine	Catapres
	Guanabenz	Wytensin
	Prazosin	Minipres
VASODILATORS	Hydralazine	Apresoline
	Minoxidil	Loniten
ACE INHIBITORS	Captopril	Capoten
	Enalapril	Vasotec

and fluid retention, minoxidil appears to cause a greater problem. Minoxidil also causes hypertrichosis (an abnormal excessive growth of hair) in patients after 3 to 6 weeks of therapy.

Angiotensin-converting enzyme (ACE) *inhibitors* decrease blood pressure by inhibiting the conversion of angiotensin I to angiotensin II. Angiotensin II is one of the most potent vasoconstrictors known. Captopril, enalapril and lisinopril are the three ACE inhibitors on the United States' market. Side effects appear to be minimal, although severe hypotension has been reported in patients receiving diuretic therapy who are volume depleted.

Many patients who are treated for hypertension may experience one or more side-effects from their medication. This is especially significant because they are being treated for an asymptomatic disease. Combination therapy with diuretics as part of most regimens is very common because many of the antihypertensives cause sodium and fluid retention. Cost becomes an important factor in the treatment of this disease. Not only are many of the medications expensive, but one has to consider that the medications will usually have to be taken for life.

Central Nervous System Drugs

ANALGESICS

Analgesics may be divided into two categories based upon their mechanism of action. The *simple* or *nonnarcotic* analgesics act peripherally, whereas the *narcotic* analgesics (and narcoticlike) analgesics have a central action.

The narcotic analgesics are derivatives of opium and many related synthetic drugs. Opium has been used for centuries to relieve pain and cause euphoria. Morphine, derived from opium, is the prototype of the narcotic analgesics, although there are many compounds available (Table 1-7). Analgesia induced by morphine may be caused by two factors. Not only does morphine elevate the pain threshold, but it also alters the reaction of the individual to the pain. It appears that narcotic analgesics act on specific receptor sites that also may be receptor sites for the body's own endogenous compounds called *endorphins*. The endorphins appear to modify the perception of, and reaction to, pain. Thus, morphine and other opiates mimic endogenous compounds.

TABLE 1-7
Narcotic Analgesics

NATURALLY OCCURRING ALKALOIDS AND SEMISYNTHETIC OPIATES
Morphine
Codeine (methylmorphine)
Oxymorphone (Numorphan)
Hydromorphone (Dilaudid)
Hydrocodone (Dicodid)
Heroin (diacetylmorphine)

MEPERIDINE AND RELATED AGENTS
Meperidine (Demerol)
Alphaprodine (Nisentil)
Anileridine (Leritine)
Diphenoxylate (in Lomotil)

METHADONE AND RELATED AGENTS
Methadone
Propoxyphene (Darvon)

BENZMORPHANS (AGONIST AND PARTIAL ANTAGONISTS)
Pentazocine (Talwin)

MORPHINAN DERIVATIVES
Levorphanol (Levo-Dromoran)
Dextromethorphan (-DM in cough syrups)

NARCOTIC ANTAGONISTS
Nalorphine (Nalline)
Naloxone (Narcan)

*Examples of trade names are given in parentheses.

In addition to producing analgesia, narcotics have other effects, some of which are useful and some of which are side-effects. Morphine and other narcotics depress respiration (respiratory depression is the cause of death in overdoses of narcotic analgesics). Morphine causes peripheral vasodilatation, reducing ventricular work and pulmonary congestion, and it is sometimes used to treat pulmonary edema. The direct effect of the narcotics on the gastrointestinal tract is constipation; in fact, several compounds are used as antidiarrheal agents. Most of the narcotic analgesics are likely to produce nausea and vomiting because of their effect on the chemoreceptor trigger zone. Another useful effect is the depression of the cough reflex by many of the narcotic agents. The narcotics also cause miosis (pupilary constriction).

Not all of the opiates are equal in potency or equally absorbed orally. The oral dose may be several times the parenteral dose. Some of the agents have narcotic antagonist activity, which may block the effects if other agents are added to the regimen. Pentazocine is one such agent. Other drugs, however, have been synthesized that are better antagonists and may be used in case of an opiate overdose or when it is desirable to decrease the activity of a narcotic previously taken.

Tolerance develops to the actions of morphine, thus increasingly larger doses of the narcotic may be needed to produce the same effect. Tolerance develops to many of the effects of morphine including analgesia, euphoria, respiratory depression, and hypotension. However, no tolerance develops to morphine-induced constipation or miosis. Narcotics also cause an abstinence syndrome in subjects physically dependent on these agents. The abstinence syndrome is characterized by CNS irritability, feeling of fatigue, autonomic hyperactivity (e.g., tachycardia, hypertension), gastrointestinal hyperactivity, insomnia, chills, and restlessness.

Analgesics that act peripherally include acetaminophen, aspirin (acetylsalicylic acid) and other salicylates, and nonsteroidal anti-inflammatory drugs (NSAIDs). In addition to their analgesic properties, these agents also have an *antipyretic* effect (reducing elevated body temperature). The salicylates and NSAIDs also have an anti-inflammatory effect that acetaminophen does not have. Although all of these agents produce their antipyretic effect centrally, other central effects, such as euphoria, are usually absent.

Acetaminophen is used for patients who cannot tolerate salicylates and NSAIDs because of adverse reactions or "allergies." Acetaminophen is also the drug of choice for children with fever because of the association of Reye's syndrome with the use of aspirin in viral illnesses.

Although aspirin is still considered by most clinicians to be the drug of choice for rheumatoid arthritis, there are many alternative nonsteroidal anti-inflammatory drugs available (Table 1-8). The different chemical classes are listed in the table. Although these agents are useful alternatives to aspirin, none of them have proved to be superior to aspirin in the treatment of rheumatoid arthritis, except for the possibility of decreased gastrointestinal side-effects. In some situations these drugs have been shown to be slightly more effective than aspirin in the treatment of pain.

ANTICONVULSANTS

Epilepsy is a chronic disorder characterized by sudden excessive discharges of neurons in the gray matter. Seizures are divided into two major categories, *generalized*

TABLE 1-8
Examples of Nonsteroidal Anti-Inflammatory Agents

Class	Drug	Trade Name
PHENYLPROPIONIC ACIDS		
	Ibuprofen	Motrin*
	Fenoprofen	Nalfon
	Naproxen	Naprosyn
	Naproxen sodium	Anaprox
	Ketoprofen	Orudis
INDOLEACETIC ACIDS		
	Tolmetin	Tolectin
	Sulindac	Clinoril
	Indomethacin	Indocin
FENAMIC ACIDS		
	Meclofenamate	Meclomen
	Mefenamic acid	Ponstel
OXICAM		
	Piroxicam	Feldene
SALICYLATES		
	Diflunisal	Dolobid
	Salsalate	Disalcid
	Aspirin	Ascriptin*
	Aspirin	Ecotrin*
	(enteric coated)	Easprin

*These drugs are also available under other trade names.

(involving the whole brain) and *partial* seizures (seizures originating in local areas). Although there may be specific causes for seizures, such as cerebral anoxia, hypoglycemia, drugs with convulsive activity, and metabolic disorders, most patients with epilepsy do not have an apparent cause.

Drugs used in the treatment of seizure disorders are listed in Table 1-9. The mechanism of action is not precisely known for all of these agents; however, it is known that phenytoin has a membrane-stabilizing effect that prevents the spread of seizure activity. Other drugs also appear to work by decreasing the spread of seizure activity or by augmenting inhibitory processes.

Most of the drugs used to treat seizure disorders are monitored with the aid of serum drug concentrations. It is known that for most of these agents a drug concentration within the therapeutic range results in maximum suppression of seizure activity with low risk of toxicity. Although this holds true for most patients, some may respond at lower or higher concentrations, and some may experience side-effects within the therapeutic range.

Side-effects of most anticonvulsants include sedation, decreased cognitive function, and nausea and vomiting. Phenytoin may also cause gingival hyperplasia, acne, peripheral neuropathy, and folate deficiency. The agents with the least sedation appear to be valproic acid and carbamazepine.

TABLE 1-9
Anticonvulsant Preferences by Seizure Type

Seizure Type	Drug	Trade Name(s)*
TONIC-CLONIC		
	Phenytoin	Dilantin
	Valproic acid	Depakene
	Carbamazepine	Tegretol
	Phenobarbital	Various names
	Primidone	Mysoline
MYOCLONIC		
	Valproic acid	Depakene
	Ethosuximide	Zarontin
	Clonazepam	Clonopin
	Corticotropin	Various names
PARTIAL		
	Carbamazepine	Tegretol
	Phenytoin	Dilantin
	Phenobarbital	Various names
	Valproic acid	Depakene
ABSENCE		
	Ethosuximide	Zarontin
	Valproic acid	Depakene

*Many of these drugs are also available under other trade names.

DRUGS FOR PARKINSON'S DISEASE

Parkinson's disease is a neurologic condition that most likely results from a deficiency of dopamine, leaving acetylcholine relatively unopposed. The symptoms that result may be divided into four separate groups: tremor, akinesia or bradykinesia, rigidity or increased muscle tone, and loss of normal postural reflexes. Parkinson's disease may have several causes, but most often it is idiopathic. Some drugs, such as the antipsychotic agents, may also cause a parkinsonian syndrome.

Drugs that are used to treat Parkinson's disease are either agents that increase dopaminergic functions or agents that decrease cholinergic activity.

Anticholinergic drugs are used to decrease cholinergic activity in an attempt to reverse the relative state of cholinergic excess. Agents that are used include trihexyphenidyl, biperiden, and benztropine. Other agents, such as diphenhydramine, are sometimes administered in the event of drug-induced parkinsonism. Side-effects to these drugs include dry mouth, blurred vision, constipation, and urinary retention.

Because it is not possible to administer dopamine into the CNS, the precursor levodopa is given. This drug is metabolized into dopamine, and it is the most frequently used drug in treating significant disease. Levodopa is usually administered as a combination with carbidopa (Sinemet) to prevent its metabolism peripherally.

Side-effects to levodopa include gastrointestinal irritation, sleep disorders, ortho-static hypotension, psychic disturbances, dyskinesias, and less commonly, arryth-mias.

Amantadine, which is used to treat, or as a prophylactic agent for, influenza type A, causes the release and blocks the reuptake of dopamine into the nerve terminal. Side-effects of amantadine include irritability, stimulation, mood distur-bances, and livedo reticularis (a "fishnet" pattern of discoloration, primarily on the legs). Amantadine may also aggravate anticholinergic side-effects.

Bromocriptine is a direct dopamine receptor agonist and is usually reserved for patients who fail to respond to levodopa and anticholinergic agents. Side-effects include psychosis, orthostatic hypotension, nausea,, dyskinesias, and rarely, cardiac arrhythmias.

PSYCHOTHERAPEUTIC AGENTS

Antidepressants

Depression is possibly the most prevalent of the psychiatric illnesses. There are sev-eral theories about the functional abnormalities involved in depression and the mechanism by which the antidepressant drugs act. The *tricyclic antidepressant drugs* (so named because of their chemical structure) can be shown to affect the reuptake of neurotransmitters, producing a greater quantity of the neurotransmit-ter in the synaptic cleft. Whether or not this is the only mechanism of action is still under debate. In any event, tricyclic and related drugs have been shown to be useful in managing depression. In most cases it takes 2 to 3 weeks for maximum effectiveness. Side-effects include anticholinergic effects (dry mouth, constipation, urinary retention) and sedation (Table 1-10). Newer agents, such as trazodone, have minimal anticholinergic effects. It should be noted, however, that these agents can be fatal if excessive doses are taken. Because of the very nature of the disease that these drugs are used to treat, it is not too suprising that a number of suicides are attempted with antidepressants. Patients must be treated for the overdose and monitored (for cardiac arrythmias) very carefully for several days.

Monoamine oxidase inhibitors (MAOIs) must be used with particular caution because of potential dangerous drug and food interactions. Drugs such as the vasoconstrictors and foods that contain tyramine can cause severe hypertension. The MAOIs may also potentiate the effects of other drugs such as amphetamines, narcotics, barbiturates, alcohol, and anticholinergic agents.

Antipsychotic Agents (Major Tranquilizers)

Drug therapy is the mainstay of treatment of the psychotic disorders. Although not all symptoms are amenable to drug treatment, many target symptoms, such as combativeness, hostility, hallucinations, and sleep disorders, are responsive. The *antipsychotic drugs* work through central dopaminergic receptor blockade. In ad-dition to their antipsychotic effects, these drugs have other pharmacologic effects. Most of these drugs have antiemetic effects, cause endocrine effects (such as gy-necomastia, impotence, and decreased libido), alter temperature regulation, have anticholinergic effects, and cause parkinsonianlike effects. The degree to which these effects are caused is somewhat related to the chemical class to which the drug belongs. Table 1-11 lists examples of antipsychotic agents. Side-effects include

TABLE 1-10
Examples of Antidepressants

Class	Drug	Trade Name*
TRICYCLICS		
	Amitriptyline	Elavil
	Imipramine	Tofranil
	Desipramine	Norpramin
	Nortriptyline	Pamelor
	Doxepin	Sinequan
	Protriptyline	Vivactil
	Trimipramine	Surmontil
TETRACYCLIC		
	Maprotiline	Ludiomil
OTHERS		
	Amoxepine	Asendin
	Trazodone	Desyrel
MONOAMINE OXIDASE INHIBITORS		
	Phenelzine	Nardil
	Tranylcypramine	Parnate

*Many of these drugs are also available under other trade names.

TABLE 1-11
Examples of Antipsychotic Agents

Chemical Class	Drug	Trade Name*
PHENOTHIAZINES		
	Chlorpromazine	Thorazine
	Thioridizine	Mellaril
	Trifluoperazine	Stelazine
	Fluphenazine	Prolixin
THIOXANTHENE		
	Thiothixene	Navane
BUTYROPHENONE		
	Haloperidol	Haldol
DIBENZOXAZEPINE		
	Loxapine	Loxitane
DIHYDROINDOLONE		
	Molindone	Moban

*Many of these drugs are also available under other trade names.

drowsiness, extrapyramidal symptoms, hypotension, dizziness, and lowering of the seizure threshold. A rare, but important, side-effect is tardive dyskinesia, which is usually irreversible even if the drug is discontinued.

Sedative-Hypnotic Agents

Both the sedatives and hypnotics depress the central nervous system, but to a different degree. *Hypnotic agents* induce sleep, whereas *sedatives* cause a milder degree of CNS depression. The four stages of CNS depression are sedation, which causes a decreased physical and mental response to stimuli; disinhibition, which is a false stimulated state of awareness; sleep; and anesthesia, which is a loss of feeling or sensation. Traditional sedatives and hypnotics include the barbiturates, alcohol, and other nonbarbiturate sedative–hypnotics.

Barbiturates are classified according to their duration of action (Table 1-12). These agents do not raise the pain threshold or have any analgesic properties but, rather, depress all areas of the CNS including the hypothalamus, vasomotor center (at anesthetic doses), and respiratory center. The barbiturates are useful as anticonvulsants (particularly phenobarbital) and as anesthetics (thiopental). Currently, they are not commonly employed as sedatives and hypnotics. Side-effects of the barbiturates include the paradoxic effect of excitement, particularly in pediatric and geriatric patients, induction of drug-metabolizing enzymes, and automatism. Automatism is a state of drug-induced confusion in which a patient forgets he has taken the drug and consumes more, potentially leading to a toxic ingestion. Because these drugs suppress rapid eye movement (REM) sleep, they are not considered the best choice for inducing sleep. Death from barbiturate ingestion is usually caused by respiratory depression through depression of the respiratory center in the brain.

The barbiturates, like the narcotic analgesics, produce tolerance and physical dependence. Withdrawal from barbiturates (and other nonbarbiturates) produces a characteristic syndrome that may result in death if not treated appropriately.

In addition to the barbiturates, there are several other drugs that continue to be marketed despite no clear-cut advantages over barbiturates or newer agents (to be discussed under antianxiety agents). These nonbarbiturate sedative–hypnotics include ethchlorvynol, methyprylon, glutethimide, and meprobamate. In addition to these, chloral hydrate (Noctec) continues to be used in certain situations to induce sleep (probably because it has little effect on REM sleep).

TABLE 1-12
Barbiturates

Drug	Examples of Trade Name	Duration of Action
Thiopental	Pentothal	Ultrashort
Methohexital	Brevital	Ultrashort
Amobarbital	Amytal	Short to intermediate
Secobarbital	Seconal	Short to intermediate
Pentobarbital	Nembutal	Short to intermediate
Phenobarbital	Luminal	Long

Ethyl alcohol is also a CNS depressant. The four stages of CNS depression can be witnessed in persons consuming large doses of alcohol. As with the agents previously discussed, death can result if enough is consumed within a short period. Withdrawal from alcohol for long-term users can also be very dangerous.

Antianxiety Agents

Anxiety is defined as a feeling of apprehension, uncertainty, and fear. Its manifestations also include nervousness, indecision, worry, tremor, restlessness, headache, nausea, diarrhea, constipation, muscle tension, and palpitations. Drugs used to treat anxiety in the past have included many of the sedative–hypnotics previously discussed. Meprobamate was considered the first modern tranquilizer, but it has some characteristics similar to the barbiturates including dependence, drug interactions, and danger from overdose. Antipsychotics have also been used to treat anxiety, but the side-effects are serious enough to prevent their use for this purpose. Antihistamines, such as hydroxyzine, continue to be used, on occasion, for anxiety.

The most commonly used drugs for anxiety are the *benzodiazepine derivatives* (Table 1-13). The mechanism of action appears to be the increased activity of γ-aminobutyric acid (GABA), which is itself an inhibitory substance. The anxiolytic effects of the benzodiazepines appear to be different from the global depression caused by the sedative–hypnotic agents. In addition to antianxiety effects, the benzodiazepines also have muscle relaxant activity, sedative effects, and anticonvulsant activity. As can be seen, there are a number of benzodiazepine derivatives. It is difficult to pick one drug for all patients because of differences in pharmacokinetic properties, such as speed of onset and duration of action. The efficacy for all of

TABLE 1-13
Antianxiety Agents

Class	Drug	Trade Name**
BENZODIAZEPINES		
	Diazepam	Valium
	Chlordiazepoxide	Librium
	Clorazepate	Tranxene
	Alprazolam	Xanax
	Lorazepam	Ativan
	Halazepam	Paxipam
	Oxazepam	Serax
	Prazepam	Centrax
	Triazolam*	Halcion
	Flurazepam*	Dalmane
	Temazepam*	Restoril
NONBENZODIAZEPINE		
	Buspirone	Buspar

*Marketed only as hypnotics.
**Some of these drugs are also available under other trade names.

these agents in the treatment of anxiety is quite similar. Some drugs are marketed especially for hypnosis, although an increased dose of the other agents will also result in sleep.

Side-effects of the benzodiazepines include drowsiness, impairment of performance (both intellectual and motor coordination), and parodoxic effects such as excitement. Some patients experience a withdrawal syndrome with prolonged use, usually at higher-than-normal doses.

The newest antianxiety agent is buspirone, a non-benzodiazepine derivative. This agent does not work at the same receptor as the benzodiazepines and appears to be a more specific anxiolytic. It has no anticonvulsant or muscle relaxant properties. It is also nearly void of sedation, may actually enhance motor coordination, and has no known withdrawal syndrome. Buspirone requires about 2 to 3 weeks to become maximally effective and is most effective in patients who have not become accustomed to the effects of benzodiazepines.

Muscle Relaxants

Most drugs that are termed skeletal muscle relaxants actually act through a CNS mechanism. Muscle relaxants are generally used to treat two categories of problems. *Spasticity*, which is seen in patients with spinal cord injury, strokes, multiple sclerosis, or cerebral palsy, may be caused by damaged inhibitory neural pathways. Drugs such as diazepam and baclofen are believed to restore some of the inhibitory tone, resulting in less spasticity. Dantrolene, another drug used for spasticity, may actually act on the muscle tissue itself.

Muscle spasms, resulting from sprains, strains, and other causes, are often treated with one of the centrally acting muscle relaxants. The mechanism of action for the skeletal muscle relaxants is not precisely known. For most of these agents, the muscle-relaxant effect appears to be related to the sedative effect.

True skeletal muscle relaxants, such as those used during surgery, are actually neuromuscular-blocking agents. These drugs decrease the response to the neurotransmitter acetylcholine at the neuromuscular junction. The neuromuscular-blocking agents work by blocking the access of acetylcholine to the receptor sites and may initially "depolarize" the cell, causing initial twitching or fasciculation of the muscle and then paralysis. These are known as *depolarizing agents*. Nondepolarizing agents also cause paralysis without the initial stimulation of the muscle (Table 1-14).

Gastrointestinal Drugs

ANTINAUSEA DRUGS

Nausea and vomiting are common complaints that almost everyone has experienced from time to time. Although there are a number of drugs available for the treatment of nausea and vomiting, none are 100% effective or void of side-effects.

The two most commonly used classes are antihistamines and phenothiazines. Antihistamines and anticholinergics appear to be more effective in the treatment of motion sickness. Table 1-15 lists several examples of specific drugs. The anticholinergic drug, scopolamine, is administered as a patch placed behind the ear. Side-effects of antihistamines are usually related to their sedative properties and

TABLE 1-14
Examples of Muscle Relaxants

Use	Drug	Trade Name**
DRUGS FOR SPASTICITY		
	Baclofen	Lioresal
	Dantrolene	Dantrium
	Diazepam	Valium
DRUGS FOR MUSCLE SPASMS		
	Carisoprodol	Soma
	Chlorzoxazone	Paraflex
	Cyclobenzaprine	Flexeril
	Diazepam	Valium
	Methocarbamol	Robaxin
	Orphenadrine	Norflex
DRUGS FOR MUSCLE SPASMS WITH ANALGESICS		
	Carisoprodol, aspirin	Soma Compound
	Chlorzoxazone, APAP**	Chlorzone Forte
	Methocarbamol, aspirin	Robaxisal
	Orphenadrine, aspirin, caffeine	Norgesic Forte
NEUROMUSCULAR-BLOCKING AGENTS		
Depolarizing agents		
	Succinylcholine	Anectine
Nondepolarizing agents		
	Pancuronium	Pavulon
	Tubocurarine	

**Many of these drugs are also available under other trade names.

anticholinergic effects. Scopolamine side-effects include dry mouth, blurred vision, and dizziness. As with other sedative medication, alcohol and other sedatives may increase sedative effects.

Phenothiazines appear to be most effective in treating toxic- or metabolic-induced vomiting. Prochlorperazine (Compazine) and promethazine (Phenergan) are two of the commonly used phenothiazines for the treatment of nausea and vomiting (see Table 1-15). Side-effects of the phenothiazines can be more severe than the side-effects of antihistamines and include drowsiness, extrapyramidal reactions, hypotension, dizziness, and lowering of the seizure threshold.

Metoclopromide (Reglan) is used for the treatment of nausea and vomiting related to delayed gastric-emptying time and in the prevention of nausea and vomiting associated with emetogenic cancer chemotherapy. This drug may have effects on the chemoreceptor trigger zone, as do the phenothiazines. Side-effects include restlessness, drowsiness, and fatigue. Although seen less commonly, patients may also develop extrapyramidal side-effects from this agent.

TABLE 1-15
Commonly Used Antiemetic Agents

Class	Drug	Trade Name*
ANTIHISTAMINES		
	Dimenhydrinate	Dramamine
	Hydroxyzine	Vistaril
	Meclizine	Antivert
PHENOTHIAZINES		
	Prochlorperazine	Compazine
	Promethazine	Phenergan
ANTICHOLINERGIC		
	Scopolomine	Transderm Scop
OTHER		
	Metoclopromide	Reglan
	Dronabinol (THC)	Marinol

*Many of these drugs are also available under other trade names.

Tetrahydrocannabinol (THC), the active ingredient in marijuana, is also used to treat the nausea and vomiting associated with chemotherapy. Side-effects include euphoria, drowsiness, panic, fear, visual hallucinations, and paranoid ideation. However, these side effects are usually associated with higher doses and usually resolve within 3 hours.

LAXATIVES

Although constipation is defined as infrequent or difficult evacuation of feces, the significance is very individualized. What one person may think of as constipation may be considered normal bowel habits for another.

Laxatives facilitate the passage and elimination of feces from the colon and rectum. Ideally, one would like to use a laxative that is nonirritating, nontoxic, and works relatively quickly (after which the bowel returns to normal). Of course, this ideal laxative does not exist, but one should begin treatment with the "safer" agents, reserving the harsh, stimulant laxatives for difficult cases. Table 1-16 classifies laxatives according to their mechanism of action.

The side-effects of laxatives are generally not serious, with the most common side-effect being diarrhea. However, long-term use of the harsh or stimulating laxatives may lead to loss of normal colonic tone, resulting in need for chronic laxative ingestion. In addition, the long-term use of mineral oil may decrease absorption of fat-soluble vitamins.

ANTIDIARRHEA AGENTS

As with nausea and vomiting, diarrhea is usually a symptom. Diarrhea is usually defined as increased frequency and fluid content of bowel movements. The etiology varies from gastrointestinal viruses to antibiotic-induced diarrhea. Treatment of

TABLE 1-16
Laxatives

Class	Agent	Example
Bulk	Methylcellulose	
	Plantago seeds	Psyllium
Emollients	Surfactants	Docusate
Lubricants	Mineral oil	
Saline	Magnesium citrate	
Stimulants	Cascara sagrada	
Miscellaneous	Castor oil	
Suppositories	Various	Glycerin
		Bisacodyl
Enemas	Various	Saline
Lactulose		Chronulac

the underlying cause is most important. In severe cases, it may be necessary to rehydrate the patient and replace lost electrolytes.

When drug treatment of mild diarrhea is necessary, several agents are available over-the-counter. These agents are listed in Table 1-17. Adsorbents, such as kaolin and pectin or bismuth subsalicylate (thought also to be an astringent), work by absorbing the causative agent and excess fluid.

Kaolin and pectin have limited toxicity, with the only known problems related to their nonspecific adsorption of nutrients and digestive enzymes. Bismuth subsalicylate, when taken in high doses or in combination with other agents containing salicylate products, may produce salicylate toxicity.

Anticholinergic agents (belladonna alkaloids) slow the gastrointestinal tract motility. These agents are used by themselves or in combination with adsorbents. Side effects, such as dry mouth and blurred vision, may be a problem with these agents when used in therapeutic doses.

Lactobacillus preparations (*L. acidophilus* and *L. bulgaricus*) are sometimes used, particularly for antibiotic-induced diarrhea. The mechanism of action of these agents is reseeding the bowel with microorganisms to replace those killed by the

TABLE 1-17
Examples of OTC Antidiarrheal Agents

Class	Ingredients	Trade Name
ADSORBENTS		
	Kaolin, pectin	Kaopectate
	Attapulgite	Diasorb
	Bismuth subsalicylate	Pepto-Bismol
ANTICHOLINERGICS		
	Belladonna alkaloids (with kaolin, pectin)	Donnagel

antibiotic. These organisms may also be effective in suppressing the growth of pathogenic microorganisms. Dietary intake of *Lactobacillus* organisms in yogurt (with live cultures), buttermilk, or sweet acidophilus milk may also be helpful.

Opiates and opiate derivatives are probably the most effective agents in the symptomatic treatment of diarrhea. Various preparations are available, including combinations with adsorbents which are sold OTC. A traditional preparation is paregoric (camphorated tincture of opium), which is usually a prescription item. The combination of atropine and diphenoxylate (Lomotil) is a prescription drug that abolishes the peristaltic reflex. Diphenoxylate is an opiate derivative similar to meperidine and causes side-effects similar to other opiates, such as nausea and vomiting, blurred vision, and constipation. Loperamide (Imodium) is an opiatelike agent that may have fewer side-effects than Lomotil. This agent has less effect on the CNS and no evidence of addition.

DRUGS FOR PEPTIC ULCER DISEASE

A *peptic ulcer* is defined as an ulceration of the mucous membrane of the esophagus, stomach, or duodenum. Patients with duodenal ulcer disease tend to have higher-than-normal secretion of acid, whereas gastric ulcer patients are likely to secrete less acid than normals. Peptic ulcer disease may actually be the result of an imbalance between defensive barriers (mucosal resistance) and acid and pepsin.

Drugs currently marketed in the United States for the treatment of duodenal ulcer disease have approximately equal efficacy on the rate of healing. These agents include antacids, H_2-receptor antagonists (cimetidine, ranitidine, famotidine, nizatidine), and sucralfate.

Antacids in dosage of 30 ml (high potency) 1 and 3 hours after meals and at bedtime have been shown to accelerate healing. This is the amount required to neutralize 140 mEq of acid, and the duration of therapy is 4 to 6 weeks. The combination of magnesium and aluminum hydroxide is recommended for several reasons. Because magnesium hydroxide causes diarrhea, aluminum hydroxide is added to help counteract this effect (aluminum hydroxide causes constipation). The other reason for this combination is to avoid calcium-containing antacids that may cause rebound acid secretion. Even with the combination product, diarrhea is still a common problem because such high doses are used. Magnesium-containing antacids should be avoided in patients with severe renal disease. The other problems with treatment with antacids are the inconvenience of carrying the large volume of liquid antacid and compliance with a seven times daily regimen. Antacid tablets are much less potent than liquid antacids. Although they may be more convenient, the lowest effective dose for antacids has not been established; therefore, one must be cautious about recommending tablets for treatment of peptic ulcer disease.

H_2-receptor antagonists have also proved to hasten healing of duodenal ulcers. These agents have the advantage of easier administration (tablets), fewer times per day. The mechanism of action is the blockade of the histamine-2(H_2) receptor which appears to be the final common pathway for acid secretion, regardless of the stimulus. There are currently four H_2-receptor antagonists on the market, cimetidine (Tagamet), ranitidine (Zantac), famotidine (Pepcid), and nizatidine (Axid). Side-effects of the H_2-antagonists are infrequent. Side-effects of cimetidine include mental disturbances, which occur primarily in the elderly and patients with renal or hepatic disease; rash; and, occasionally, headache. Drug interactions appear to be much more likely with cimetidine because it has the ability to inhibit the metabolism of other drugs. Drug interactions with cimetidine include warfarin, theophylline, diazepam, chlordiazepoxide, phenytoin, propranolol, carbamazepine, and others.

Another agent useful for the treatment of peptic ulcer disease is sucralfate (Carafate). Although the mechanism of action is unclear, sucralfate forms a protective coating over the ulcer, inactivates pepsin, binds bile salts to a certain degree, and may stimulate local prostaglandin synthesis. The efficacy of this agent is essentially the same as for antacids and H_2-receptor antagonists. The drug is not absorbed to any appreciable degree, thus it has very few side-effects. The most frequently reported side-effect is constipation, which is related to the drugs chemical composition (an aluminum salt of a sulfated disaccharide).

Hormones

ADRENAL STEROIDS

The *glucocorticoids* (corticosteroids) and *mineralocorticoids* are hormones secreted from the adrenal glands. The glucocorticoids regulate carbohydrate, protein, and fat metabolism, exert some effect on electrolyte and water metabolism, and exert an anti-inflammatory effect. The mineralocorticoids (*e.g.*, fludrocortisone) affect water and electrolyte metabolism to a much greater extent than glucocorticoids. The primary steroid excreted from the adrenals is *cortisol* (also known as hydrocortisone). Release of this hormone is through stimulation of the adrenal by adrenocorticotropic hormone (ACTH) which is released from the anterior pituitary by corticotropin-releasing factor (CRF). Administration of ACTH must be by injection to have any pharmacologic effect. Its duration of action is very short and the release of cortisol, with its longer duration, accounts for its pharmacologic activity.

Other preparations of the glucocorticoids exist (Table 1-18). Most of these drugs are available for oral and parenteral administration. There are also a number of these and other glucocorticoid drugs available for topical use. These drugs are most commonly used for their anti-inflammatory effect and for adrenal insufficiency. Continued use of the glucocorticoids may result in Cushing's syndrome (excess adrenal steroids), including moon face, muscle wasting, osteoporosis, electrolyte

TABLE 1-18
Examples of Glucocorticoids

Drug	Trade Name*
Cortisol (hydrocortisone)	Solu-Cortef
Prednisolone	Delta-Cortef
Prednisone	Deltasone
Methylprednisolone	Medrol
Dexamethasone	Decadron

*These drugs are also available under other trade names.

problems, hypertension, acne, and aggravation of diabetes mellitus. Extended use may also result in adrenal insufficiency because the administration of exogenous glucocorticoids decreases production of ACTH through a negative-feedback mechanism. Short-term administration of the glucocorticoids (1 to 2 weeks) is usually not associated with serious problems.

ANTIDIABETIC AGENTS

Insulin

Diabetes mellitus is a disease in which glucose levels in the blood are elevated because of an absolute or relative shortage of insulin. There are two main types of diabetes, Type I, or insulin-dependent diabetes mellitus, and Type II, or non-dependent diabetes mellitus. Although both types may be treated with insulin, Type I patients must have insulin injections.

Insulin is essential for glucose utilization. It not only promotes the uptake of glucose by cells, but also aids in conversion of fatty acids, amino acids, and glucose into storage forms. Without insulin, blood glucose increases, but the patient cannot utilize it. As a result the body detects a relative shortage of glucose and begins to break down fatty acids and proteins to glucose.

Several different insulin preparations are available. In the past, insulin was derived from animal sources, beef and pork. With today's technology, human insulin is being synthesized and most new diabetics begin therapy with human insulin. Differences between preparations are related to onset and duration of action. Insulin is usually administered subcutaneously, at least once daily (in many cases twice daily), with long-acting insulin (Table 1-19). The dosage of insulin is given in units as opposed to milligrams or grams. The most common side-effect of insulin is hypoglycemia; however, some patients develop local reactions at the site of injection.

Oral Hypoglycemic Agents

Patients who are not insulin-dependent diabetics may be treated with orally administered antidiabetic agents. These drugs work by stimulating insulin release from the pancreas and causing the insulin receptor to become more sensitive to the insulin already present. A number of drugs are available in the United States, all of which belong to the chemical class, sulfonylureas (Table 1-20). Side-effects include hypoglycemia and, less commonly, rash, hyponatremia, and alcohol-induced flushing.

TABLE 1-19
Examples of Insulin Preparations

Insulin	Onset (hr)	Duration (hr)
Regular	1.5–1	5–7
Semilente	1–2	12–16
Lente	1–2.5	24+
NPH	1–1.5	24+
Ultralente	6	36+

TABLE 1-20
Examples of Oral Hypoglycemic Drugs

Drug	Trade Name*
Tolbutamide	Orinase
Tolazamide	Tolinase
Chlorpropamide	Diabenese
Glipizide	Glucotrol
Glyburide	Diabeta, Micronase

*Some of these drugs are available under other trade names.

THYROID AND ANTITHYROID AGENTS

Thyroid

The thyroid gland controls many body functions. A deficiency is manifested by a slowing down of physical and mental functions. Replacement of the thyroid hormone is usually accomplished by replacing the thyroid hormone, thyroxine (T_4). Triiodothyronine (T_3) is occasionally used; however, it usually is not necessary to replace T_3 because the body converts adequate amounts of T_4 to T_3. Levothyroxine (synthetic T_4) has a long half-life and may take several weeks to reach steady-state levels, but it is usually the preferred agent. Therapy is generally started with a low dose and gradually increased until the appropriate levels are reached. Several thyroid preparations are available (Table 1-21). Side-effects of too much thyroxine include weight loss, nervousness, abdominal cramps, sweating, tachycardia, and other symptoms consistent with hyperthyroidism.

Antithyroid Drugs

Drugs that are useful to treat hyperthyroidism include the thioamides (propylthiouricil and methimazole), iodides, and radioactive iodine. Thioamides block hormone synthesis and peripheral conversion of T_4 to T_3. The iodides decrease release of thyroxine from the thyroid gland. Radioactive iodine causes destruction of the thyroid gland itself. The side-effects of the thioamides include rashes, gastrointesti-

TABLE 1-21
Examples of Thyroid Preparations

Drug	Composition	Trade Name(s)
Thyroid, USP	Dessicated thyroid	Various names
Levothyroxine	Synthetic T_4	Synthroid, Levothroid
Liothryonine	Synthetic T_3	Cytomel
Liotrix	T_4:T_3 (4:1)	Euthroid, Thyrolar

nal symptoms, and possible blood dyscrasias. Iodides may cause rashes, ulcers on mucous membranes, anaphylaxis, and runny nose. Radioactive iodine often causes hypothyroidism and, possibly, radiation sickness. Patients who become hypothyroid while receiving any of these treatments will need to be treated with thyroid replacement.

SUMMARY

This chapter presents a basic introduction to pharmacology and is not to be viewed as an all-encompassing reference. Readers are urged to consult the specific references for additional information. It behooves the practicing clinician and developing therapist to become knowledgeable about this area as they become more active participants in the total rehabilitation of their patients. This will become increasingly important as therapists become more independent and are required to see an increasing percentage of their patients on an outpatient/home-care basis.

BIBLIOGRAPHY

Drug Therapy

Katcher BS, Young LY, Koda-Kimble MA: Applied Therapeutics: The Clinical Use of Drugs, 3rd ed. San Francisco, Applied Therapeutics, 1983
Rakel RE: Conn's Current Therapy. Philadelphia, WB Saunders, 1987

Pharmacology

American Medical Association: Drug Evaluations, 6th ed. Chicago, American Medical Association, 1986
Gilman AG, Goodman LS, Rail TW: Goodman and Gilman's The Pharmacological Basis of Therapeutics, 7th ed. New York, Macmillan, 1985
American Society of Hospital Pharmacists: Drug Information 87. Bethesda, American Society of Hospital Pharmacists, 1987

Drug Interactions

Drug Interaction Facts. St Louis, JB Lippincott
Hansten PD: Drug Interactions, 5th ed. Philadelphia, Lea & Febiger, 1985

Adverse Effects

Dukes MNG: Meyler's Side Effects of Drugs, 10th ed. Amsterdam, Excerpta Medica, 1984

Over-The-Counter Drugs

American Pharmaceutical Association: Handbook of Nonprescription Drugs, 7th ed. Washington, American Pharmaceutical Association, 1982

Neuropharmacologic Implications in Management of the Rehabilitation Patient

2

Clyde B. Killian

In this chapter, selected neurophysiologically active pharmacologic agents are discussed in light of their importance to the therapy evaluation and treatment of dysfunctional muscle tone, postural fixation and adjustment, movement, and function. Rehabilitation therapists evaluate and treat individuals who have specific musculoskeletal, neuromuscular, cardiopulmonary problems, or any combination thereof. Patient goals may include pharmacologic management of medical/surgical problems, as well as therapy goals that may not be related to the pharmacologic history of the individual patient. The therapy practitioner must be cognizant of a patient's pharmacologic history when determining the rehabilitative therapy plan of care. For example, an elderly patient with a cerebral vascular accident may be taking medications for hypertension and diabetes that could act on the central nervous system, produce side-effects, and interact with each other to affect muscle tone, postural fixation and adjustment, mobility, and functional motor performance.

Although therapists do not prescribe pharmacologic agents and, thus, do not need an extensive knowledge of therapeutics and pharmacodynamics, they do need to recognize the following in light of the total person whom they treat: the direct effects of the pharmacologic agents; the indirect effects or side-effects associated with pharmacologic agents; the unwanted effects and potential toxicities associated with pharmacologic agents; and interactions among pharmacologic agents. Figure

I would like to acknowledge Rosalind Sprague Hickenbottom, Ph.D., and Carol Voegle, Pharm.D., for their editorial assistance and their contributions as resource individuals to this chapter.

2-1 offers a paradigm for integrating pharmacologic agents into therapy assessment and treatment.

The following examples of neurologic problems for which pharmacologic protocols exist will be used: pain as an example of neurophysiologic input and processing; parkinsonism and spasticity as examples of disorders of movement and postural adjustment. These examples, as illustrated in Figure 2-2, will emphasize integrating pharmacologic and therapy treatment goals.

PAIN MANAGEMENT

Understanding human pain perception poses a major problem for all health professionals in returning patients with pain to a functional life-style. Pain management is a "key" to successful treatment of many rehabilitation patients. Therefore, all therapists need to understand the basic pharmacologic principles of pain management and neural mechanisms for pain processing.

Myelinated type III and unmyelinated type IV axons are the primary axons conveying pain impulses to the central nervous system. These axons usually have free nerve endings that respond to intense mechanical, thermal, and chemical stimuli. Such stimuli depolarize free nerve endings (nociceptors), and an action potential is propagated along the axon into the central nervous system.[2,8]

In the central nervous system, A δ and C fibers make synaptic connections in the substantia gelatinosa in the spinal cord dorsal horn and in the trigeminal

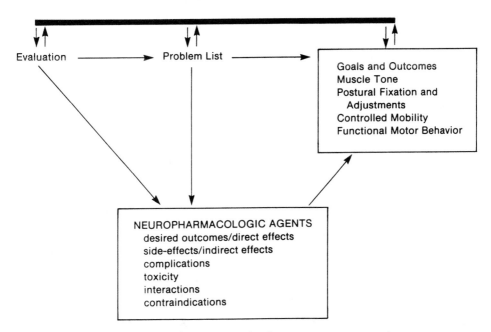

FIGURE 2-1. Neuropharmacologic agents in therapy assessment and treatment.

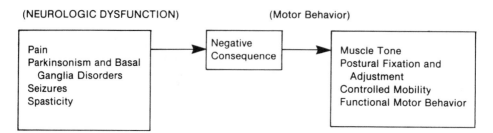

FIGURE 2-2.   Negative consequence of neurologic dysfunction on motor behavior.

spinal nucleus in the brain stem. Through these synaptic connections, multiple interneuronal pathways conveying pain information travel in the spinal cord, brain stem, thalamus, and cerebral cortex. These neuronal pathways provide for conscious awareness of pain relative to location, intensity, and frequency, along with the emotional/affective overlay associated with conscious pain perception.[2]

Pathways that transmit pain can effect such motor responses as muscle spasm and muscle guarding through activation of upper and lower motor neurons. Pain pathways can also activate the sympathetic component of the autonomic nervous system. In addition, pain activates the neuroendrocine system through connections with the limbic system, hypothalamus, brain stem, and spinal cord. Experiencing pain over a long period can result in personality and behavioral changes, manifesting themselves as depression, anxiety, and alteration of the sleep–wake cycles. These personality and behavior problems associated with pain may prove more disabling than the original problem.

The perception of pain is modulated internally by specific biochemical compounds and membrane-bound molecular receptors within the brain and spinal cord. Endorphins are examples of endogenous biochemical mediators of pain suppression. In the brain, endorphins bind to specific receptor sites called opiate receptors. Opiate receptor sites in the central nervous system, if activated by binding to endorphin molecules or to exogenous narcotic compounds, help to diminish pain perception. Opiate receptor sites are found in the dorsal horn of the spinal cord, the trigeminal spinal nucleus, the periaqueductal gray region of the brain stem, and throughout much of the limbic system and basal ganglia. Serotonin pathways from the brain stem also play a major role in blocking pain perception.[1,2,8]

In addition to the endogenous biochemical-receptor mechanism of pain modulation, the perception of pain can be modified by the perception of nonpain perception. Activation of sensory nonpain A β peripheral axons diminish pain transmission by coactivating interneuronal pathways shared among pain and nonpain sensations. The activation of A β fibers functionally blocks the spread of pain transmission of A δ and C fibers. Stimuli compete with painful sensation by using such physical modalities as heat, cold, graded electrical impulses, buoyancy, and exercise to diminish pain perception. These therapeutic strategies act centrally as well as peripherally by activating central pathways within the brain. The pathways that are activated probably include the endogenous enkephalin and endorphin system, the serotoninergic pathways from the brain stem; and, nonpain sensory pathways that block pain transmission.[2,8,11]

Pharmacologic management of pain may accompany therapy protocols for pain control. Drugs used in the pharmacologic management of pain may act peripherally or centrally or they may have combined sites and mechanisms of action. For example, peripherally acting drugs may control pain by inhibiting the chemical activation of free nerve endings, or they may diminish axonal transmission of impulses from free nerve endings. Centrally acting pharmacologic agents probably activate endorphin and serotoninergic systems. Still other drugs used in the pharmacologic management of pain act both peripherally and centrally.[5,7,10]

Nonnarcotic Analgesics

Analgesics diminish or eliminate pain without causing loss of consciousness.[3] Nonnarcotic analgesics are used to reduce mild to moderate pain(analgesic), to reduce inflammation (anti-inflammatory) in arthritis, and to reduce elevated body temperature (antipyretic). Aspirin and acetaminophen are the major examples of nonnarcotic analgesics. Aspirin and acetaminophen both have antipyretic and analgesic effects. Inhibition of prostaglandin synthesis may be the mechanism for the analgesic effect.

Aspirin (acetylsalicylate) decreases body temperature by inhibiting synthesis and release of prostaglandin in the hypothalamus and by causing vasodilation of peripheral vessels. Acetaminophen decreases body temperature by direct action of the hypothalamic heat-regulating center, resulting in vasodilation and sweating.

Aspirin diminishes inflammation by inhibiting prostaglandin synthesis. Inhibition of prostaglandin synthesis partially explains the analgesic effect of aspirin because peripheral pain sensory receptors are stimulated by prostaglandin. Aspirin, therefore, blocks pain perception at the peripheral and central nervous system. Other effects of aspirin include decreasing platelet aggregation and increasing prothrombin time, both of which contribute to the constant aspirin user's tendency to easily bruise. The effect of aspirin on platelet aggregation is utilized for patients with coronary artery disease such as infarction, angina, or transient ischemic attacks. Aspirin has a mild uricosuric effect, and decreases uric acid secretion.[3,5,10]

Nonnarcotic analgesics are indicated in the treatment of mild to moderate pain, arthritic and rheumatic conditions involving musculoskeletal pain, and fever and discomfort caused by viral and bacterial infections. Acetaminophen is indicated in patients who have aspirin allergy or gastrointestinal ulcers, but it is not as effective as aspirin in decreasing inflammation. Acetaminophen lacks anti-inflammatory action but has pain-relieving properties from its site of action in the central nervous system through inhibition of prostaglandin synthesis.

Acetaminophen is relatively free of adverse effects. Aspirin is contraindicated in patients receiving anticoagulant therapy and in persons with gastric ulcers. Adverse reactions to aspirin include nausea, dyspepsia, occult blood loss, and anaphylactic or allergic reactions. Large doses of aspirin can result in dizziness, tinnitus, and mental confusion. Aspirin should be taken with a large glass of water to minimize gastrointestinal effects. The use of aspirin and alcoholic beverages should be avoided.[6] Table 2-1 lists the more common drugs classified as nonnarcotic analgesics.

TABLE 2-1
Nonnarcotic Analgesics

Drug	Trade Name(s)
Acetaminophen	Anacin-3, Tempra, Tylenol, Valadol, Phenaphen, Datril
Aspirin	Ascripin, Bufferin, Emperin, Ecotrin, Encaprin, Zoprin
Choline salicylate	Arthropan
Magnesium salicylate	Magan
Salicylate combination	Trilisate
Diflunisal	Dolobid

Nonsteroidal Anti-Inflammatory Agents

Nonsteroidal anti-inflammatory agents (NSAIDs) produce their analgesic and anti-inflammatory effects through inhibition of prostaglandin synthesis. Prostaglandin sensitizes peripheral pain receptors to chemical mediators such as bradykinin and histamine and produces many of the signs and symptoms of inflammation. Inhibition of the peripheral synthesis of prostaglandin diminishes tissue swelling, tissue exudates, and pain. The NSAIDs are also antipyretic in addition to being anti-inflammatory and analgesic.

Nonsteroidal anti-inflammatory drugs are frequently used in the pharmacologic treatment of rheumatoid arthritis, osteoarthritis, mild to moderate pain, ankylosing spondylitis, acute inflamed soft-tissue injuries, gout, and fever. Adverse reactions to this drug group include nausea, vomiting, diarrhea, and abdominal distress. The incidence of gastrointestinal side-effects is higher with indomethacin (Indocin) and meclofenamate (Meclomen). The recommendation that NSAIDs should be given with food is a rule that is even more important when dealing with the patient in a rehabilitation environment.

Adverse reactions of the CNS to NSAIDs include dizziness, headache, light-headedness, vertigo, paresthesia, peripheral neuropathy, and muscle weakness. Caution should be observed when driving and other tasks requiring alertness because of the possible side-effects of dizziness, drowsiness, and blurred vision. Adverse reactions have also been noted in the cardiovascular, renal, hematologic, respiratory, and endocrine system.[5,6,9] Generic and trade (proprietary) names for the common NSAIDs are referenced in Table 2-2.

Steroidal Agents

Corticosteroids are normally synthesized endogenously in the adrenal cortex. Naturally occurring and synthetic corticosteroids administered in greater than physiologic amounts decrease inflammation and suppress the immune response. Glucocorticoids are the class of steroids used for inhibition of the inflammatory process. Corticosteroid therapy diminishes pain indirectly, but these agents do not cure the

TABLE 2-2
Generic and Trade Names of NSAIDs

Drug	Trade Name(s)
Aspirin	Bufferin, Empirin, and others
Suprofin	Suprol
Fenoprofen	Nalfon
Ibuprofen	Motrin, Rufen, Nuprin
Naproxen	Naprosyn, Anaprox
Sulindac	Clinoril
Indomethacin	Indocin
Tolmetin	Tolectin
Piroxicam	Feldene
Meclofenamate	Meclomen
Mecfenamic acid	Ponstel
Diflunisal	Dolobid

disease process or the cause of the inflammation. Long-term administration of ex-ogenous steroids results in inhibition of endogenous steroid production, with subse-quent atrophy of the adrenal cortex.[5] Therefore, use of steroids should be carefully monitored, and they should be used with caution. Steroid therapy proves useful for acute short-term episodes, with adverse side-effects being minimal. In patients for whom extended use of steroids is required, alternate-day dosage is frequently uti-lized to minimize adrenal gland suppression. Long-term use is common with some rehabilitation patients.

Adverse reactions to steroid therapy are numerous. Muscle myopathy, osteo-porosis, diminished tensile strength of connective tissue, and inhibition of wound healing are all of primary concern for therapists. Increased risk of peptic ulcer de-velopment, hyperglycemic reactions in diabetic patients, decreased resistance to infection, and potential mental disturbance also pose major problems in therapy.[1,5] Table 2-3 categorizes the common glucocorticosteroids.

TABLE 2-3
Classification of Corticosteroids

Duration	Drug	Trade Name(s)
Short-acting	Cortisone	Cortef
	Hydrocortisone	Cortef
Intermediate-acting	Prednisolone	Delta-Cortef
	Prednisone	Deltasone, Orasone
	Methylprednisone	Medrol
	Triamcinolone	Aristocort, Kenacort
Long-acting	Paramethasone	Haldrone
	Dexamethasone	Decadron
	Betamethasone	Celestone

Local Anesthetics, Peripheral Nerve Blocks, and Cold

Local anesthetics inhibit the propagation of action potentials along axons by blocking sodium conductance. Sensory input and motor output are diminished and pain transmission is thus nonselectively blocked. Local anesthetics are utilized to block pain perception during surgical procedures. In certain instances, local anesthetics are used to relieve severe chronic pain.

Lidocaine (Xylocaine), mepivacaine (Carbocaine), and prilocaine (Citanest) are frequently used local anesthetics. In addition to sensation loss, local anesthetics can also block motor and autonomic peripheral nerves. Convulsive seizures, in rare instances, can occur from administration of local anesthetics.[1,2,7]

Peripheral nerve surgical transection and phenol injections of peripheral nerve blocks are used to block severe cases of intractable pain. The peripheral nerve is irreversibly damage by these procedures and cannot conduct nerve impulses. Therapists frequently use cold as a local anaesthetic. Cold blocks sodium conductance which, in turn, blocks sensory transmission to the central nervous system. Cold also helps block pain through inhibition of the inflammatory reaction, diminished anoxic by-products, and diminished tissue deformation by decreasing swelling.[2,11]

Narcotic Analgesics

Narcotic analgesics relieve moderate to severe pain without loss of consciousness, but potentially produce physical and psychologic dependence. Narcotics resemble opium in action and are, therefore, referred to as *opiates*. Morphine, meperidine (Demerol), and codeine are examples of narcotic analgesics prescribed for pain control.

Narcotic analgesics diminish pain perception by direct action on the central nervous system. They do not alter threshold or responsiveness of afferent nerve endings to noxious stimuli, nor do they affect the conduction of nerve impulses in the peripheral nervous system. These drugs alter pain perception at the spinal cord and higher centers within the central nervous system along with affecting the patient's emotional response to pain. In addition to analgesia, opiates cause suppression of the cough reflex, respiratory depression, drowsiness, sedation, change in mood, euphoria, dysphoria, mental clouding, and EEG changes.[2,5]

Narcotics are used to provide temporary relief of moderate to severe pain such as that caused by renal or biliary colic, myocardial infarct, acute trauma, surgical pain, and cancer. Narcotics are utilized in the treatment of chronic intractable pain where nonopiate analgesics have failed. Administration of narcotics requires careful titration that is based on a patient's individualized response to medication.

The primary adverse reaction to narcotics is respiratory depression. Other adverse reactions include circulatory collapse, dizziness, visual disturbance, mental clouding, depression, sedation, coma, euphoria, dysphoria, fainting, agitation, restlessness, nervousness, and seizures. Gastrointestinal effects of narcotics include increased smooth-muscle tone of the large and small intestine and decreased motility, both of which result in constipation.[7] Rehabilitation patients are at risk for these reactions, and careful monitoring is thus required.

Compound analgesics are compounds that contain aspirin or acetaminophen combined with a narcotic. These compounds, because of their synergistic effects, are able to reduce the amount of narcotic required to effectively control pain. Caffeine is used in some compounds to increase the potency of aspirin or acetaminophen. Amphetamines, antipsychotics, antianxiety agents, and antidepressants potentiate the effects of narcotic agonists and are being utilized in the pharmacologic management of patients with chronic pain.[1,2,5,9] Refer to Table 2-4 for a list of the more common opiate agonists and partial opiate agonists. Refer to Table 2-5 for a listing of the compound analgesic agents.

Agents Used to Treat Vascular Headaches

Pharmacology plays an integral role in managing patients with vascular headaches. Vascular headaches occur when cerebral blood vessels are overly dilated. These dilated vessels stimulate nociceptors which, in turn, cause headache pain. Medication in vascular headaches is used to abort an existing headache or to prevent future vascular headaches.[12]

Ergotamine tartrate and related substances are used to reverse a headache in progress. This approach is used when headaches are infrequent and when the patient is not placed at risk with this medication.

Ergotamine tartrate is a vasoconstrictor of blood vessels throughout the body. This action purportedly limits the swelling and inflammation associated with vasodilation during the "headache" phase. Adverse reactions to this drug can include diminished cerebral circulation, which may increase the risk of stroke, irregular heart beats, gastrointestinal upset, and numbness or tingling in the extremities.[2,5,12]

Isometheptene mucate (Midrin), phenothiazine drugs, and prednisone are other agents used in aborting vascular headaches. Propranolol (Inderal) is indicated for migraine prophylaxis. This drug is a β-adrenergic blocking agent that may have associated reactions of weight gain, fluid retention, and fatigue. Methysergide (Sansert) is also used on a limited basis to prevent migraine headaches. This drug blocks serotonin, which is thought to be the causative agent in the dilation phase of the vascular headache.[5,12]

TABLE 2-4
Opiate Agonists and Partial Agonists

Drug	Trade Name
AGONISTS	
Meperidine	Demerol
Hydromorphone	Dilaudid
Oxymorphone	Numorphan
Methadone	Dolophine
Codeine	
Morphine	
PARTIAL AGENTS	
Butorphanol	Stadol
Pentazone	Talwin
Nalbuphine	Nubain

TABLE 2-5
Compound Analgesic Agents

Trade Name	Compounds
Tylenol #1–4	Acetaminophen and codeine
Empirin #1–4	Aspirin and codeine
Percodan	Aspirin and oxycodone
Tylox	Acetaminophen and codeine
Darvon Compound	Aspirin, caffeine, and propoxyphene
Darvocet	Acetaminophen, propoxyphene

Miscellaneous Agents Utilized in Pain Management

General anesthetics and psychotropic drugs also may be useful in diminishing pain perception. Anesthetics, as a group, block sensation. Psychotropic drugs deal with the emotional overlay strongly associated with pain perception. Tryptophan, a metabolic precursor to serotonin, is effective in increasing pain relief.[2,8]

Central-acting muscle relaxants are sometimes used to relieve pain related to muscle spasm and postural muscle guarding. These agents are thought to act within the central nervous system on polysynaptic interneuronal pathways that indirectly effect α motor neurons, γ motor neurons, and upper motor neurons to decrease muscle spasm and muscle guarding.[2,7]

Adverse reactions to muscle relaxants are drowsiness, dizziness, blurred vision, fainting, dry mouth, difficulty with urination, constipation, headache, and gastrointestinal upset. Medication should be taken with food if gastrointestinal upset occurs. Pain perception can increase with administration of muscle relaxants and, therefore, careful monitoring of patient response to these drugs is indicated. The use of alcohol and other CNS depressants should be avoided because they potentiate the effects of the drugs.[9]

The more common centrally acting muscle relaxants are carisoprodol (Soma, Rela), chlorphenesin carbonate (Maolate), chlorzoxazone (Paraflex), cyclobenzaprine (Flexeril), metaxalone (Skelaxin), methocarbamol (Robaxin), orphenadrine (Norfex), diazepam (Valium), and baclofen (Lioresal). Central-acting muscle relaxants are often also classified sedatives and hypnotics.[7]

Implications for Therapists

Patients who have been treated pharmacologically over a period for pain may develop tolerance to the effects of the drugs and require larger doses to maintain pain control compared with those required for the pain associated with acute disease or injury onset. In addition, the long-term pain patient may become less responsive to therapeutic management strategies than the pain-naive individual. Therapy practitioners need to be familiar with a patient's history of pain management and with pharmacologic protocols used in pain management to determine if therapy intervention is effective.

Adjunctive therapeutic procedures can decrease the amount of pain medication required for an effective dose. Diazepam, codeine, narcotics, and steroids are thought to diminish the effectiveness of transcutaneous electrical nerve stimulation (TENS). However, TENS appears to be effective in getting these patients off the medication that diminishes the effectiveness of TENS.[8,11]

Therapists will employ physical agents and motor behavioral modification to return their patients to maximum functional independence. Motor behavioral changes include postural correction, development of movements that are ergonomically sound, and avoidance of tasks that exacerbate pain and biomechanical stress. The following case study with pharmacologic considerations will help emphasize the physical therapist's role in treating patients in pain.

CASE 1   A 35-year-old man, who is 40-lb overweight, has been referred to physical therapy with low-back pain and generalized pain in the right gluteal region, right hip, and right anterior thigh. He has a slight scoliosis in the thoraco-lumbar region, with the convexity to the right. Apparent leg length is 1/2-in. shorter on the left, but true leg lengths are equal. The lumbar curve is flattened. Abdominal muscle strength is poor. The patient lacks pelvic motor control to hold the pelvic girdle and lumbar spine in neutral position during functional activities.

All active and passive movements of the lumbar spine are limited with the greatest limitations in forward bending, right lateral bending, and left rotation. The patient reports pain upon active and passive movement with the greatest pain in active forward bending. Isometric resistive exercises are painful and strong in back muscles.

A straight-leg raise test on the left results in pain in the low-back region. A straight-leg test on the right results in pain in the right gluteal region, right hip, and right anterior thigh. The Lasegue's sign is positive on the right, the Kernig test is positive, and the Valsalva maneuver is positive.

Palpation of the supraspinous and intraspinous ligaments indicates thickening in the L4-L5 and L5-S1 regions. Subcutaneous fibrositic nodules are present throughout the lumbar region. Muscle spasm and increased temperature are present throughout the lumbar region.

The patellar and Achilles deep tendon reflexes are equal and normal. Epicritic and protopathic sensations are intact in the lower extremities. Thigh and calf circumference measurements are equal and symmetric. Muscle power is normal in all muscle groups in the lower extremities. There is no evidence of structural abnormality in the lower extremities. Serologic laboratory reports indicate absence of autoimmune disease and systemic infection.

Patient history reveals a sudden onset of back pain after falling while mowing the back yard. Previous to this incident there was no history of back pain. The patient indicates that his symptoms are not changing. Activity appears to aggravate the patient's symptoms, and rest appears to relieve the symptoms. The patient reports feeling depressed and anxious related to his inability to return to work. He feels that his being unable to work will jeopardize his job and, furthermore, that his health insurance will not adequately cover his medical expenses.

Medications include oxycodone (Percodan) for pain and inflammation; naproxen (Naprosyn) for inflammation; and cyclobenzaprine (Flexeril) for muscle spasm and anxiety. This patient is being seen within 3 days of his back injury at the hospital as an inpatient.

The patient's pain likely contributes to muscle spasm, postural guarding, and inability to perform functional movements with the low back and pelvis maintained in the neutral position. Medication will help control patient pain during this acute stage. The amount of Percodan needed for pain relief may be decreased by the patient using TENS and through the use of physical agents in physical therapy. The patient's depression, anxiety, and nervousness can be consequences of ingestion of narcotic analgesics as well as a result of his injury.[5]

Naprosyn, Flexeril, and rest potentially contribute to decreasing inflammation, decreasing muscle spasm, and diminishing postural guarding. Gentle mobilization techniques and other physical therapy adjuncts should work in concert with medications to decrease inflammation, decrease muscle spasm, decrease postural guarding, and to restore pain-free motion. Medication should be used judiciously to prevent drug dependency and to minimize adverse drug reactions while allowing increased function. In addition, combined medication can mask patient symptoms, which can result in further injury.[2,5]

Once the patient is in the subacute stage of recovery, therapeutic exercises to gain pelvic and lumbar motor control in functional activities should be instituted. The patient will require instruction in how to avoid movements that exacerbate pain and biomechanical stress. Postural correction and development of movements that are ergonomically sound are the long-term goals of therapy so that the liklihood of a recurrence of back pain is diminished. Long-term medication is unable to substitute for the benefits of properly prescribed exercises in therapy. Patient education about the problem and its management is an absolute requirement for successful therapy of the rehabilitation population.

MANAGEMENT OF BASAL GANGLIA DISORDERS

Basal ganglia movement disorders can be classified into positive phenomena, reflecting abnormal increase of motor activity, and negative phenomena, reflecting abnormal decrease or absence of motor activity. Positive phenomena include, rigidity, tremor, chorea, hemiballismus, athetosis, dystonia, and dyskinesia. Negative phenomena include diminished equilibrium reactions; diminished protective extension reactions; decreased automatic postural fixation and adjustment; difficulty with initiation, speed, and cessation of movement; and paucity of movement. These disorders result in severe impairment of muscle tone, postural fixation and adjustment, controlled mobility, and functional motor performance. To appreciate the pharmacologic and therapy implications in the management of basal ganglia disorders, a discussion of basal ganglia components and function is warranted.[5,13,14]

The basal ganglia and associated structures include the caudate nucleus and putamen, globus pallidus, substantia nigra, subthalamic nucleus, and neural pathways connecting the basal ganglia with the thalamus, cerebral cortex, and brain stem. The cerebral cortex, thalamus, and substantia nigra provide neural input to the caudate nucleus and putamen. The greatest influence on the caudate nucleus and putamen is thought to come from the cerebral cortex. The caudate nucleus and putamen, in turn, project neural pathways to the globus pallidus and substantia nigra. Processed output from the substantia nigra and globus pallidus to the cerebral cortex and thalamus provides feedback primarily to assist in the regulation of muscle tone, posture, and movement.[13]

The basal ganglia have an indirect influence on α and γ motor neurons. Processed output from the basal ganglia to the cerebral cortex, thalamus, and brain stem results in activation of upper motor neurons. Upper motor neuron activation subsequently influences α and γ motor neuron excitation, thus controlling the desired type of skeletomotor contraction. Figure 2-3 depicts a schematic representation of the basal ganglia, their associated structures, and their indirect influence on motor output. Clinical and animal studies indicate that the basal ganglia likely function in the appropriate gain (amplification or dampening) of neural input before the expression of the activity to ensure proper temporal coordination of a given motor task.[14]

Dopamine (DA), γ-aminobutyric acid (GABA), and acetylcholine (ACh) are the primary neurotransmitters in the basal ganglia. Dopamine is transmitted by neurons from the substantia nigra to the caudate nucleus and putamen. γ-Aminobuteric acid is transmitted by neurons from the caudate nucleus and putamen to the substantia nigra and globus pallidus. Acetylcholine is transmitted by neurons within the caudate nucleus and putamen. Refer to Figure 2-3 which represents neurotransmitter pathways within the basal ganglia.

Lack of dopamine and high levels of ACh within the basal ganglia are associated with Parkinson's disease. High levels of dopamine and low levels of ACh within the basal ganglia are associated with dyskinesia. Dopamine is thought to inhibit ACh activity and ACh is thought to inhibit dopamine activity within the basal ganglia. Diminished levels of GABA and increased dopaminergic activity is associated with chorea. In Huntington's chorea, autopsy studies have revealed a decrease of GABA- and ACh- releasing neurons. Proper functioning of the basal ganglia is presumed to require a balance of appropriate levels of dopamine, ACh, and GABA. Pharmacologic management of basal ganglia disorders is, therefore, targeted at establishing a proper balance of these neurotransmitters.[5,13,14]

Parkinsonism

In Parkinson's disease in which the disease is primarily the result of degeneration of the substantia nigra, dopaminergic agents and anticholinergic/antihistamine agents can be used to decrease rigidity, tremor, bradykinesia, poverty of movement, postural alterations, and abnormal gait. Dopaminergic agents include dopamine pre-

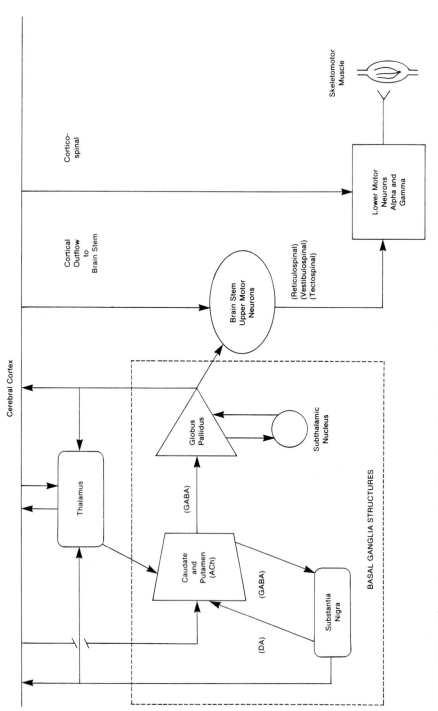

FIGURE 2-3. Schematic representation of basal ganglia, their associated structures, and their indirect influence on motor output.

cursors, such as levodopa, and dopamine-releasing agents, such as amantakine. Levodopa (Dopar, Bendopa, Larodopa) is a metabolic precursor to dopamine. It is able to cross the blood–brain barrier where in the brain it is decarboxy-lated into dopamine for action in the corpus striatum. Levodopa is contraindi-cated in narrow-angle glaucoma, melanoma, patients on monoamine oxidase (MAO)-inhibitor therapy, and acute psychosis.[6,7,9]

There are significant adverse reactions to levodopa therapy for parkinsonian pa-tients. Choreiform or dystonic movements occur in 90% of the patients, nausea and vomiting occurs in 80%, and anorexia occurs in 50% of the patients. Cardiac arrhyth-mias, orthostatic hypotension, loss of drug efficacy, psychiatric disturbances, sleep disturbances, and "on–off" symptoms are also other significant adverse reactions to levodopa. On–off symptoms are characterized by fluctuation of normal movement, chorea, and rigidity within a span of a few minutes.[7,11] Even though there are sig-nificant adverse reactions in levodopa therapy, long-term studies on parkinsonian patients clearly demonstrate the effectiveness of this therapeutic regimen.[14]

Carbidopa is frequently used in a combined form with levodopa (Sinemet) in the treatment of Parkinson's disease. This combination helps prevent decarbox-ylation of peripheral levodopa. Carbidopa does not cross the blood–brain barrier. Peripheral levodopa is, therefore, able to effectively cross the blood–brain barrier at therapeutic levels with lower doses than when levodopa is administered without carbidopa. As a consequence, peripheral adverse reactions, such as nausea and vomiting, cardiac arrhythmias, and orthostatic hypotension, are reduced.[7,9]

Amantadine (Symmetrel) is thought to either enhance the release of dopamine from intact dopaminergic presynaptic neuron terminals or to inhibit the reuptake of dopamine within the synaptic cleft. Amantadine is usually administered in con-junction with levodopa to maximize dopamine concentration in the putamen and caudate nucleus. Drug efficacy usually decreases over time but may remain effec-tive for a period of several months to several years. Adverse reactions are relatively mild and are reversible.[6,7,9]

Central nervous system-acting anticholinergic agents are used to decrease rest-ing tremor, rigidity, and drooling, but they have little effect on bradykinesia, and diminished postural reactions associated with Parkinson's disease. Anticholinergics suppress cholinergic activity. Anticholinergics are frequently used in conjunction with dopaminergic drugs for the treatment of parkinsonism. This drug combination is designed to decrease the concentration of ACh and increase the concentration of dopamine within the caudate nucleus and putamen (striatum). Parkinsonism with its low levels of dopamine and high levels of ACh within the striatum are ostensibly brought into a more normal balance with this drug combination regimen.[9,14]

Contraindications to anticholinergic agents are myasthenia gravis; angle-closure glaucoma; pyloric, duodenal obstruction; and prostatic hypertrophy. Adverse reac-tions to these drugs are blurred vision, muscle weakness and cramping, dry mouth, dizziness, nausea, nervousness, and urinary retention. These agents should be taken with food. Alcohol and central nervous system depressants should be avoided when the patient is taking anticholinergic agents. Patients should exercise caution when performing tasks that require alertness. Table 2-6 lists the more frequently used anticholinergic agents in the treatment of parkinsonism.[11]

Bromocriptine (Parlodel), an ergot derivative, is used in limited instances for the treatment of parkinsonism. It is designed to act directly on dopamine recep-tors in conjunction with other antiparkinsonian drugs.[8] The benefits of levodopa

---

TABLE 2-6
Anticholinergic Agents for Treatment of Parkinsonism

Agent	Trade Name(s)
Benztropine	Cogentin
Biperiden	Akineton
Diphenhydramine	Benadryl
Ethopropazine	Parsidol
Orphenadrine	Disipal
Procyclidine	Kemadrin
Trihexyphenidyl	Artane, Tremin, Trihexidyl

---

therapy diminish over time. A suggested pharmacologic approach in the treatment of parkinsonism is to begin with amantadine and anticholinergic drugs during the initial stages of the disease and introduce levodopa at a later point when parkinsonian symptoms are more severe. Introduction of bromocriptine on a trial basis in conjunction with levodopa can help minimize complications of long-term levodopa therapy.[8,14]

Chorea and Hemiballismus

Chorea, another type of basal ganglia disorder, is characterized by uncoordinated, dancelike, jerky, and stereotypic movements. Chorea can occur from infection (Sydenham's), from an autosomal-dominant pattern (Huntington's), from pharmacologic agents (dopamine, amphetamine, neuroleptics, and reserpine), and can occur spontaneously in the elderly. Chorea is associated with increased levels of dopamine, decreased levels of ACh, and decreased levels of γ-GABA. In Huntington's disease, there is striatal deterioration and deterioration of the cerebral cortex.[13,14]

Pharmacologic management of chorea includes dopaminergic antagonists (perphenazine, haloperidol, metyrosine, and reserpine), cholinergic agonists (choline chloride) and agents that enhance GABA (isoniazid with pyridoxine). Dopamine antagonists are now the most effective in controlling non–drug-induced chorea. Side-effects from dopamine antagonists include depression, dyskinesia, parkinsonianlike symptoms, and drowsiness.

In drug-induced chorea, the pharmacologic management involves reducing or eliminating the medication causing the chorea. For example, a parkinsonian patient taking dopamine will likely develop chorea while on a levodopa medication regimen. The physician will attempt to establish a balance between the symptoms of parkinsonism and chorea through the reduction of levodopa medication. Most patients, however, prefer some degree of choreiform movement over the bradykinesia found in parkinsonism.[14]

The biochemical basis for hemiballismus is not understood but the pharmacologic management of this movement disorder is the same as that for chorea. It is treated with haloperidol, phenelzine, and other dopaminergic blocking agents. Disruption of input and output of neural pathways between the globus pallidus and the subthalamic nucleus results in hemiballismus on the contralateral side to the lesion (Refer to Figure 2-3 for a representation of the relationship between the globus pallidus and subthalamic nucleus). This movement disorder is characterized by large-scale involuntary movements of the extremities and trunk. Stereotactic surgery of basal ganglia structures and thalamic nuclei have had some success in the treatment of this condition.[3,8]

Dystonia and Athetosis

Dystonia is characterized by slow, mass movements of the trunk and extremities that often result in abnormal postural fixation. Athetosis is characterized by slow, writhing movements observed particularly in the hands and feet. The fingers and toes tend to forcibly contort into hyperextension. The biochemical and anatomic basis of these basal ganglia disorders are not well understood. Pharmacologic intervention for these disorders are frequently unsuccessful in resolving the movement disorder. Dopamine agonists, dopamine antagonists, anticholinergics, and other drugs that may effect the basal ganglia are administered on a trial basis to determine effectiveness. Stereotactic surgery has also been utilized in the treatment of these conditions.[3,8,14]

Wilson's Disease

Wilson's disease is a recessively inherited disorder of copper metabolism. Toxic levels of copper affect particularly the basal ganglia, cerebellum, and liver and, thus, Wilson's disease is also referred to as hepatolenticular degeneration. If the disease is untreated, dystonia, cerebellar signs, seizures, dementia, and personality disorders become pronounced. Management is geared toward removal of excess copper through medication and diet. Penicillamine (dimethylcysteine) is a chelating agent that effectively removes copper from the body. With treatment, the disease process is arrested and the patient often shows substantial recovery of motor function.[8,11,13,14]

Iatrogenic Movement Disorders

Iatrogenic movement disorders are drug-induced disorders that have their effect on the basal ganglia. The major categories of movement disorders are drug-induced parkinsonism, tardive dyskinesia, dopamine agonist-induced chorea, and neuroleptic-induced dystonia. These disorders are related to the effects that pharmacologic agents have on the dopaminergic pathways within the basal ganglia.[8,14]

The major tranquilizers (phenothiazines and butyrophenones), collectively referred to as neuroleptics, are dopamine antagonists. They interfere with dopamine interaction within the striatum and can, therefore, result in drug-induced parkinsonism. This condition can be effectively counteracted with anticholinergic drugs when necessary. Drug-induced parkinsonism, however, is a temporary condition.

Over a period of months, dopamine pathways within the striatum are thought to overcome the receptor blockade of neuroleptics, with the resolution of parkinsonism symptoms.

Tardive dyskinesia, however, is a serious consequence of long-term neuroleptic medication. The movements are choreiform and believed to be due to heightened striatal dopaminergic activity. Extended administration of neuroleptics is believed to cause denervation supersensitivity of dopaminergic receptors. This condition is not reversible in over 50% of patients with tardive dyskinesia. Anticholinergics in conjunction with neuroleptics increases the likelihood of developing tardive dyskinesia. Pharmacologic management to prevent tardive dyskinesia should limit the dose and duration of neuroleptic therapy, avoid use of anticholinergics with neuroleptics, institute drug holidays in which patient is taken off of medication, and monitor the patient closely for signs of abnormal movement.

Dopamine agonist-induced chorea occurs frequently (90%) in patients with parkinsonism. Dopamine agonists increase concentration of dopamine within the striatum. The degeneration of dopamine-releasing interneurons that occurs in Parkinson's disease produces denervation supersensitivity of dopamine receptors. This condition is reversible with reduction of dopamine agonist medication. Parkinsonian movement disorders become worse, however, upon reduction of dopamine agonists. As discussed in the section of this chapter on Parkinson's disease, most parkinsonian patients would prefer to have choreiform movement over parkinsonian rigidity and bradykinesia.

Neuroleptic-induced dystonia occurs primarily in adolescents and young adults. Within a few days of neuroleptic administration, the patient becomes immobile with fixation in dystonic postures. The pharmacologic mechanism for this disorder is not known, but it is believed to be related to the dopaminergic system within the basal ganglia. Patients with this condition respond favorably to anticholinergic agents.[8,9,14]

Implications for Therapy

Basal ganglia disorders present the therapist with the difficult task of teaching these patients to control abnormal muscle tone, postural adjustment, and movement in functional patterns. When there is lack of movement and postural reactions, the therapist introduces exercises to increase mobility and to balance reactions and righting reactions. Where there are exaggerated extraneous movements, the therapist introduces stability and controlled mobility exercises. Dementia in Huntington's disease and in the later stages of parkinsonism will impair the patient's ability to learn motor skills in therapy.

In the progressive diseases of parkinsonism and Huntington's chorea, the patients will develop secondary complications related to inactivity imposed by the disease process. These complications could include, osteoporosis, pneumonia, muscle and joint deterioration, bowel and bladder dysfunction, and skin breakdown. Although therapists cannot arrest the progression of these diseases, they can help these patients maintain their maximal psychomotor independence and thus enhance their quality of life.[13]

Pharmacologic agents play a major role in the management of basal ganglia movement disorders. The therapist should be aware of how medications are enhancing or hindering motor performance. A therapist's ongoing feedback on patient motor performance to physicians, nurses, and patients can prove invaluable in the proper adjustment of medication for treatment. The following case study helps to highlight the therapy implications in the treatment of basal ganglia disorders:

CASE 2   A 60-year-old man with a 7-year history of parkinsonism is referred to therapy for evaluation and treatment. He had just completed a "drug holiday" within a hospital where he was taken off his antiparkinsonian medications for 6 days to diminish undesired effects and reestablish the effectiveness of the medications at lower doses. Over this 6-day period, he became rigid and unable to move. He presently is receiving lower doses of levodopa/carbidopa than he did before admission.

During the first 3 years of the disease, the patient's symptoms were successfully managed with anticholinergics and amantadine. During the last 4 years, he has required higher doses of levodopa, in combination with carbidopa, for the management of his parkinsonian symptoms. This past year, on a regimen of levodopa therapy, the patient has developed choreiform dyskinesia, on–off phenomena, periods of paranoia and hallucinations, and nausea and vomiting. These undesirable effects were felt to be a consequence of medication. The patient was also exhibiting signs of dementia, which was thought to be related to the progression of the disease. The patient's condition has regressed to a point at which the family (his daughter, son-in-law, and grandchildren) question whether he should remain living with them or seek placement in a nursing home.

Therapy assessment revealed that the patient was exhibiting overall kyphotic flexion posture with an inability to extend his neck or trunk to a neutral upright posture. Joint limitations restricted full shoulder elevation, hip extension, and knee extension. He had moderate cogwheel rigidity and resting tremor. He had difficulty with volitional pronation and supination and was impaired in fine motor tasks. His speech was monotone and slightly difficult to understand. His ability to show facial expressions was diminished, but he was capable of most self-care activities, although movements were slow.

He had difficulty with dynamic and static balance reactions. He performed reciprocal movements with great difficulty, and he lacked volitional rotation in his trunk and extremities. He required slight assistance in assuming a standing from a sitting posture. He could maintain a standing posture but had a tendency to fall without the use of a walker in gait. His step and stride lengths were diminished, and he had difficulty in starting, stopping, and negotiating turns when walking.

He complained of generalized muscle and joint soreness. His kyphotic posture limited chest expansion which made him susceptible to pulmonary complications. He had seborrhea and diminished gastrointestinal motility. With the lower dosages of levodopa, the patients' appetite has improved, as well as his motor skills since the prehospital admission. He no longer demonstrates choreiform dyskinesia and the on-off symptoms. His parkinsonian symptoms, although severe, appear to have diminished as a result of medication and therapy. His overall mentation has also improved.

In this case, the patient gained the ability to physically care for himself but required supervision because of the onset of dementia. From the improvement the patient gained through therapy and medication, he was capable of remaining within the home environment. However, he required placement in a geriatric day-care center during the day when the family was out of the home.

Discussion

Moist heat often reduces muscle and joint soreness associated with parkinsonism. The following therapy exercises should assist in the patient maintaining maximum motor function:

1. Mobility and gentle stretching exercises to maintain maximum movement within available joint range
2. Rotation and reciprocal movements within the patient's ability, to enhance more normal movement patterns
3. Postural righting and balance activities, to encourage more-normal postural reactions and controlled mobility
4. Activities to encourage initiation, cessation, and speed of movement
5. Oral facial exercises to enhance speech, eating, drinking, and facial expression
6. Pregait and gait exercises to improve balance and ability to stop, start, and negotiate turns when walking
7. Trunk extension exercises and chest expansion exercises, as tolerated, to retard progression of flexion posture and pulmonary congestion
8. Adaptive equipment and functional exercises, to maintain maximum independence in daily self-care

Therapy funding is limited for parkinsonian patients. Therefore, it is incumbent upon the therapist to integrate the preceding exercises into a home-treatment program in which the patient, family, and other health professionals can provide care at reduced costs. The therapist, with the implementation and follow-up of this exercise and home program, can enhance the quality of the parkinsonian patient's life.

SPASTICITY

Spasmolytic Agents

Spasticity as seen in spinal cord injury, multiple sclerosis, cerebral vascular accidents, and traumatic head injury, interferes with the patient's ability to control muscle tone, postural fixation and adjustment, controlled mobility, and functional motor behavior. Consequently, therapists are very much involved in treating patients who have spasticity. Therapists frequently use therapeutic exercise, serial casting, splinting, orthotics, ice, and electrical stimulation in the management of this disorder.

Pharmacologic agents can be useful in the reduction of spasticity. Therapists, therefore, require a basic understanding of the clinical application of these pharmacologic agents. Central nervous system-acting agents include diazepam and baclofen (Lioresal). Diazepam is thought to facilitate the action of γ-aminobutyric acid within the central nervous system. This facilitation of GABA is thought to reduce spasticity through activation of presynaptic inhibition within interneurons contained in the spinal cord and brain stem. Unfortunately, this drug frequently causes sedation at dose levels necessary to reduce spasticity.[7]

Baclofen, on the other hand, reduces spasticity and does not cause the same degree of sedation as diazepam. Baclofen can, however, cause lethargy and confusion. It is thought to reduce spasticity through inhibition of neurotransmitters within the spinal cord. Baclofen is considered the centrally acting drug of choice in treating spasticity; however, patients with impaired cognition may not be candidates for this drug. Also, seizure activity may be increased in the epileptic patient.[8,15]

Dantrolene sodium (Dantrium) reduces spasticity through interference with skeletal muscle excitation. Dantrolene acts directly on skeletomotor muscle through inhibition of the release of calcium from the sarcoplasmic reticulum. Sedation from dantrolene is mild in comparison with diazepam and baclofen. Dantrolene is often the drug of choice in treating spastic patients with impaired cognition, and it is effective in treating patients who have pain associated with their spasticity.

Generalized muscle weakness is a frequent negative occurrence in patients taking dantrolene. Dantrolene also can cause liver damage which, therefore, requires close medical monitoring of liver function.[7,8,15]

Peripheral nerve blocks can effectively reduce spasticity when more traditional therapy interventions have failed to control spastic-induced postural fixation and contracture formation. Phenol is applied percutaneously to a given nerve and, in turn, destroys a portion of the axons within that nerve bundle, reducing the spasticity. In mixed nerves, this results in both sensory and motor loss. Local pain, swelling, and edema are frequent short-term complications of phenol injections. Central nervous system depression, cardiovascular collapse, and thrombophlebitis are infrequent complications of this procedure. An advantage of applying phenol nerve injections over systemic medications is that there is no impairment of cognitive function and other systemic effects.[16]

Therapy Implications

Therapists work with spastic patients in helping them learn to inhibit the reflex nature of their spasticity while teaching them to move in more normal patterns and postures. Positioning, splinting, serial casting, range-of-motion, electrical stimulation, and exercises help to reduce spasticity, increase the range-of-motion, and prevent muscle contractures. Learning to incorporate volitional functional movement while controlling spasticity is the next stage in the patient's recovery.

Therapists should be aware of when antispastic agents enhance or hinder patient function. Systemic drugs can cause varied degrees of cognitive impairment.

The therapist should be cognizant of patient responses and notify the physician if antispastic medication is causing drug-induced cognitive impairment. Dantrolene can cause generalized weakness and may interfere with the patient's ability to move and sustain antigravity postural control. Phenol injection can selectively reduce spasticity along given nerve distributions. This procedure causes denervation of selected axons with varied degrees of motor or sensory loss. This procedure should be applied when the more traditional therapy interventions have failed to reduce spasticity.

CASE 3   A 25-year-old patient had an intracranial bleed from a ruptured aneurysm of the right middle cerebral artery. She had successfully tolerated surgery in which the middle cerebral artery had been clipped. It has been a month since surgery without any subsequent bleeding into the subarachnoid space. She was considered medically stable and was transferred to a rehabilitation unit. She was referred to therapy for evaluation and treatment.

She had left hemiplegia, left hemianesthesia, left hemianopsia, difficulty with space perception, position, and some impairment in ability to maintain attention and memory. Her left upper extremity postured in flexion with severe spasticity in the shoulder girdle, elbow flexors, and forearm pronators. The range-of-motion was limited in shoulder elevation, elbow extension, and forearm supination. She demonstrated left upper extremity volitional movement in synergy through partial range. Left-hand function showed instinctive grasp without volitional release.

The patient could roll to her right, to her left, and assume a short sitting posture independently. She could shift weight and scoot while sitting, but balance reactions were absent when the center of gravity was displaced in left lateral flexion and rotation. She was independent in wheelchair mobility and negotiated transfers under supervision.

She assumed a standing posture by shifting weight onto her right lower extremity. Her left plantar flexion spasticity was severe, which limited the ankle dorsiflexion range. Lower extremity volitional movements were in synergy through a partial range. She could not ambulate without assistance. She had limited ability to bear weight and maintain balance on her left lower extremity. Her gait was not functional, which required her to rely on her wheelchair for mobility.

Progressive serial casting, electrical stimulation to the triceps, and prolonged ice to the shoulder girdle helped reduce spasticity and allow full upper extremity range of motion. Baclofen helped reduce her spasticity but, unfortunately, the medication caused confusion and difficulty with maintaining her attention in therapy. Baclofen, thus, had to be discontinued. Dantrolene sodium proved effective in decreasing spasticity, but it also had to be discontinued because of the elevation of liver enzymes, indicating hepatotoxicity. Therapeutic exercise allowed the patient to learn to move her left upper extremity independent of synergy and to functionally use her arm for protective extension and postural support. Trunk balance concomitantly improved in sitting balance, in lateral flexion, and in rotation. Because therapy intervention controlled spasticity and helped the patient to regain limited functional recovery of her left upper extremity, it was determined that a phenol injection for control of upper extremity spasticity would not be warranted.

Serial casting and prolonged ice helped decrease plantar flexion spasticity and increase her ankle dorsiflexion range. Plantar flexion, however, continued to present a barrier to the development of a functional gait. A phenol injection to the posterior tibial nerve reduced flexion spasticity to a manageable level. The patient learned to bear weight on her left leg and dorsiflex the foot to the neutral position. An ankle–foot orthosis helped improve ankle stability. With gait training and the use of a quad cane, the patient developed a functional gait and no longer required a wheelchair for mobility.

This chapter has focused on selected patient problems that the neurologic therapist would likely encounter in clinical practice. The neurologic therapist helps treat patients with dysfunctional muscle tone, postural fixation and adjustment, controlled mobility, and functional motor behavior. Pharmacologic agents can enhance or hinder therapy treatment progressions. It is hoped that this chapter with its selected case studies will help the clinician in integrating pharmacologic agents into therapy assessment and treatment.

REFERENCES

1. Becker DE: Pharmacology for the Health Professional. Reston, Reston Publishing Co, 1985
2. Bond MR: Pain: Its Nature, Analysis and Treatment, 2nd ed. New York, Churchill Livingston, 1984
3. Brodal A: Neurological Anatomy in Relation to Clinical Medicine, 3rd ed. New York, Oxford University Press, 1981
4. DiPalma JR (ed): Basic Pharmacology in Medicine. New York, McGraw-Hill, 1976
5. Duvoisin R: Parkinsonism. Clin Symp, 28:1, 1976
6. Goodman LS, Alford G: The Pharmacological Basis of Therapeutics, 6th ed. New York, Macmillan, 1980
7. Kastrup EK (ed): Facts and Comparisons. St Louis, JB Lippincott, 1986
8. Katzung B: Basic and Clinical Pharmacology. Los Altos, CA Lange Medical Publications, 1982
9. Malseed RT: Pharmacology: Drug Therapy and Nursing Considerations. Philadelphia, JB Lippincott, 1982
10. Mannheimer JS, Lampe GN: Clinical Transcutaneous Electrical Nerve Stimulator. Philadelphia, FA Davis, 1984
11. McEvoy GK, McQuarrie GM (eds): American Hospital Formulary Service Drug Information 86. Bethesda, American Society of Hospital Pharmacists, 1986
12. Melmen KL, Marelli HF: Clinical Pharmacology—Basic Principles in Therapeutics, 2nd ed. New York, Macmillan, 1978
13. Umphred DA (ed): Neurological Rehabilitation. St Louis, CV Mosby, 1985
14. Weiner WJ, Goetz CG (ed): Neurology for the Non-Neurologist. Philadelphia, Harper & Row, 1981
15. Wroblewski B, Glenn MB: Antispasticity medication in the patient with traumatic brain injury. Jl Head Trauma Rehabil 1(2):71–72, 1986
16. Glenn, MB; Nerve blocks in the treatment of spasticity. Jl Head Trauma Rehabil 1(3):72–74, 1986

Cardiovascular Medications   3

Lawrence P. Cahalin

Therapists, whether practicing general therapy or specializing in cardiopulmonary care, must be familiar with the commonly prescribed cardiovascular medications. This is imperative because approximately 30% to 40% of potential therapy patients have coexisting cardiovascular disease, and a substantial number have had cardiovascular medications prescribed.[13,54,57] The therapist must be knowledgeable about cardiovascular medications to accurately assess the cardiovascular responses occurring during exercise and to appropriately design individual therapeutic exercise programs. Depending upon the medication used, significant effects may be observed in one or more of the clinically monitored exercise responses including heart rate and rhythm, blood pressure, electrocardiographic measurements, and symptoms. Furthermore, a therapist with a thorough understanding of cardiovascular medications is able to obtain objective information pertaining to the efficacy and side-effects of a given medication during functional or therapeutic activities. As a result, the therapist can provide information that can be extremely useful to the physician in making decisions about the medical management of a given patient.

The major purpose of this chapter is to provide information on the most commonly prescribed cardiovascular medications. The clinical pharmacology, indications, contraindications, and side-effects of antihypertensive, antiarrhythmic, and antianginal medications will be discussed. β-Adrenergic blockers and calcium antagonists will be reviewed in detail because they are the two most commonly prescribed classes of cardiovascular medications. Part of this detailed description includes information on the effects of exercise training in patients receiving β-blockers. A brief review of cholesterol-lowering agents will also be included because the use of these medications will increase substantially in the future (perhaps to be used as frequently as antihypertensive medications)[43] and because their use has demonstrated favorable effects upon lipid levels and atherosclerosis in those with and without existing coronary artery disease (CAD).[5,7,58-60,87]

Finally, case studies of patients evaluated and treated in our clinic will be included to illustrate the significance of the preceding information. Before discussing each class of medication, background information on the pathophysiology will be presented so that the clinician will better understand the rationale for the use of each medication.

HYPERTENSION

Probably the most common cardiovascular disease that therapists encounter is hypertension. As many as one-third of all people over 65 have systolic hypertension,[36] and approximately two-thirds of all strokes occur in individuals who were previously hypertensive.[76] "In the United States, hypertension has become the most frequent reason for visits to physicians as well as the leading indication for prescription drugs."[50]

The pathogenesis of hypertension is a slow and gradual process, the probability of which increases as one ages. Hypertension is diagnosed when blood pressure readings are repeatedly above 140/90 mm Hg.[94] The primary determinants of blood pressure (BP) are the cardiac output (CO) and peripheral vascular resistance (PVR) (BP = CO × PVR). Changes in CO and PVR have been observed during the pathogenesis of hypertension. Early in this disease process, CO *appears* to be normal or slightly increased, whereas PVR is normal, but as hypertension progresses, CO falls and PVR increases.[62,90] The expected response to an increase in CO is peripheral vasodilatation, resulting in a decreased PVR. Therefore, a "normal resistance in the presence of a high cardiac output is actually abnormally elevated, constituting the primary mechanism of hypertension."[51] The possible mechanisms producing the preceding changes include autoregulation; genetic predisposition; sympathetic nervous activation; renal pressure–natriuresis; intracellular sodium and calcium exchange; the renin–angiotensin–aldosterone system; vasopressin; vasodepressor deficiency; excesses or deficiencies of various minerals and changing ratios among dietary sodium, calcium, and potassium; the percentage of fast-twitch and slow-twitch muscle fibers throughout the body; and the "sodium transport" hypothesis.[46,51]

Many of the aforementioned mechanisms are responsible for hypertension, but the *sodium transport hypothesis* is most widely accepted because it encompasses many of the other hypotheses (autoregulation, renal pressure–natriuresis, sympathetic stress, and renin–angiotensin). This hypothesis indicates that an inherited defect in renal sodium excretion causes an increase in intracellular sodium. An increased intracellular sodium concentration increases the peripheral vascular tone and reactivity which increases PVR and produces hypertension (Fig. 3-1). The increase in vascular tone and reactivity that increases PVR is the result of (1) increased fluid volume; (2) increased intracellular calcium (from an increased sodium–calcium exchange) that binds to myofilament regulatory proteins, stimulating myosin phosphorylation and increasing the resting tone of vascular smooth muscles; or (3) autoregulation (an intrinsic property of resistance vessels which increases vasoconstriction because of an increased blood flow).[51] Emotional stress

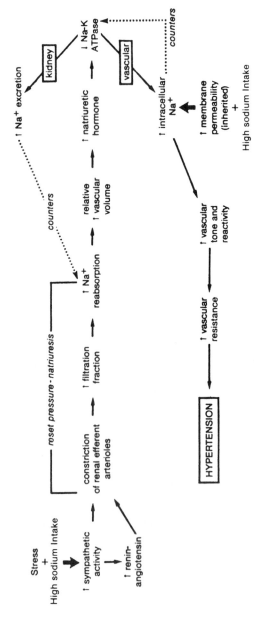

FIGURE 3-1.   Hypothesis for the pathogenesis of primary (essential) hypertension, starting from two points, shown as heavy arrows. One, starting on the top left, is the combination of stress and high sodium intake, which induces an increase in natriuretic hormone and thereby inhibits sodium transport. The other, starting at the bottom right, invokes an inherited defect in sodium transport plus a high sodium intake to induce an increase in intracellular sodium. (Kaplan NM: Systemic Hypertension: Mechanisms and Diagnosis. In Braunwald E (ed): Heart Disease, 3rd ed, Vol I, p 833. Philadelphia, WB Saunders, 1987)

can also be a contributing factor to the pathogenesis of hypertension by increasing sympathetic activity, which not only increases CO and causes arteriolar and venous constriction but, also, increases renin–angiotensin levels. Renin, a proteolytic enzyme, liberates angiotensin I, which is converted into angiotensin II by a converting enzyme. Angiotensin II is a powerful arterial constrictor and also increases renal retention of salt and water. This may result in an increased resistance within the renal efferent arterioles, increasing the filtration fraction, which increases peritubular oncotic pressure and, finally, increases reabsorption of tubular sodium. This process (pressure-natriuresis) is a major factor in the pathogenesis of hypertension.

The various medications used to treat hypertension are classified according to their mode of action. The major classes of antihypertensive agents are diuretics, antiadrenergic agents (central and peripheral acting), vasodilators, angiotensin-converting enzyme (ACE) inhibitors, calcium-channel blocking agents, and β-adrenergic blockers. These medications are used after other methods of blood pressure control have failed (exercise, weight loss, dietary sodium restriction, and stress reduction).

Antihypertensive Medications

DIURETICS

Diuretics are often the first medications used to treat hypertension. These drugs enhance the excretion of sodium, chloride, and water and correct or prevent the retention of excessive fluid in various tissues. Diuretics, in essence, improve the normal function of the kidney by increasing the glomerular filtration rate, decreasing the rate at which sodium is reabsorbed from the glomerular filtrate by the renal tubules, and promoting the excretion of sodium, chloride, and water from the kidney. The most commonly prescribed diuretics are the thiazides and related drugs, a few of which are hydrochlorothiazide (HydroDIURIL), chlorothiazide (Diuril), chlorthalidone (Hygroton), and bendroflumethiazide (Naturetin). The most common side-effect of the thiazides is hypokalemia. This is why the potassium-sparing diuretics were introduced: hydrochlorothiazide/triamterene (Dyazide, Maxzide), hydrochlorothiazide/spironolactone (Aldactazide), spironolactone (Aldactone), amiloride/hydrochlorothiazide (Moduretic), spironolactone with hydrochlorothiazide, amiloride (Midamor), and triamterene (Dyrenium). Another common diuretic is furosemide (Lasix), which is classified as a loop diuretic. Loop diuretics inhibit the reabsorption of sodium and chloride in the ascending loop of Henle, resulting in the excretion of sodium, chloride, and to a lesser degree, potassium and bicarbonate ions. Furosemide has a slight antihypertensive effect but is used primarily for the treatment of edema associated with congestive heart failure, nephrotic syndrome, hepatic cirrhosis, pulmonary edema, and severe hypercalcemia. Side-effects include hypokalemia, severe dehydration, gout, and metabolic alkalosis. All diuretics are contraindicated when renal function is impaired.

ANTIADRENERGIC AGENTS

Antiadrenergic agents are then added if maximal doses of diuretics fail to control BP. Diuretics are usually continued to provide synergistic effects and to prevent secondary fluid accumulation, which may occur with the use of antiadrenergic agents alone. The antiadrenergic agents depress the activity of the sympathetic nervous system centrally and peripherally. The centrally acting agents include methyldopa (Aldomet), clonidine (Catapres), and guanabenz (Wytensin), all of which appear to lower arterial pressure by the stimulation of central inhibitory α-adrenergic receptors, thus decreasing sympathetic outflow from the brain.

The peripherally acting agents include reserpine (Hydropres, Salutensin, Diupres) and the numerous other rauwolfia derivatives, guanethidine (Esimil, Ismelin), guanadrel (Hylorel), prazosin (Minipress), and terazosin (Hytrin), of which the first three exert their antihypertensive effects by depleting norepinephrine in the post-ganglionic adrenergic nerve ending, which causes relaxation of vascular smooth muscle and decreases total PVR. Prazosin lowers arterial BP by selectively blocking postsynaptic α-adrenergic receptors, which dilates both arterioles and veins.

Because the central and peripheral adrenergic agents are such potent antihypertensives, the most common side-effect is hypotension associated with dizziness, headache, drowsiness, and fatigue. The antiadrenergic agents are contraindicated in the presence of active hepatic disease (methyldopa) or hypersensitivity to any of the above-mentioned medications.

VASODILATORS

Vasodilators are often initiated if BP control is inadequate with a combination of the preceding medications. The vasodilators include hydralazine (Apresoline), minoxidil (Loniten), and nitrates (see antianginals). Hydralazine reduces arterial BP by directly relaxing vascular smooth muscle in arterioles, which produces a peripheral vasodilatation. Minoxidil also relaxes vascular smooth muscle, but the exact mechanism of action is unknown. Contraindications of minoxidil are pheochromocytoma, acute myocardial infarction, and dissecting aortic aneurysm. Minoxidil may produce serious adverse effects including pericardial effusion, occasionally progressing to tamponade, and exacerbation of angina pectoris.

Hydralazine is contraindicated when hypersensitivity exists and in patients with CAD or mitral valvular heart disease. The most common adverse reactions include headache, anorexia, nausea, vomiting, diarrhea, palpitations, tachycardia, and angina pectoris. In a few patients, hydralazine may produce a clinical picture simulating acute systemic lupus erythematosus.

Although nitrates are used primarily for the relief of angina, their mode of action is similar to the foregoing medications. Relaxation of vascular smooth muscle dilates both arterial and venous beds. In addition, intravenous nitroglycerin is used to control BP in perioperative hypertension and to produce controlled hypotension during surgical procedures.

ANGIOTENSIN-CONVERTING ENZYME (ACE) INHIBITORS

The ACE inhibitors are initiated when BP control is resistant to other medications, or when the foregoing medications produce intolerable side-effects. The ACE inhibitors consist of captopril (Capoten), enalapril maleate (Vasotec), and lisinopril (Zestril, Prinivil). These medications appear to suppress the renin–angiotensin–aldosterone system; however, the exact mechanism of action has not been fully determined. Both captopril and enalapril are contraindicated when hypersensitivity exists. The side-effects of both medications are few, the most common being proteinuria, neutropenia/ agranulocytosis, hypotension, and angioedema.

CALCIUM-CHANNEL BLOCKING AGENTS

The calcium-channel blockers have many uses, one of which is to control hypertension. Those currently available are nifedipine (Procardia), verapamil (Calan, Isoptin), and diltiazem (Cardizem). These agents reduce arterial BP at rest and at a given level of exercise by dilating peripheral arterioles and reducing the total PVR. Nifedipine is contraindicated when hypersensitivity exists, and verapamil and diltiazem when sick sinus syndrome, second-degree AV block, systolic hypotension ($<$ 90 mm Hg), cardiogenic shock, or congestive heart failure exist. The most common side-effects associated with these medications include peripheral edema (nifedipine), light-headedness, dizziness, weakness, nausea, and headache. Nifedipine often produces the greatest percentage of adverse reactions.

β-ADRENERGIC BLOCKERS

The β-adrenergic blockers are similar to the calcium-channel blockers in that hypertension is just one of their many uses. The β-blockers used for the treatment of hypertension include acebutolol (Sectral), atenolol (Tenormin), metoprolol (Lopressor), nadolol (Corgard), timolol (Blocadren), propranolol (Inderal), and pindolol (Viskin). β-blocking agents compete with β-adrenergic agonists for available β-receptor sites. Metoprolol, acebutolol, and atenolol are cardioselective and preferentially inhibit β_1-adrenoreceptors located primarily in cardiac muscle and adipose tissue. Cardioselective β-blockers inhibit the chronotropic response (rate) and inotropic response (force of contraction) of the heart, as well as conduction through the atrioventricular (AV) node. Lipolysis in adipose tissue is also inhibited by cardioselective β-blockade. Propranolol, nadolol, timolol, and pindolol inhibit both β_1- and β_2-receptors (which are located primarily in the bronchial and vascular musculature). These drugs are nonselective and inhibit the foregoing β_1-responses of the heart and adipose tissue as well as the vasodilator responses to β-adrenergic stimulation in the bronchial and peripheral vascular musculature. In addition, nonselective β-blockers inhibit the release of insulin from the pancreas, as well as glycogenolysis in the liver and muscles. The hemodynamic effects of β-blockers include decreased heart rate, stroke volume, and CO; increased end-diastolic volume and end-diastolic pressure; and decreased myocardial oxygen requirement. Arterial BP, therefore, is lowered primarily because of a decreased CO. Pindolol and acebutolol provide a slight stimulation of the blocked receptor, which preserves adequate β-adrenergic sympathetic tone, particularly maintaining CO. This partial agonist effect is called *intrinsic sympathomimetic activity.*

Contraindications to the use of β-blockers include (1) sinus bradycardia, (2) greater than a first-degree heart block, (3) cardiogenic shock, (4) congestive heart failure, (5) hypersensitivity to β-blocking agents, and (6) bronchial asthma or bronchospasm, including severe chronic obstructive pulmonary disease (for the nonselective β-adrenergic blockers). The most common side-effects are bradycardia, worsening of angina, dizziness, fatigue, mental depression, dyspnea, peripheral vascular insufficiency (cold extremities, paresthesias of hands), congestive heart failure, and conduction disturbances.

DYSRHYTHMIAS

Cardiac dysrhythmias are common, occurring frequently in healthy individuals[28] as well as those with CAD.[6] Some dysrhythmias are benign, whereas others are life-threatening. Antiarrhythmic agents are used to control both life-threatening and benign, symptomatic dysrhythmias. To understand the clinical pharmacology, indications, contraindications, and side-effects of the many antiarrhythmics, it is necessary to first understand the normal cardiac cycle, the abnormalities of the cardiac cycle, and the causes of abnormal cardiac cycles.

The normal electrical events that occur during a cardiac cycle are best understood with the use of a normal single-lead electrocardiogram (ECG) (Fig. 3-2). During sinus rhythm, the cardiac impulse originates in the sinoatrial (SA) node and travels through the right and left atria, which causes the atria to depolarize and contract, generating a P wave. This wave of depolarization next travels through the atrioventricular (AV) node, bundle of His, and bundle branches (right, left anterosuperior fascicle, and left posteroinferior fascicle), producing the P-R interval. As conduction continues through the bundle branches and Purkinje fibers, the ventricles depolarize and contract, producing the QRS complex. The S-T segment, immediately following the QRS complex, represents ventricular repolarization, which is completed with the presence of the T wave.

To better understand dysrhythmias and the effects of antiarrhythmic agents, the action potential that initiated the previous ECG tracing must be examined. Each area of the heart possessing automaticity (SA node, parts of the atria, AV node, and His-Purkinje system) has the ability to spontaneously initiate an action potential. The resultant action potential has five phases: phase 0 (rapid depolarization), phase 1 (early repolarization), phase 2 (the plateau phase of repolarization, which corresponds to the S-T segment of the ECG), phase 3 (absolute refractory period and relative refractory period corresponding to the T wave of the ECG), and phase 4 (return of the action potential to its resting value, or "diastolic depolarization"; Fig. 3-3). The action potentials of the SA node, Purkinje fibers, and portions of the specialized conduction system differ from those of atrial and ventricular muscle. The primary difference between these areas is the slope of phase 4, which is steepest

FIGURE 3-2. Electrical pattern of cardiac cycle. (Adpated with permission from Andreoli KG, Zipes DP, Wallace AG, Kinney MR, Fowkes VK: Comprehensive Cardiac Care, 6th ed; p 133. St. Louis, CV Mosby, 1987)

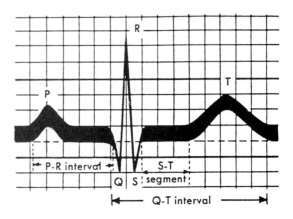

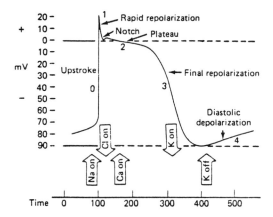

FIGURE 3-3. Diagrammatic representation of a cardiac action potential, emphasizing characteristics of the Purkinje fiber (false tendon) action potential. Each distinctive phase is labeled where the ionic events related to it are discussed. The arrows below the diagram refer to the approximate time when the indicated ion is influencing membrane potential. They point in the direction of the effect on the membrane potential, upward for depolarization and downward for repolarization (reproduced, with permission, from Fozzard HA, Gibbons WR: Action potential and contraction of heart muscle. *Am J Cardiol* 31:182,1973; and Bigger JT Jr: Antiarrhythmic drugs in ischemic heart disease. *Hosp Pract* 7:69,1972).

in the SA node, allowing its threshold potential to be reached first, making it the pacemaker of the heart.

Cardiac dysrhythmias occur in any condition that enhances impulse formation (automaticity) or impairs impulse conduction (unidirectional block and reentry), or a combination of these factors. The sinus node is normally the pacemaker of the heart because it spontaneously discharges faster than the other previously mentioned pacemakers. If the discharge rate of one of the other pacemakers is greater than that of the sinus node, then the heart will be controlled by the overriding pacemaker. This is a disorder of impulse formation and probably produces the dysrhythmias noted in Table 3-1.

Dysrhythmias may also be the result of conduction abnormalities. The normal electrical conduction of the heart may become depressed unevenly by blocks or diseased tissue, stopping or slowing the conduction of impulses along the previously described route. Such blocks cause some areas of the myocardium to depolarize and repolarize faster than others. Because of this unevenness in the conduction system, impulses originating from the SA node may reenter an area of myocardium that is no longer refractory and cause a retrograde (backward) impulse from the blocked segment to reenter the unblocked segment of the conduction system. This is a reentry circuit, and for it to occur the following must be present: an impaired conduction in one system (area) and a unidirectional block in the other system. Such reentry is best understood by the example in Figure 3-4 and probably produces the dysrhythmias noted in Table 3-1.

Other causes of dysrhythmias exist, including electrolyte imbalance (hyperkalemia or hypokalemia), acid–base disorders, thyrotoxicosis, hypotension, hypoxia,

TABLE 3-1
Probable Electrophysiologic Mechanism Responsible for Various Cardiac Arrhythmias

AUTOMATICITY
Escape beats—atrial, junctional, or ventricular
Atrial rhythm
Atrial tachycardia with or without AV block
Junctional rhythm
Nonparoxysmal AV junctional tachycardia
Accelerated idioventricular rhythm
Parasystole

REENTRY
AV nodal reentry
AV reciprocating tachycardia using an accessory (WPW) pathway
Atrial flutter
Atrial fibrillation
Ventricular tachycardia
Ventricular flutter
Ventricular fibrillation

AUTOMATICITY OR REENTRY
Premature systoles—atrial, junctional, or ventricular
Flutter and fibrillation
Ventricular tachycardia

Adapted with permission from Andreoli KG, Zipes DP, Wallace AG, Kinney MR, Fowkes VK: Comprehensive Cardiac Care, 6th ed, p 136. St Louis, CV Mosby, 1987

hypercapnia resulting from poor ventilation in chronic lung disease or after pulmonary surgery, and adverse effects of certain cardiovascular medications.

Antiarrhythmic Agents

Antiarrhythmic agents alter the abnormal electrophysiologic causes of dysrhythmias and are classified according to their effects on the action potential of cardiac cells and their presumed mechanism of action. Antiarrhythmic agents may be categorized into four classes.

CLASS I AGENTS

Class I agents consist of local anesthetics or membrane-stabilizing agents that depress phase O by blocking membrane sodium channels. These agents are further divided into IA, including quinidine (Quinaglute), procainamide (Procan-SR), disopyramide (Norpace); IB, including tocainide (Tonocard), lidocaine (Xylocaine), phenytoin (Dilantin), and mexiletine (Mexitil); and IC, including encainide (Enkaid) and flecainide (Tambocor). The IA agents depress phase O and prolong the action potential duration, whereas IB agents depress phase O slightly and may shorten the

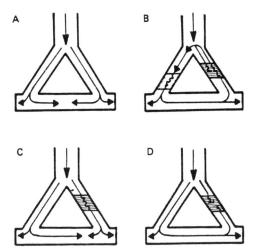

FIGURE 3-4. Schematic diagram of reentrant pathway and means for its modification. (*A*) Normal propagation through the distal conducting system to the ventricle. Conduction proceeds with equal velocity through both limbs of a terminal Purkinje fiber bundle and then activates the myocardium. (*B*) Shaded area on right indicates diseased tissue, including partially depolarized Purkinje fibers. Antegrade activation through the site is blocked. Activation is slowed (shaded area on left) but proceeds normally through the other limb to the myocardium and then activates the depressed segment (which is no longer refractory) in a retrograde direction. This impulse succeeds in propagating slowly through the depressed segment and reenters the proximal conducting system. (*C*) If physiologic changes occur or appropriate pharmacologic agents are administered (see text), conduction may improve through the depressed segment and result in reestablishment of antegrade activation and abolition of reentry. (*D*) If changes occur (or are induced) that result in block of retrograde activation as well as antegrade activation, then bidirectional conduction block occurs. This condition, too, would suppress a reentrant arrhythmia (modified and reproduced, with permission, from Rosen MR et al: Electrophysiology and pharmacology of cardiac arrhythmias. 5. Cardiac antiarrhythmic effects of lidocaine. *Am Heart J* 89:526,1975.

action potential. Flecainide and encainide profoundly slow conduction, significantly depressing phase O of the action potential and slightly affecting repolarization.

Class I agents are used to treat premature ventricular contractions, ventricular tachycardia, and ventricular fibrillation; quinidine and procainamide also treat supraventricular tachycardia and atrial fibrillation.

Contraindications for the class I agents include (1) hypersensitivity to any of the medications, (2) digitalis toxicity manifested by dysrhythmias or AV conduction disorders, (3) myasthenia gravis (procainamide), (4) Stokes-Adams or Wolff-Parkinson-White syndrome (lidocaine), and (5) cardiogenic shock (disopyramide, mexiletine, and flecainide). The side-effects associated with these medications are many, with dizziness and light-headedness, headache, nausea, blurred or double vision, dysrhythmias, and hypotension being the most common.

CLASS II AGENTS

Class II agents consist of the β-adrenergic blockers that depress phase 4 depolarization. Three of these agents (propranolol, acebutalol, and esmolol) have been extensively studied and are indicated to have antiarrhythmic properties. By depressing phase 4 depolarization, class II agents (1) reduce the slope of the pacemaker action potential, either sinus or ectopic, by blocking β-adrenergic sympathetic stimulation; and (2) stabilize myocardial cell membranes by increasing the threshold of excitability and the effective refractory period, which decreases conduction velocity. In addition, class II agents possibly alter the effects the central nervous system may have upon dysrhythmias. Class II agents are used to treat most dysrhythmias, including supraventricular tachycardia, atrial fibrillation, premature ventricular contractions, and ventricular tachycardia.

Contraindications and side-effects of these agents were previously described.

CLASS III AGENTS

Class III agents include bretylium tosylate (Bretylol) and amiodarone hydrochloride (Cordarone). Class III agents prolong phase 3 of the action potential (repolarization), which causes a uniform prolongation of the action potential duration and refractory period. Bretylium tosylate is available only for intravenous therapy of ventricular fibrillation and related rhythms. Amiodarone is a potent but toxic antiarrhythmic with a complex electropharmacology. Both medications are used in the treatment of life-threatening ventricular arrhythmias that have failed to respond to first-line antiarrhythmic agents (such as lidocaine). Sotalol, a β-blocker that exhibits class III activity, has undergone extensive clinical trials and may be approved in the near future for the management of ventricular and supraventricular dysrhythmias.

Bretylium tosylate produces the foregoing effects by depressing adrenergic nerve terminal excitability, which inhibits norepinephrine release. Adrenergic nerve terminal excitability is depressed by an early release of norepinephrine from the adrenergic postganglionic nerve terminals, which may cause transient catecholamine effects (increased heart rate and BP) shortly after administration. These effects, as well as hypotension, bradycardia, nausea and vomiting, light-headedness, and dizziness, are among the most common side-effects of bretylium tosylate. Because this medication is used for the treatment of life-threatening ventricular dysrhythmias, no contraindications for its use exist.

The pharmacologic actions of amiodarone hydrochloride are less understood. Its antiarrhythmic effect may be due to a prolongation of the myocardial cell action potential duration and refractory period, as well as noncompetitive α- and β-adrenergic inhibition. Contraindications include severe sinus node dysfunction, marked sinus bradycardia, and second- or third-degree heart block. Adverse reactions are common with dosages greater than 400 mg/day and include numerous neurologic problems, exacerbation of dysrhythmias, congestive heart failure, pulmonary inflammation or fibrosis, and abnormal liver function tests. Because of its unique pharmacokinetic properties, difficult dosing schedule, and severity of side-effects, amiodarone must be administered carefully with routine monitoring of the effectiveness and side-effects.

CLASS IV AGENTS

The class IV agents consist of calcium-channel blockers (primarily verapamil) and digoxin (Lanoxin), a cardiac glycoside. The calcium-channel antagonists depress phase 4 depolarization and lengthen phases 1 and 2 of repolarization, which decreases SA and AV node conduction and prolongs the AV node effective and functional refractory periods. Calcium-channel blockers are generally indicated for supraventricular dysrhythmias and are used only occasionally for ventricular dysrhythmias. Digoxin is also used for supraventricular dysrhythmias (primarily atrial fibrillation/flutter) and produces its effects by decreasing the maximal diastolic potential and action potential duration, as well as increasing the slope of phase 4 depolarization. These effects indirectly increase parasympathetic tone in the sinus and AV nodes, thereby slowing conduction.

The contraindications and side-effects associated with the use of calcium-channel blockers were previously described. Digoxin is contraindicated when hypersensitivity exists or ventricular fibrillation is present. It should be given cautiously in patients with renal impairment or with an acute myocardial infarction. In addition to the aforementioned actions, digoxin also increases the force and velocity of myocardial contraction. Hence, it is indicated in congestive heart failure and must be given cautiously to individuals with acute myocardial infarction. A few of the most common side-effects include ECG abnormalities (S-T segment changes and P-R interval prolongation), weakness, and visual disturbances. Anorexia, nausea, and vomiting are commonly associated with overdosage.

ANGINA

Angina is *usually* a manifestation of CAD and occurs because of an inadequate supply of oxygen and substrate to myocardial tissue. This produces myocardial ischemia and is often the result of a limitation of oxygen delivered by narrowed coronary arteries, increased CO, increased myocardial demands for oxygen, or coronary spasm.[84] The clinical patterns of angina pectoris are chronic stable angina, unstable angina, Prinzmetal's variant angina, and silent myocardial ischemia.

Chronic stable angina is further divided into classic exertional angina and mixed angina. *Classic exertional angina* is the result of a fixed atherosclerotic obstruction alone, whereas *mixed angina* occurs because of an "increase in coronary vasomotor tone superimposed on a fixed atherosclerotic obstruction."[37] *Unstable angina* is of recent onset; is more severe, prolonged, and frequent (crescendo); and occurs at rest or during minimal exertion.[37] The development of unstable angina often indicates a progression in the severity of CAD.[68] *Prinzmetal's variant angina* is best described as a "syndrome of episodic myocardial ischemia" occurring because of coronary artery vasospasm.[37]

Recently, *silent* or *asymptomatic myocardial ischemia* has been a subject of great interest and scientific study. Perhaps the most important finding is that in patients with symptomatic CAD, episodes of silent ischemia appear to be two to five times as frequent as episodes of symptomatic ischemia.[9,17,82] The absence of anginal pain "is of no value in predicting the absence of coronary disease,"[24] because studies have shown that only small percentages of individuals with positive stress tests experience angina.[25] Silent ischemia appears to be related to either a transient increase in myocardial oxygen demand or a transient reduction in coronary blood flow.[37]

Although angina itself is an unreliable variable for CAD, the Framingham data indicate that one-third of men and two-thirds of women experience it as the first manifestation of CAD.[49] It is for these individuals that antianginal medications are prescribed.

Antianginal Agents

The antianginal agents include rapid-acting nitrates (for prompt relief of acute angina) and long-acting nitrates (for prophylaxis or to decrease the frequency and severity of angina pectoris). Dipyridamole (Persantine), calcium-channel blockers, and β-adrenergic blocking agents are also effective in the prophylaxis of chronic angina.

NITRATES

The rapid-acting nitrates are amyl nitrate, an inhalant, and nitroglycerin, which is available intravenously, sublingually, or as a translingual spray. The long-acting nitrates consist of (1) nitroglycerin (transmucosal, oral-sustained release, topical ointment, transdermal); (2) isosorbide dinitrate (Isordil, Sorbitrate; sublingual and chewable, oral, oral-sustained release); (3) erythritol tetranitrate (Cardilate; sublingual and chewable, oral); and (4) pentaerythritol tetranitrate (Peritrate; oral, oral-sustained release).

All of the nitrates have similar actions, relaxing vascular smooth muscle in both arterial and venous beds. Dilation of the small and large veins produces peripheral pooling of blood and decreases venous return to the heart, which reduces left ventricular end diastolic pressure (preload). Dilation of the arterioles decreases PVR and arterial pressure (afterload). The reductions in preload and afterload cause myocardial oxygen consumption to decrease and improve perfusion to ischemic myocardium by redistributing blood to collateral arteries.

The contraindications to nitrates include hypersensitivity, severe anemia, acute myocardial infarction with hypotension, head trauma or cerebral hemorrhage, hypotension, constrictive pericarditis, and pericardial tamponade. The most common adverse reactions are headache, dizziness, tachycardia, hypotension, cutaneous vasodilation, and flushing.

DIPYRIDAMOLE

Dipyridamole acts as an antianginal agent by dilating the coronary arteries, thus increasing coronary blood flow. It appears that the dilation is a result of an accumulation of potent vasodilators (adenosine, adenine nucleotides, and cyclic AMP). Dipyridamole should be used cautiously in patients with hypotension because excessive doses can produce peripheral vasodilatation. Adverse reactions are minimal and transient, but headache, dizziness, nausea, flushing, and weakness have been noted.

CALCIUM-CHANNEL BLOCKING AGENTS

The calcium-channel blockers perform an antianginal role in (1) angina pectoris because of coronary spasm, (2) chronic stable angina, and (3) unstable, crescendo, preinfarction angina (oral verapamil). As previously described, these medications dilate the peripheral arterioles. This effect also occurs in the coronary arteries and arterioles in both normal and ischemic areas and inhibits coronary spasm, thus increasing myocardial oxygen delivery to patients with vasospastic (Prinzmetal's or variant) angina and possibly classic angina.

Calcium-channel blockers provide further antianginal effects by reducing myocardial energy and oxygen requirements. These effects are the result of peripheral arteriolar dilation which reduces the total PVR (afterload) against which the heart works, both at rest and at a given level of exercise. The contraindications and side-effects have been described.

β-ADRENERGIC BLOCKING AGENTS

The β-blocking agents (primarily propranolol and nadolol) are also used for the treatment of angina pectoris because they reduce myocardial oxygen requirements at any given level of effort by blocking catecholamine-induced increases in heart rate, systolic BP, and the velocity and extent of myocardial contraction. The contraindications and side-effects of β-blockers have been previously described.

Conclusion

The preceding sections on antihypertensive, antiarrhythmic, and antianginal agents are by no means complete. The most commonly used medications, as well as a brief description of the pharmacology, primary contraindications, and most frequent adverse reactions, were presented. In view of the many medications presented, it is difficult to assign any one a greater importance over another. However, the most versatile, and probably the most commonly prescribed medications, are the β-adrenergic blockers and calcium-channel blockers. Their many indications and minimal adverse reactions allow them such popularity. A complete and thorough understanding of these medications should enhance every therapist's practice and, thus, provide patients with quality care.

EXERCISE TRAINING AND β-ADRENERGIC BLOCKADE

As previously described, β-adrenergic receptor-blocking agents compete with β-adrenergic agonists for available β-receptor sites. Some β-blockers are selective and block only β_1-receptor sites (becoming less selective with higher doses), reducing heart rate, myocardial force of contraction, lipolysis, and plasma values of nonesterified free fatty acids. Others are nonselective and block both β_1- and β_2-receptors, producing the aforenoted effects, as well as inhibiting vasodilatation in the capillary beds, muscle relaxation in the bronchial tracts, glycogenolysis in the liver and muscles, and the release of insulin from the pancreas. Because of these effects, many cardiovascular, pulmonary, muscular, and metabolic values are reduced. Reductions have been observed in (1) resting and exercise heart rates, (2) BP, (3) skeletal muscle and coronary blood flow, (4) CO at rest and during exercise, (5) myocardial oxygen requirements, (6) exercise-induced lipolysis, (7) translocation of lactate from the muscle cell to the blood, (8) peripheral blood flow, and (9) carbon dioxide production.[10,32,83] With such reductions, it is questionable if individuals taking β-blockers can achieve a training effect. Many studies have investigated this, and the results have been inconsistent. Nevertheless, many individuals are exercising while taking β-blockers and are doing so without confidence that they are conditioning their bodies. To better understand this matter, two questions must be answered: What effect does endurance exercise training have on the body, and can the effects of training occur during β-blockade?

Endurance exercise training produces many physiologic changes, the most obvious of which is an increased physical work capacity (PWC). This is the result of both central and peripheral adaptations occurring in response to the demands of physical exercise. The central adaptations include (1) improved lung function (a decrease in the transit time index during submaximal exercise),[12] and (2) improved heart performance (increased stroke volume and CO; increased parasympathetic activity which decreases resting and exercise heart rates; improved myocardial metabolic response; and decreased myocardial oxygen consumption during submaximal exercise).[11,77] The peripheral adaptations include (1) an increase in the number and size of mitochondria, (2) improved extraction of oxygen from circulating blood to the exercising muscles, (3) increased muscle strength, (4) a two- to threefold increase in mitochondrial enzyme activity, (5) proliferation of capillaries, (6) an increase in the mean transit time of blood through the muscle capillaries, (7) a lowering of PVR, and (8) an increased arteriovenous oxygen (A-VO$_2$) difference.[3,38,79,80] Both central and peripheral adaptations increase aerobic performance (VO$_2$max), thus allowing for an increased PWC.

The central and peripheral changes previously mentioned occur not only in normal individuals but also in cardiac patients. Even after a myocardial infarction, individuals who exercise regularly at moderate to high intensities for appropriate durations can improve the heart's stroke volume, CO, and coronary circulation.[20-22,33,40] Many of these individuals who made central adaptations were taking β-adrenergic blockers. These studies indicate that for many with CAD, the central adaptations occurring in response to vigorous exercise do occur in the presence of β-blockade.

The real questions, then, are: Do central and peripheral adaptations occur in those without CAD who are taking β-adrenergic blockers? Do peripheral adaptations to physical exercise occur in those with CAD who are taking β-adrenergic blockers? To answer these questions, we must further discuss the peripheral adaptations occurring in response to endurance exercise training as well as review the literature on exercise training of individuals with and without CAD who are taking β-blockers.

Human skeletal muscle contains a mixture of two types of muscle fiber: *slow-twitch* (ST) or type I, and *fast-twitch* (FT) or type II. Each individual appears to be genetically provided with specific proportions of each type.[3] The ST fibers perform endurance-type activity requiring "high combustive potential and recruitment during moderate activity."[52] The FT fibers perform "sprintlike" activity, or high-intensity exercise for short periods. These FT fibers have a "high capacity for phosphate splitting and lactate formation," making them more fatigable.[52]

The contractile tissues in both FT and ST fibers depend upon calcium to trigger muscle contraction. The FT fibers have large intracellular concentrations of calcium, whereas ST fibers depend more on extracellular sources. The ST and FT muscle fibers differ in many other ways besides intracellular calcium concentrations. Another difference between the two muscle fibers is enzyme activity. Slow-twitch muscle fibers have low-activity levels of myofibrillar ATPase (resulting in a relatively slow contraction time) and glycogenolytic enzyme, but high levels of mitochondrial enzymes, allowing for prolonged work. Fast-twitch muscle fibers have high-activity levels of myofibrillar ATPase (resulting in a more rapid contraction time) and glycogenolytic enzyme, but low activity levels of mitochondrial enzymes, allowing for short bursts of maximal activity. These muscle fibers also have a low myoglobin content and small capillary density compared with the ST muscle fibers, which have a high content of myoglobin and a great capillary density.

Endurance exercise training produces changes in all of the aforementioned areas. As a result of training, FT muscle fibers begin to function like ST muscle fibers, promoting "the fast-twitch fibers' aerobic metabolism" as well as the aerobic function of ST fibers.[3] Needle biopsy and electron microscopic studies have discovered that the number and size of mitochondria increase in response to endurance exercise.[3] This increases the concentration of mitochondrial proteins, which enhances mitochondrial enzyme activity. Increased enzyme activity allows trained muscle cells to oxidize pyruvate and long-chain fatty acids more efficiently, thus increasing the capacity for aerobic metabolism. Glycogen synthesis is also improved by exercise training as glycogen synthetase and glycogen-branching enzyme activities are increased.[3] Exercise training also increases the number of capillaries in skeletal muscle.[3]

These peripheral adaptations occurring in both FT and ST muscle fibers have been observed in individuals both with and without CAD.[3,38,79,80] However, only a few studies have evaluated the peripheral adaptations occurring in response to exercise training in those taking β-adrenergic blockers. Most of these studies have evaluated the metabolic effects of β-blockade and conclude that both lipolysis and glycolysis are impaired,[61] fat utilization is significantly restricted,[61] and neither β_1- nor β_1/β_2-blockade inhibits muscle glycogenolysis, but the translocation of lactate from the muscle cell to the blood is impaired.[32] This impaired release of lactate from exercising muscles is probably the result of β-blockade that alters the capillary blood flow and muscle cell metabolism.[45] Additionally, increased levels of muscle lactate appear to be related to both capillary density and plasma concentration of the drug, thus showing the important role of β_2-governed, sympathetic-induced vasodilatation during exercise in normal muscle metabolism.[47] Therefore, those with a high percentage of ST muscle fibers demonstrate more impairment in PWC than do individuals rich in FT muscle fibers after treatment with a nonselective β-blocker. This impairment in the individual with a high percentage of ST muscle fibers is due to the high capillary/fiber ratio (with less sympathetic-induced vasodilatation) that, associated with a decreased heart rate (because of the β-blockade), decreases oxygen transport capacities and accumulates more muscle lactate, producing fatigue. This can be reduced by administering a β_1-selective agent as opposed to a nonselective agent.[53]

β-adrenergic blockers, therefore, affect the metabolic function of exercising muscles by altering the availability of substrates necessary for the production of energy.[71] The free fatty acid supply is suppressed, which increases glucose uptake. Less oxygen is required to oxidize glucose; therefore, oxygen consumption may be lower in those who are taking β-blockers.[86] During exercise, muscle glycogenolysis is not inhibited by β-blockade but is actually enhanced and, as demonstrated in previous studies, it does not require sympathetic stimulation.[85] Muscle contraction itself activates phosphorylation, and treatment with a specific versus a nonspecific β-blocker has shown no higher degree of glycogenolysis.[32]

It is surprising that no needle biopsy studies have been conducted to evaluate the number and size of mitochondria in individuals who are training while taking β-blockers since it has been suggested that a reduction or loss of sympathetic activity in muscle fiber may lead to a reduction in the number of ST muscle fibers.[53] Because of this lack of information and the relatively small amount of information on peripheral adaptations to training, we must *assume* that many of the studies that have shown improved Vo_2max do so because of the peripheral adaptations (primarily an increase in the number and size of mitochondria) occurring in response to exercise training. The equation for oxygen consumption (Vo_2 = heart rate $\times$ stroke volume $\times$ A-Vo_2 difference) helps us realize that significant improvements in Vo_2 can occur only with a widening of the A-Vo_2 difference.

Such a widening must have occurred when Pratt and coworkers observed a 30% and 46% increase in Vo_2max when cardiac patients trained while taking 30–80 mg/day and 120–240 mg/day of propranolol, respectively.[75] Obma and coworkers also demonstrated a significant increase in estimated oxygen consumption after an 8-week, 30–60-min, 5–7-days/week exercise program, during which patients with stable angina were taking 40–240 mg/day (mean dosage of 128.8 mg/day) of propranolol.[72] Vanhees and associates compared two groups of postmyocardial infarction patients without angina.[89] Fifteen patients were treated with atenolol (100–200 mg/day), metoprolol (75–200 mg/day), or propranolol (120–300 mg/day), whereas 15 other patients were treated with medications other than β-blockers. Exercise training consisted of cycling, rowing, running, and calisthenics for 75 min 3 days/week at an intensity of 60% to 80% of each patient's maximal capacity. After 3 months, peak measured Vo_2 was similar in the patients with, and without, β-blocker therapy, increasing approximately 35%. Other studies evaluating the effects of exercise training on patients with CAD taking β-blockers have also demonstrated training effects.[4,8,19,35,44,66,88]

Not all investigations have shown such favorable results. Malborg and coworkers were the first to investigate the effect of β-blockade on physical training in patients with CAD.[64] Twenty-nine patients were divided into four groups. Group 1 received a placebo alone. Group II received a placebo and physical training. Group III received β-blockade therapy. Group IV received β-blockade therapy and physical training. Patients were administered 5 mg t.i.d. of pindolol and exercised intermittently for 18 min twice a week at an intensity of approximately 70% of each patient's maximal working capacity. No training effect was observed after 2 or 4 months. This is not surprising because the exercise frequency and duration were minimal, and previous studies have demonstrated training effects only after continuous aerobic exercise is performed for approximately 30 min three times a week.[70,74] Even though some studies were unable to demonstrate significant improvements in Vo_2max, many other clinical values improved including PWC, magnitude of S-T segment depression, and the number of anginal attacks.[4,8,19,35,44,66,88]

Controversy still exists over the effects of β-adrenergic blockade on obtaining a trained exercise state in normal subjects without CAD. Ewy and colleagues demonstrated an increase in Vo_2max in β-blocked individuals but only after β-blockade was discontinued.[27] Twenty-seven healthy adult men (mean age 24 years) were randomly assigned to either a β-blocking group (sotalol 320 mg/day) or a placebo group. Subjects exercised 45 min/day, 5 days/week, at an intensity of 75% of their measured Vo_2max for 14 weeks. The placebo group demonstrated a 6.7% to 8.3% increase in VO_2 after training. The β-blocked group demonstrated no change in Vo_2max after training when compared with the pretraining unblocked state, but 1 week after the cessation of medication, Vo_2max increased 6.1% to 11.7%. Such findings suggest that "stroke volume had attained its maximum physiologic capacity during β-adrenergic blockade and that the reduction in maximal heart rate with β-blockade did not allow cardiac output to attain its potential for increase following training."[27] When the β-blockers were discontinued, the subjects were able to increase maximal heart rate and stroke volume, which produced an increased maximal CO and oxygen consumption.

Sable and coworkers also investigated normal men aged 21 to 35 years, before and after 5 weeks of aerobic conditioning during which high levels of β-blockers (160–640 mg/day of propranolol) were administered.[78] Seventeen subjects were separated into pairs with similar maximal oxygen consumptions. One member of each pair was randomly administered propranolol, whereas the other received a placebo. Aerobic conditioning was performed for 45 min/day, 5 days/week, at intensities of 75% maximal heart rate for 5 weeks. Exercise tests performed before and after exercise training revealed no significant change in Vo_2max but a slight increase in exercise duration in those taking β-blockers, and a 21% increase in Vo_2max and 29% increase in exercise duration in those not taking β-blockers. It has been implied that the unchanged Vo_2max observed in those taking β-blockers may be due to an inadequate period of training, suggesting "that obtaining a training effect may take longer in individuals receiving β-adrenergic blockade."[27] Additionally, Vo_2max may have been unchanged because of the high doses of propranolol administered during this study. This appears to be of little significance because Marsh and associates demonstrated similar effects with *relatively* low dosages of propranolol (approximately 80 mg/day).[65]

Anderson and coworkers investigated the effects of cardioselective and nonselective β-adrenergic blockade on the performance of highly trained runners.[1] This study demonstrated a decrease in maximal heart rate, Vo_2max, maximal ventilation, maximal respiratory exchange ratio, treadmill time, and slower 10-km race times during β-blockade. Propranolol caused greater decreases than atenolol in each of these areas. These results support Furberg's hypothesis that highly trained individuals cannot fully compensate for the decreased maximal heart rate to maintain Vo_2max as do normal subjects or those with disease.[35] Other studies involving normal and slightly hypertensive subjects have also shown significant decreases in exercise tolerance, Vo_2max, or both.[8,23,26,29,30,73,92] Many of these investigations have evaluated the effects of short-term β-blockade to determine if maximal effort is attenuated, but they did not study training effects nor the effects of extended β-blockade.

It is evident from the previous discussion that many discrepancies exist concerning the effects of exercise training during β-adrenergic blockade therapy. These discrepancies are probably the result of the type of β-adrenergic blocker used, the method of medication administration, the timing of the tests with respect to peak medication effect, the length of time on the medication regimen, the dosage level, the exercise protocol, the motivation and age of subject, and the type of statistical analysis used.[93] Even with these problems, the consensus of some of the foremost authorities on exercise training is that "the hemodynamic and performance consequences of exercise training occur in persons on either nonselective or selective β-blockers."[34]

Summary

In view of the available data, particular training effects (both central and peripheral) can occur in those with or without CAD when (1) the training stimulus is appropriate (adequate frequency, intensity, and duration); (2) dosages of β-blockers are not extreme (when the peak heart rate is reduced less than 40 beats per minute);[27] (3) the initial cardiorespiratory fitness is not extreme, as suggested by Davies and

Knibbs who state that "the magnitude of Vo$_2$max increase during training depends on its starting value";[16] and (4) the percentage of ST muscle fibers to FT muscle fibers is relatively equal.[53]

Exercise conditioning appears to be unaffected by the type of β-adrenergic blocker used. Training with selective and nonselective β-blockers have produced similar central and peripheral adaptations. It is possible that the unchanged Vo$_2$max observed in some studies was due to changes in substrate utilization during exercise. During β-blockade, free fatty acid utilization decreases, whereas glycogenolysis increases, which requires less oxygen for oxidative phosphorylation.[86]

HYPERLIPIDEMIA

The use of antihyperlipidemic agents has recently increased because many studies have demonstrated that lowering cholesterol reduces the frequency of CAD.[5,7,58–60,87] Additionally, a few investigations have shown that reduced cholesterol levels, achieved through the use of cholesterol-lowering agents or prudent life-style changes, may actually regress CAD in *particular* patients.[2,55,69,81] The diagnosis of hyperlipidemia (hypercholesterolemia and hypertriglyceridemia) is made when repeated total cholesterol and triglyceride measurements are elevated. *Hypercholesterolemia* exists when total cholesterol values are higher than 220 mg/dl (or the 75th percentile), as suggested by the Consensus Conference.[14] The diagnosis of *hypertriglyceridemia* is less defined and exact, but levels higher than 180 mg/dl are often considered abnormal.[31] These elevations may be the result of inherited disorders or related to life-style and diet. Therefore, antihyperlipidemic agents are used only after dietary means (which may reduce cholesterol levels 10% to 15%)[39] and other methods (exercise, weight loss, etc.) have failed. Plasma lipoprotein disorders have been classified by phenotype (Table 3-2), which categorizes the inherited hyperlipidemias and provides necessary information for medical therapy, such as the type of medication indicated.

Antihyperlipidemic Agents

Antihyperlipidemic agents that decrease cholesterol alone are cholestyramine (Questran), colestipol (Colestid), probucol (Lorelco), and dextrothyroxine (Choloxin). Both cholesterol and triglycerides are decreased by clofibrate (Atromid-S), gemfibrozil (Lopid), nicotinic acid or niacin (Nicobid), and lovastatin (Mevacor). The two primary antihyperlipidemic groups are bile acid sequestrant resins and fibric acid compounds. The former consist of cholestyramine and colestipol, both of which act by binding bile acids (secreted by the bile from the liver and gallbladder) in the intestine to form an insoluble complex which is excreted in the feces. The increased fecal loss of bile acid leads to an increased oxidation of cholesterol to bile acids because cholesterol is the major precursor of bile acids. This, in effect, decreases low-density lipoproteins (LDL) and serum cholesterol levels. These compounds are generally regarded as first-choice agents in the treatment of hypercholesterolemia and can be used with other cholesterol-lowering agents. Total cholesterol and LDL can be expected to decrease approximately 20% if full doses can be tolerated. This is difficult for some patients because the major side-effects are nausea and constipation, which may lead to poor compliance. Hypersensitivity to bile acid sequestrant resins and complete biliary obstruction are the only contraindications to these medications.

The fibric acid compounds include clofibrate and gemfibrozil, both of which have many adverse reactions and should be used only in special circumstances when other medications have failed. The exact mechanism of action of these medications is unknown, but the triglyceride-lowering effect appears to be due to accelerated catabolism of very low-density lipoprotein (VLDL) to LDL and decreased hepatic synthesis of VLDL, thus decreasing plasma triglycerides by 40% to 55%. In addition to lowering triglycerides and cholesterol, gemfibrozil may increase high-density lipoprotein (HDL) levels. As mentioned earlier, these medications have many adverse reactions, most commonly nausea, diarrhea, and flatulence; abdominal and epigastric pain; headache, dizziness, and blurred vision; and fatigue. In addition, the results of two major studies have demonstrated that treatment with clofibrate was associated with an increased incidence of nonfatal pulmonary emboli, angina pectoris, intermittent claudication, gallstones, and gastrointestinal malignancies.[15,91] Both medications enhance the pharmacologic effect of anticoagulants, which requires maintenance of the prothrombin time to prevent bleeding complications. Contraindications to these medications include hepatic or severe renal dysfunction including primary biliary cirrhosis, preexisting gallbladder disease, and hypersensitivity to either medication.

Probucol and dextrothyroxine are two other antihyperlipidemic agents that lower serum cholesterol alone. Probucol lowers cholesterol by increasing the catabolism of LDL, inhibiting the early stages of cholesterol synthesis, and slightly inhibiting the absorption of dietary cholesterol. Unfortunately, besides reducing total cholesterol and LDL, probucol also decreases HDL levels. The only contraindication to probucol is hypersensitivity. The side-effects are minimal: headaches, dizziness, paresthesias, and eosinophilia.

The antihyperlipidemic effect of dextrothyroxine is the result of the liver's increased catabolism and excretion of cholesterol and its degradation products by the biliary route into the feces. This medication is contraindicated in euthyroid patients with organic heart disease, advanced liver or kidney disease, or a history of iodism. The side-effects of dextrothyroxine are primarily the result of an increased metabolism and may be minimized by following the recommended dosage schedule.

The antihyperlipidemic effects of nicotinic acid (niacin) have been very promising. The exact mechanism of action is unknown, but it is known that nicotinic acid inhibits lipolysis in adipose tissue, decreasing the esterification of triglycerides in the liver and increasing lipoprotein lipase activity. Nicotinic acid is contraindicated in hepatic dysfunction, active peptic ulcer disease, severe hypotension, and hemorrhaging. The most common adverse reaction is cutaneous flushing with a sensation of warmth. This is transient and usually subsides with continued therapy.

Another antihyperlipidemic agent, which has recently gained Food and Drug Administration (FDA) approval, is lovastatin. Several studies evaluating the effectiveness of lovastatin have demonstrated significant reductions in total cholesterol, LDL, and triglycerides, as well as significant increases in HDL levels. This medication has recieved much attention because these improvements are obtained with minimal side-effects, of which liver dysfunction, myositis, and cataracts are the most common. Lovastatin alters lipids by inhibiting 3-hydroxy-3-methylglutaryl coenzyme A (HMG-CoA) reductase, an enzyme that catalyzes the conversion of in-

(Text continues on p. 80)

TABLE 3-2
Hyperlipoproteinemia Phenotype Definitions and Their Association with Genetic and Other Disorders

Phenotype	Common Name	Laboratory Definition	Associated Genetic Disorders	Conditions Associated with Secondary Hyperlipoproteinemia
Type I	Exogenous hyperlipidemia	Hyperchylomicronemia and absolute deficiency of lipoprotein lipase or postheparin lipolytic activity Cholesterol normal Triglycerides greatly increased	Familial LPL deficiency ApoC-II deficiency	Dysglobulinemia, pancreatitis, poorly controlled diabetes mellitus
Type IIa	Hypercholesterolemia	LDLs increased Cholesterol increased Triglycerides normal	Familial hypercholesterolemia LDL receptor abnormal Familial combined hyperlipidemia Polygenic hypercholesterolemia	Hypothyroidism, acute intermittent porphyria, nephrosis, idiopathic hypercalcemia, dysglobulinemia, anorexia nervosa
Type IIb	Combined hyperlipidemia	LDLs increased VLDLs increased Cholesterol increased Triglycerides increased	Familial hypercholesterolemia Familial combined hyperlipidemia	

Type	Name	Features	Familial syndrome	Secondary causes
Type III	Dysbeta-lipoproteinemia	Floating β-lipoproteins; VLDL cholesterol/VLDL triglyceride >0.35; ApoE-II homozygote on isoelectric focusing; Cholesterol increased; Triglyerides increased	Familial dysbeta-lipoproteinemia	Diabetes mellitus, hypothyroidism, dysglobulinemia (monoclonal gammopathy)
Type IV	Endogenous hyperlipidemia	VLDLs increased; Cholesterol normal or increased; Triglycerides increased	Familial hypertriglyceridemia; Familial combined hyperlipidemia	Glycogen storage disease, hypothyroidism, disseminated lupus erythematosus, diabetes mellitus, nephrotic syndrome, renal failure, ethanol abuse
Type V	Mixed hyperlipidemia	Chylomicrons and VLDLs increased; LDLs present but reduced; Cholesterol increased; Triglycerides greatly increased	Familial hypertriglyceridemia; Familial multiple lipoprotein-type hyperlipidemia	Poorly controlled diabetes mellitus, glycogen storage disease, hypothyroidism, nephrotic syndrome, dysglobulinemia, pregnancy, estrogen administration (either contraceptive or therapeutic) in women with familial hypertriglyceridemia

LDL = low-density lipoprotein; VLDL = very low-density lipoprotein.
(From Gotto AM. Practical approach to phenotyping hyperlipoproteinemia. In Kligfield PD [ed]: Cardiology Reference Book, pp 46–47. New York, CoMedica, 1984)

tracellular acetate to cholesterol. Contraindications to lovastatin are active liver disease, unexplained persistent elevations of serum transaminases, and hypersensitivity to any component of lovastatin.

Neomycin, a relatively old antibiotic, has recently been reintroduced as a cholesterol-lowering agent, although it has not yet been approved by the FDA as an antihyperlipidemic. Its exact mechanism for lowering cholesterol is unknown, but it appears to suppress cholesterol absorption in the gut. Side-effects are minimal with small doses (mild nausea and loose stools), but when large doses are used, severe otic and nephrotoxicity may occur. However, these effects were observed in patients with preexisting hepatic coma, which may have contributed to neomycin toxicity. Neomycin, therefore, is contraindicated for those with liver or kidney dysfunction.

Many of the antihyperlipidemic agents are used in combination with another, which has been demonstrated to dramatically alter lipids and reduce the incidence of CAD (Tables 3-3 and 3-4).

CASE 1   A 53-year-old obese man with a 3-year history of hypertension [treated with clonidine (Catapres) 0.1 mg b.i.d. and hydrochlorothiazide/triamterene (Dyazide) 25 mg q.d.] and a long history of hy-

---

TABLE 3-3
Trials of Combined Drug Therapy for Hypercholesterolemia

Author	Drugs Administered	Patients (N)	Average Cholesterol Levels (mg/dl)		Average Reduction (%)
			Pre- treatment	*Post- treatment*	
Miettinen (1979)	Neomycin + cholestyramine	9	403	252	38
Kane et al (1981)	Colestipol + niacin	18	420	231	45
Mabuchi et al (1983)	Colestipol + compactin	10	356	217	39
Hoeg et al (1984)	Neomycin + niacin	14	350	223	36
Hoeg et al (1985)	Neomycin + cholestyramine	18	334	240	28
Kuo et al (1986)	Colestipol + probucol	44	415	215	48
Dujovne et al (1986)	Colestipol + probucol	47	323	226	30

N = number of patients.

Udall JA: Hypercholesterolemia and Coronary Heart Disease: New Approaches to an Old Problem. Cardiovas Reviews and Reports, Vol 8, No 7, p 19, 1987

TABLE 3-4
**Percent Changes in Lipoprotein Cholesterol Concentrations and Total
High-Density Lipoprotein Cholesterol Ratios with Different
Drug Regimens (11 Patients)**

Regimen	% Change from Baseline			TC/HDL
	Total	*LDL*	*HDL*	
Baseline	. . .	. . .	. . .	8.0
Neomycin	−25	−24	−4	6.2
Neomycin + niacin	−37	−39	+16	4.3
Cholestyramine	−32	−38	+21	4.2
Cholestyramine + neomycin	−39	−39	+2	4.8
Lovastatin	−32	−34	+16	4.6
Lovastatin + neomycin	−40	−42	−9	5.2

HDL = high-density lipoprotein cholesterol; LDL = low-density lipoprotein cholesterol;
TC/HDL = ratio of total cholesterol to HDL cholesterol.
Hoeg JM, Maker MB, Bailey KR, Brewer HB: Comparison of Six Pharmacologic Regimens
for Hypercholesterolemia. Am J Cardiol 59:813, 1987

percholesterolemia (240 mg/dl) began experiencing exertional chest "pressure" in May 1988. Catapres was discontinued and nefedipine (Procardia) 10 mg t.i.d. initiated, which decreased the frequency of chest "pressure" and improved the blood pressure control. The result of a treadmill stress test, performed in June 1988, was positive for angina, ischemia, poor diastolic BP control, and frequent PVCs (occasional coupled PVCs and a three-beat salvo of ventricular tachycardia). Atenolol (Tenormin) 25 mg b.i.d. therapy was started immediately after the test, and a subsequent cardiac catheterization revealed 75% occlusion of the left anterior descending artery, 50% to 60% of the obtuse marginal artery, and 75% of a dominant circumflex artery.

The patient began weekly cardiac rehabilitation sessions during which PVCs were rare, BP was adequately controlled, and angina was very rare. During this time dipyrimadole (Persantine) 75 mg t.i.d., aspirin 1 tablet q.d., and cholestyramine (Questran) 8 g b.i.d. were initiated and Dyazide discontinued. The patient began training for 30 min daily at heart rates approximately 50 beats faster than the resting heart rate.

Approximately 3 months later, the patient underwent another treadmill stress test that revealed an increased treadmill duration (> 2 min), absence of angina but similar S-T segment changes, diastolic hypertension, and dysrhythmias (three-beat salvo of ventricular tachycardia). Tenormin was increased to 50 mg b.i.d., after which a subsequent treadmill stress test revealed similar duration, absence of angina, and good control of BP and rhythm (no ventricular tachycardia). Repeat lipid determinations revealed that total cholesterol had decreased 40 mg, yielding a total of 200 mg/dl.

Discussion

This individual, who was initially treated for hypertension with Catapres and Dyazide, benefited not only from the antihypertensive effects of Procardia but also the antianginal effects. Because of the June 1988 treadmill stress test results of angina, ischemia, poor diastolic BP control, and frequent PVCs (with three-beat salvo of ventricular tachycardia), the patient was started on a regimen of Tenormin 25 mg b.i.d. that provided antianginal, antihypertensive, and antiarrhythmic effects. This, however, was inadequate until an increased dosage of Tenormin was initiated. This individual with CAD did exhibit training effects while taking a β-blocker (Tenormin). Prudent life-style changes and cholestyramine decreased total cholesterol levels approximately 40 mg/dl, thus decreasing the likelihood for further progression of his CAD.

CASE 2   This 66-year-old man is status post-inferolateral myocardial infarction complicated by ventricular tachycardia, ventricular fibrillation requiring defibrillation, and cerebrovascular accident with right hemiparesis on 5/19/88. On 5/22/88, junctional bradycardia occurred causing loss of consciousness. His past medical history is unremarkable except for a transient ischemic attack in 1983. The patient was transferred to CIGNA Medical Center on 5/27/88 with the following medications: Transderm nitroglycerin 10 mg q.d., atenolol (Tenormin) 25 mg q.d., diltiazem (Cardizem) 30 mg t.i.d., quinidine 300 mg b.i.d., and dipyridamole (Persantine) 75 mg t.i.d.

> *5/28/88:* Initial cardiac rehabilitation assessment included evaluation of muscle strength and functional activities followed by approximately 500 feet of hallway ambulation. The patient ambulated with minimal assistance of 1 (exhibiting right lower extremity weakness) without complaint, complication, or significant dysrhythmias (very rare PVCs).
>
> *5/29/88:* Patent ambulated on a treadmill at 1.3–1.8/miles for 12 min, terminated secondary to mild fatigue. Very rare PVCs were again observed.
>
> *5/30/88:* Low-level treadmill stress test was performed while on the preceding medication regimen. The patient completed the post-myocardial infarction protocol of 9 min (3 min of the Bruce protocol) without angina, ischemia, or significant dysrhythmias (rare PVCs).
>
> *6/20/88:* Cardiac catheterization was performed, revealing 70% narrowing of the proximal circumflex artery and 25% narrowing of the proximal left anterior descending artery. Left ventricular size and function were normal.
>
> *6/27/88:* Initial outpatient cardiac rehabilitation consisted of

treadmill ambulation for 15 min, terminated because of dizziness and a hypoadaptive systolic BP response. The primary physician was contacted, who decreased Transderm nitroglycerin to 5 mg q.d.

7/2/88: Outpatient cardiac rehabilitation consisted of treadmill ambulation for 35 min without complaint, complication (no hypoadaptive systolic BP response), or dysrhythmia.

7/11/88: Primary physician discontinued the Tenormin.

7/18/88 through 8/18/88: During weekly outpatient cardiac rehabilitation visits, there were no complications or medicine changes.

8/21/88: Maximal treadmill stress test was performed with the patient on the following medication regimen: quinidine 300 mg b.i.d., Cardizem 30 mg t.i.d., Persantine 75 mg t.i.d., Transderm nitroglycerin 5 mg q.d. The patient completed 5 min 35 sec of the Bruce protocol which was terminated secondary to frequent ventricular ectopy (bigeminy) associated with a hypoadaptive systolic BP response. The primary physician was contacted, who restarted therapy with Tenormin 25 mg q.d., increased quinidine to 300 mg q.i.d., and discontinued Transderm and Cardizem. Persantine was unchanged.

9/3/88: Outpatient cardiac rehabilitation consisted of treadmill ambulation terminated after 17 min because of a hypoadaptive systolic BP response without dysrhythmias. The primary physician was contacted, who decreased Tenormin to 12.5 mg b.i.d.

9/11/88: Outpatient cardiac rehabilitation consisted of treadmill ambulation for 35 min without complication or dysrhythmia but with complaints of extreme fatigue during exercise and throughout the day. The primary physician was contacted, who discontinued Tenormin.

12/15/88: Maximal treadmill stress test was performed while on a regimen of quinidine 300 mg q.i.d. and aspirin. The patient completed 9 min of Bruce protocol, terminated secondary to fatigue without angina or ischemia. Rare PVCs occurred with one episode of paired PVCs during exercise. Systolic BP response was adaptive.

Discussion

This individual with a recent complicated myocardial infarction (ventricular tachycardia, ventricular fibrillation, cerebrovascular accident, and junctional bradycardia with loss of consciousness) was started on a regimen of Transderm nitroglycerin and Persantine for prophylactic treatment of angina and myocardial ischemia. Tenormin and Cardizem also provided some antianginal effect as well as antiarrhythmic effect. Quinidine was given for its antiarrhythmic effect (ventricular ectopy). Dizziness and hypotension were eliminated with a reduction in transderm nitroglycerin. Tenormin was discontinued on 7/11/88 because of the patient's excellent status, but a maximal treadmill exercise test revealed frequent ventricular ectopy associated with a hypoadaptive systolic BP response. Tenormin 25 mg q.d. was readministered for its antiarrhythmic effect. In addition, quinidine was increased from 300 mg b.i.d. to q.i.d. for added control of ventricular ectopy. Transderm nitroglycerin and Cardizem were discontinued to prevent hypotension because it was previously a problem. Hypotension and fatigue made it necessary to first decrease, then discontinue, Tenormin. This, however, did not adversely affect the control of ventricular ectopy because only rare PVCs (one episode of paired PVCs) were observed during a maximal exercise test. The increased dosage of quinidine adequately controlled the patient's rhythm.

The foregoing case studies demonstrate the indications, contraindications, and side effects of some of the most commonly used cardiovascular medications. The effects of these pharmacologic agents upon underlying disease processes make treating the cardiac patient an ongoing challenge. Most cardiac patients take several cardiovascular medications that may interact, thus requiring careful and persistent monitoring. The effectiveness of treatment, whether it be endurance exercise training, isometric strengthening after a total knee replacement, or gait training after a CVA, is often directly related to the appropriateness of pharmacologic control of the underlying disease processes. Therefore, it is imperative for rehabilitation professionals to work as a team to carefully assess the progression of activities in view of the cardiovascular responses. Only through such an effort will appropriate care be provided.

REFERENCES

1. Anderson RL, Wilmore JH, Joyner MJ et al: Effects of cardioselective and nonselective β-adrenergic blockade on the performance of highly trained runners. Am J Cardiol 55:149D-154D, 1985
2. Arntzenius AC, Kromhout D, Barth JD et al: Diet, lipoproteins, and the progression of coronary atherosclerosis: The Leiden Intervention Trial. N Engl J Med 312:805-811, 1985
3. Astrand P, Rodahl K: Textbook of Work Physiology, 2nd ed. New York, McGraw-Hill, 1977
4. Battler A, Ross J Jr, Slutsky R et al: Improvement of exercise-induced left ventricular dysfunction with oral propranolol in patients with coronary heart disease. Am J Cardiol 44:318-324, 1979
5. Blankenhorn DH, Nessim SA, Johnson RL et al: Beneficial effects of combined cholestipol-niacin therapy on coronary atherosclerosis and coronary venous bypass grafts. JAMA 257:3233-3240, 1987
6. Bleifer SB et al: Diagnosis of occult arrhythmias by Holter electrocardiography. Prog Cardiovasc Dis 16:569, 1974
7. Brensike JF, Levy RI, Kelsey SF et al: Effects of therapy with cholestyramine on progression of coronary arteriosclerosis: Results of the NHLBI Type II Coronary Intervention Study. Circulation 69:313-324, 1984
8. Bruce RA, Hossack KF, Kusumi F et al: Acute effects of oral propranolol on hemodynamic responses to upright exercise. Am J Cardiol 44:132-140, 1979
9. Cecchi AC, Dovellini EV, Marchi F et al: Silent myocardial ischemia during ambulatory electrocardiographic monitoring in patients with effort angina. J Am Coll Cardiol 1:934-939, 1983
10. Ciske PE, Dressendorfer RH, Gordon S et al: Attenuation of exercise training effects in

patients taking beta blockers during early cardiac rehabilitation. Am Heart J 112:1016, 1986

11. Clausen JP: Circulation adjustment to dynamic exercise and effect of exercise training in normal subjects and patients with ischemic heart disease. Prog Cardiovasc Dis 18:459–495, 1976

12. Clausen JP: Effect of physical training on cardiovascular adjustments to exercise in man. Physiol Rev 57:779–815, 1977

13. Conant RG, Perkins JA, Ainley AB: Stroke morbidity, mortality, and rehabilitative potential. J Chronic Dis 18:397–403, 1965

14. Consensus Conference: Lowering blood cholesterol to prevent heart disease. JAMA 253:2080–2090, 1985

15. Coronary Drug Project Research Group. Am J Cardiol 42:489, 1978

16. Davies CTM, Knibbs AV: The training stimulus: The effects of intensity, duration and frequency of effort on maximum aerobic power output. Int Z Angew Physiol 5:29, 1971

17. Deanfield JE, Shea M, Ribiero P et al: Transient ST-segment depression as a marker of myocardial ischemia during daily life. Am J Cardiol 54:1195–1200, 1984

18. Dujovne CA, Krehbiel P, Chernod SB: Controlled studies of the efficacy and safety of combined probucol-colestipol therapy. Am J Cardiol 57:36H–42H, 1986

19. Dwyer EM, Wiener L, Cox JW: Effects of β-adrenergic blockade (propranolol) on left ventricular hemodynamics and the electrocardiogram during exercise-induced angina pectoris. Circulation 38:250–260, 1968

20. Ehsani AA: Altered adaptive responses to training by nonselective β-adrenergic blockade in coronary artery disease. Am J Cardiol 58:220–224, 1985

21. Ehsani AA, Biello DR, Schultz J et al: Improvement of left ventricular contractile function by exercise training in patients with coronary artery disease. Circulation 74:350–358, 1986

22. Ehsani AA, Martin WH III, Heath GW et al: Cardiac effects of prolonged and intense exercise training in patients with coronary artery disease. Am J Cardiol 50:246–254, 1982

23. Ekblom B, Goldbarg AN, Kilbom A et al: Effects of atropine and propranolol on the oxygen transport system during exercise in man. Scand J Clin Lab Invest 30:35–42, 1972

24. Ellestad MH: Stress Testing. Principles and Practice, 2nd ed. Philadelphia, FA Davis, 1980

25. Ellestad MH et al: Maximal treadmill stress testing for cardiovascular evaluation. One year follow-up of physically active and inactive men. Circulation 39:517, 1969

26. Epstein SE, Robinson BF, Kahler RL et al: Effects of β-adrenergic blockade on the cardiac response to maximal and submaximal exercise in man. J Clin Invest 44:1745–1753, 1965

27. Ewy GA, Wilmore JH, Morton AR et al: The effect of β-adrenergic blockade on obtaining a trained exercise state. J Cardiac Rehab 3:25–29, 1983

28. Fleg JL, Kennedy HL: Cardiac arrhythmias in a healthy elderly population: Detection by 24-hour ambulatory electrocardiography. Chest 81:302, 1982

29. Folgering H, van Bussel M: Maximal exercise power after a single dose of metoprolol and of slow release metoprolol. Eur J Clin Pharmacol 18:225–229, 1980

30. Franciosa JA, Johnson SM, Tobian LJ: Exercise performance in mildly hypertensive patients. Chest 78:291–299, 1980

31. Fredrickson DS, Levy RI, Lees RS: Fat transport in lipoproteins—an integrated approach to mechanisms and disorders. N Engl J Med 276:34, 1967

32. Frisk-Holmberg M, Jorfeldt L, Juhlin-Dannfelt A: Metabolic effects in muscle during antihypertensive therapy with β-1 and β-1/β-2-adrenoceptor blockers. Clin Pharmacol Ther 30:611–618, 1981

33. Froelicher V, Jensen D, Genter F et al: A randomized trial of exercise training in patients with coronary heart disease. JAMA 252:1291–1297, 1984

34. Froelicher V, Kelly J et al: Workshop III: Pharmacologic differences among β blockers: Implications for exercise training. Am J Cardiol 55:170D–171D, 1985

35. Furberg C: Adrenergic β blockade and physical working capacity. Acta Med Scand 182:119–127, 1967

36. Gifford RW Jr: Isolated systolic hypertension in the elderly. JAMA 247:781, 1982
37. Goldschlager N: Angina pectoris. A three-article symposium. Postgrad Med 80:148, 1986
38. Gollnick PD, Armstring RB, Saubert CW IV et al: Enzyme activity and fiber composition in skeletal muscle of untrained and trained men. J Appl Physiol 33:312–319, 1972
39. Grundy SM: Comparison of monounsaturated fatty acids and carbohydrates for lowering plasma cholesterol. N Engl J Med 314:745–748, 1986
40. Hagberg JM, Ehsani AA, Holloszy JO: Effect of 12 months of intense exercise training on stroke volume in patients with coronary artery disease. Circulation 67:1194–1199, 1983
41. Hoeg JM, Maher MH, Bailey KR et al: Effects of combination cholestyramine-neomycin treatment on plasma lipoprotein concentrations in type II hyperlipoproteinemia. Am J Cardiol 55:1282–1286, 1985
42. Hoeg JM, Maher MB, Boj E et al: Normalization of plasma lipoprotein concentrations in patients with type II hyperlipoproteinemia by combined use of neomycin and niacin. Circulation 70:1004–1011, 1984
43. Hulley SB, Martin MJ: Health policy for treating hyperlipidemia: Analogy with hypertension and prospects for the next decade. Am J Cardiol 57:3H–6H, 1986
44. Jackson G, Schwartz J, Kates RE et al: Atenolol: One-daily cardioselective β blockade for angina pectoris. Circulation 61:555–560, 1980
45. Jorfeldt L, Juhlin-Dannfelt A, Karlsson J: Lactate release from human skeletal muscle during exercise. J Appl Physiol 44:350–352, 1978
46. Juhlin-Dannfelt A, Frisk-Holmberg M, Karlsson J et al: Central and peripheral circulation in relation to muscle fibre composition in normo- and hypertensive man. Clin Sci Mol Med 56:335–340, 1979
47. Kaiser P, Tesch PA: Effekten av β-adrenerg blockad pa mjolksyrametabolismen under submaximalt arbete. Lakarsallskapets Riksstamma 1M 15, 1981
48. Kane UP, Malloy M, Tun P et al: Normalization of low-density lipoprotein levels in heterozygous familial hypercholesterolemia with a combined drug regimen. N Engl J Med 304:251–258, 1981
49. Kannel WB, Sortie P, McNamara PM: Prognosis after myocardial infarction. Am J Cardiol 44:53–59, 1979
50. Kaplan NM: Systemic hypertension: Mechanisms and diagnosis. In Braunwald E (ed): Heart Disease, Vol. I, 3rd ed. p 819. Philadelphia, WB Saunders, 1987
51. Kaplan NM: Systemic hypertension: Mechanisms and diagnosis. In Braunwald E (ed): Heart Disease, Vol. I, 2nd ed. p 849. Philadelphia, WB Saunders, 1984
52. Karlsson J: Metabolic adaptations to exercise: A review of potential β-adrenoceptor antagonist effects. Am J Cardiol 55:48D–58D, 1985
53. Karlsson J, Dlin R, Kaiser P et al: Muscle metabolism, regulation of circulation and beta blockade. J Cardiac Rehab 3:404–420, 1983
54. Kuller L, Anderson H, Petterson D et al: Nationwide cerebrovascular disease morbidity study. Stroke 1:86–98, 1976
55. Kuo PT, Hayase K, Kostis JB et al: Use of combined diet and colestipol in long-term (7–7 1/2 years) treatment of patients with type II hyperlipoproteinemia. Circulation 59:199–211, 1979
56. Kuo PT, Wilson AC, Kostis JB et al: Effects of combined probucol–colestipol treatment for familial hypercholesterolemia and coronary heart disease. Am J Cardiol 57:43H–48H, 1986
57. Kyei-Mensah K, Somanathan S: Medical disease and the anesthetist. Proc R Soc Med 69:731–736, 1976
58. Levy RI, Brensike JF, Epstein SE, et al: The influence of changes in lipid values induced by cholestyramine and diet on progression of coronary artery disease: Results of the NHLBI Type II Coronary Intervention Study. Circulation 69:325–337, 1984
59. Lipid Research Clinics Program: The Lipid Research Clinics Coronary Primary Prevention Trial results. I. Reduction in incidence of coronary heart disease. JAMA 251:351–364, 1984

60. Lipid Research Clinics Program: The Lipid Research Clinics Coronary Primary Prevention Trial results. II. The relationship of reduction in incidence of coronary heart disease to cholesterol lowering. JAMA 251:365–374, 1984

61. Lundborg P, Astrom H, Bengtsson C et al: Effect of β-adrenoceptor blockade on exercise performance and metabolism. Clin Sci 61:299–305, 1981

62. Lund-Johansen P: Hemodynamic alterations in hypertension—spontaneous changes and effects of drug therapy. Acta Med Scand Suppl 603:1, 1977

63. Mabuchi H, Sakai T, Sakai Y et al: Reduction of serum cholesterol in heterozygous patients with familial hypercholesterolemia: Additive effects of compactin and cholestyramine penod. N Engl J Med 308:609–613, 1983

64. Malborg R, Isaccson S, Kallivroussis G: The effect of β-blockade and/or physical training in patients with angina pectoris. Curr Ther Res 16:171–183, 1974

65. Marsh RC, Hiatt WR, Brammell HL et al: Attenuation of exercise conditioning by low dose β-adrenergic receptor blockade. J Am Coll Cardiol 2:551–556, 1983

66. McAllister RM, Lee SJK: The effects of exercise training in patients with coronary artery disease taking β blockers. J Cardiopulm Rehabil 6:245–250, 1986

67. Miettinen TA: Effects of neomycin alone and in combination with cholestyramine on serum cholesterol and fecal steroids in hypocholesterolemic subjects. J Clin Invest 64:1485–1493, 1979

68. Moise A, Theroux P, Taeymans Y et al: Unstable angina and progression of coronary atherosclerosis. N Engl J Med 309:685–689, 1983

69. Nash DT, Gensini G, Esente P: Effect of lipid-lowering therapy on the progression of coronary atherosclerosis assessed by scheduled repetitive coronary arteriography. Int J Cardiol 2:43–55, 1982

70. Naughton J, Nagle F: Peak oxygen intake during physical fitness program for middle-aged men. JAMA 191:899–901, 1965

71. Nazar K, Brzezinska S, Lyzczarz J et al: Sympathetic control of the utilization of energy substrates during long term exercise in dogs. Arch Int Physiol Biochem 79:873–880, 1971

72. Obma RT, Wilson PK, Goebel ME et al: Effect of conditioning program in patients taking propranolol for angina pectoris. Cardiology 64:365–371, 1979

73. Pearson SB, Banks DC, Patrick JM: The effect of β-adrenoceptor blockade on factors affecting exercise tolerance in normal man. Br J Clin Pharmacol 8:143–148, 1979

74. Pollock ML, Cureton TK, Greniger L: Effects of frequency of training on working capacity, cardiovascular function, and body composition of adult men. Med Sci Sports 1:70–74, 1969

75. Pratt CM, Welton DE, Squired WG Jr et al: Demonstration of training effect during chronic β-adrenergic blockade in patients with coronary artery disease. Circulation 64:1125–1129, 1981

76. Roberts WC: The hypertensive diseases. Evidence that systemic hypertension is a greater risk factor to the development of other cardiovascular diseases than previously suspected. Am J Med 59:523, 1975

77. Rowell LB: Human cardiovascular adjustments to exercise and thermal stress. Physiol Rev 54:75, 1974

78. Sable DL, Brammell HL, Shehan MV et al: Attenuation of exercise conditioning by β-adrenergic blockade. Circulation 65:679–684, 1982

79. Saltin B: Hemodynamic adaptations to exercise. Am J Cardiol 55:42D–47D, 1985

80. Saltin B, Nazar K, Costill DL et al: The nature of the training response: Peripheral and central adaptations to one-legged exercise. Acta Physiol Scand 96:289–305, 1976

81. Sanmarco ME, Selvester RH, Brooks SH et al: Risk Factor Reduction and Changes in Coronary Arteriography. Circulation 54 (Supple II):11–140 (Abstr) 1976

82. Schang SJ Jr, Pepine CJ: Transient asymptomatic S-T segment depression during daily activity. Am J Cardiol 39:396–402, 1977

83. Shepherd JT: Circulatory response to β-adrenergic blockade at rest and during exercise. Am J Cardiol 55:87D–94D, 1985

84. Sokolow M, McIlroy MB: Clinical Cardiology, 3rd ed. Los Altos, CA, Lange Medical Publications, 1981

85. Stull JI, Mayer S: Regulation of phosphorylase activity in skeletal muscle in vivo. J Biol Chem 246:5716–5723, 1971

86. Tesch PA, Kaiser P: Effects of β-adrenergic blockade on O_2 uptake during submaximal and maximal exercise. J Appl Physiol 54:901–905, 1983

87. The Coronary Drug Project Research Group: Clofibrate and niacin in coronary heart disease. JAMA 231:360–381, 1975

88. Turner GG, Nelson RR, Nordstrom LA et al: Comparative effect of nadolol and propranolol on exercise tolerance in patients with angina pectoris. Br Heart J 40:1361–1370, 1978

89. Vanhees J, Eagard R, Amery A: Influence of β adrenergic blockade on effects of physical training in patients with ischaemic heart disease. Br Heart J 48:33–38, 1982

90. Weiss YA, Safar ME, London GM et al: Repeat hemodynamic determinations in borderline hypertension. Am J Med 64:382, 1978

91. WHO Cooperative Trial. Lancet 2:600, 1984

92. Wilmore JH, Ewy GA, Morton AR et al: The effect of β-adrenergic blockade on submaximal and maximal exercise performance. J Cardiac Rehab 3:30–36, 1983

93. Wilmore JH, Freund BJ, Joyner MJ et al: Acute response to submaximal and maximal exercise consequent to β-adrenergic blockade: Implications for the prescription of exercise. Am J Cardiol 55:135D–141D, 1985

94. Working Group on Risk and High Blood Pressure: An epidemiological approach to describing risk associated with blood pressure levels. Hypertension 7:641, 1985

Pharmacologic Implications for the Rehabilitation Professions in Obstetrics and Gynecology

4

Anne L. Harrison

As women are learning and understanding more about their health, they are becoming wiser in their role as consumers in the health care system. Rehabilitative therapists are applying their knowledge and skills in the areas of obstetrics and gynecology in an effort to offer more choices and improve the quality of care for women. One area that is difficult to gain a firm understanding about is pharmacology in obstetrics and gynecology. Some of the roles of the obstetric–gynecologic therapist involve providing alternatives or adjuncts to drug use. The therapist may also be the person who can give initial guidance to the woman who has questions about pharmacologic issues. Included in this chapter is basic information about these issues.

OBSTETRIC PHARMACOLOGY

According to Fofar and Nelson, the average woman consumes four to five different drugs during pregnancy, including prescription and over-the-counter (OTC) medications.[9] Drugs are currently believed to be responsible for 4% to 5% of fetal malformations.[18] However, a large percentage of fetal malformations and deaths go unexplained. In addition, the etiology of emotional and learning disabilities as they are related to drug intake during pregnancy is an unexplored field. It is known that most drugs freely cross the placental barrier.

Research and experimentation to determine the effects of drugs on the fetus began to grow after the thalidomide tragedy in the early 1960s. Thalidomide, which had been found safe for pregnancy in animal studies, was linked to such abnormalities as amelia and phocomelia in humans. Because of differences between species' responses to drugs, it is not always reliable to transfer conclusions from animal studies to humans. In addition, ethical and practical considerations make this a difficult field to study. The problem is compounded by such factors as drug interactions, and womens' individual responses to particular drugs. Some authorities term the area of obstetrics a "therapeutic orphan" of pharmacology; active research on new drugs is hard to justify to companies because costs outweigh benefits. As a result, most new drugs will carry a warning about unknown risks to the fetus if taken during pregnancy.

Obstetric pharmacology must be studied in terms of interactions between the mother, the placenta, and the fetus. In the pregnant woman, drug physiologic action is altered from the prepregnant state by several factors. Increased extracellular and intracellular fluid volume and increased uterine blood flow alter the plasma concentration and distribution of a drug. Decreased plasma protein levels in pregnancy cause decreased protein binding of drugs, resulting in an increase in the amount of unbound drug available for placental transfer. Decreased gastric-emptying time because of decreased gastric motility, can cause delayed absorption of a drug. Increased renal plasma flow will cause increased renal excretion of drugs that are primarily cleared through this system. The influence of each of these factors depends on the individual physiologic responses of the woman, as well as the individual properties of the drug.

Transfer across the placenta is primarily by simple diffusion and is dependent on concentration gradients. The fact that many drugs are lipid-soluble also encourages transfer across the placenta. The amount of drug transfer will increase as the surface area of the placenta increases. Most researchers agree that almost any drug in sufficient concentration will cross the placenta, particularly if the drug is administered for an extended period.

Drugs that cross the placenta usually reach fetal levels of 50% to 100% of the maternal blood level. In the fetus, blood is shunted with a bias toward the heart and brain, and the permeability of the blood–brain barrier is increased. In addition, it is thought that the fetus has decreased ability to metabolize and excrete drug agents. In general, the severity of abnormal effects from a drug increases with decreasing gestational age. In an embryo of 0 to 30 days, toxicity of an introduced drug may result in spontaneous abortion. The same drug may result in major organ malformation or physical deformity if introduced in a fetus of 3 to 10 weeks. After the 10th week, such introduction may result in prematurity, growth delays, abortions, or behavioral and learning dysfunctions. In any of these examples, it is quite possible for the mother to have no overtly negative effects.

After the child is born, the placenta is no longer available to assist in detoxifying and excreting drugs. The renal and hepatic systems may not be fully mature for up to 6 weeks after birth. This can result in the prolonged presence in the newborn of drugs introduced to the mother before or during labor and delivery. This also has implications for the nursing mother. With the properties of lipid solubility, affinity toward protein binding, and low molecular weight, many drugs freely pass into breast milk. At this time, the long-term consequences of infants being fed breast milk containing drugs and other chemicals is largely unknown. Some of the drugs that reportedly reach levels of concern in breast milk are phenacetin, antibiotics, antiepileptics, antihypertensives, hypnotics, narcotics, metals, laxatives, nicotine, steroid hormones, caffeine, anticoagulants other than heparin, and large amounts of vitamins.[17]

The obvious conclusion is that many variables exist, and must be weighed when determining the benefit to the mother versus the risk to the fetus or the child, in administering drugs. Given the lack of resolve on the subject, it is safe to say that only necessary drugs should be introduced to the pregnant or nursing woman.

Nonprescription Drugs

The unsuspecting woman may have no knowledgeable guidance on the use of nonprescription drugs or of medications not normally considered drugs by many people. Once again, conclusive information is rarely available.

One of the most commonly used nonprescription drugs in the second and third trimester is the antacid. The most popular preparations contain sodium. Increased sodium intake is related to increased blood pressure and edema, which is related to a preeclamptic state. Conservative measures such as avoiding bending over; eating small, frequent meals; decreasing smoking; and practicing relaxation techniques, should always be tried first.

Laxatives and stool softeners are often desired throughout pregnancy because increased progesterone levels result in decreased colonic tone. These drugs frequently contain phenolphthalein or docusates, both of which should be avoided in pregnancy. Some enemas contain high sodium concentrations and should be avoided. The *Handbook of Nonprescription Drugs* warns that excessive cathartic use may promote labor.[13] Conservative measures such as increased fruits, bran, and fluids, as well as exercise, should start early in pregnancy in anticipation of this problem.

Caffeine appears in many foods, as well as in some diuretics and diet pills. In a questionnaire study, Weathersbee and coworkers found a higher incidence of abortion, stillbirth, or premature birth associated with excessive caffeine ingestion.[30] Collins and associates found skeletal variations in fetal rats exposed to high doses of caffeine.[4] It appears best to avoid caffeine or to ingest only small, infrequent amounts.

There are several studies on the effects of carbon monoxide and nicotine on the developing fetus. Both have been associated with delayed fetal growth.[20] Effects on behavior and intellectual development have not been adequately studied.

Vitamin deficiencies or surpluses can have adverse effects on the fetus. Excessively large doses of vitamins A and D, for prolonged periods, have been found to be toxic to the fetus.[21] Oral iron should be taken with guidance in early pregnancy because of its association with increased gastrointestinal disturbance.

Nonprescription analgesics, such as aspirin, are frequently taken for the aches and pains experienced by pregnant women. Aspirin, as with other nonsteroidal anti-inflammatory drugs, is very useful in treating joint inflammation and pain, but these drugs inhibit prostaglandin synthesis. Prostaglandins have important functions in the reproductive process, and they also affect fetal homeostasis. Fidler and Ellis reported that prostaglandin inhibitors may interfere with uterine contractility and with fetal vascular structure. They may also interfere with maternal, fetal, and neonatal platelet functions.[8] The intensity of the effect is dependent on the frequency and the dose. It is particularly recommended that aspirin not be taken during the week before delivery because of the possibility of impaired platelet function in the fetus.[28] The therapist can offer alternative treatments, using mobilization, massage, posture and body mechanics education, and therapeutic exercise to treat joint inflammation and pain.

Studies exist that conclude that children born to mothers who are actively alcoholic have increased risk of fetal abnormalities. A full fetal alcohol syndrome, involving consistent abnormalities in these children, has been described.[16] It has been reported that 10% of children born to women who drink 30 ml to 60 ml of alcohol daily, exhibit intrauterine growth retardation, with the possibility of congenital anomalies.[14]

In mothers addicted to heroine or methadone, infant withdrawal after birth is well documented. It can be life-threatening to the fetus if withdrawal from the drug occurs before birth. Studies conflict about whether the newborn is best weaned from the drug through a heroin or a methadone program, or through no drugs at all. A common conclusion, however, is that this infant needs increased attention to catch problems as they arise in the process.

Prescription Drugs

Prescription drugs are an area in which the therapist will have less input. However, women will continue to question therapists with whom they work. Once again, researchers have found it difficult to draw firm conclusions in this area, and physicians must weigh many factors in determining the risk/benefit ratio.

Antiemetics for the woman with persistent vomiting are most commonly used during the first trimester. Antihistamines are widely used as antiemetics. It is reported that in cases of prolonged high doses, blocking of histamines can have a negative fetal or embryonic effect.[26]

Children born to women with epilepsy who are using drug therapy, have a two- to threefold increase in congenital anomalies.[24] It is difficult to separate the teratogenic effects of the disease from those of the drugs that are being used for therapy. A physician may try to decrease or withdraw medication before pregnancy, but it is dangerous to the mother and fetus to do so during pregnancy. This danger is enhanced by the estimation that half of pregnant women with epilepsy will experience an increase in seizure activity because of altered physiologic responses and changing therapeutic levels.[19] It is the physician's challenge to closely monitor the situation and use anticonvulsive medications that have the least risk to the fetus and to the mother.

Hypertension is termed by Lewis, "the most common, preventable cause of both maternal and perinatal mortality in the Western world."[10] After the sixth month of pregnancy, a pre-eclamptic state is said to exist when hypertension, proteinuria, and edema are present. The goal of the physician must be to prevent maternal stroke, cardiac problems, and death, all of which are possible if this condition progresses. The best treatment of preeclampsia is through prevention by close monitoring, proper diet, and use of relaxation skills. Mild exercise to decrease edema may also aid in prevention. Many hypertensive drugs are considered unhealthy for the fetus, but conclusions differ on the risk/benefit ratio of these drugs.

For the pregnant woman with diabetes, insulin remains the drug of choice for treatment. Although children born to these women exhibit an increased rate of congenital malformations, the alternative drugs show even greater fetal risk factors.[6] Serum glucose levels must be closely monitored because insulin requirements fluctuate with the changing physiologic responses and demands of pregnancy.

All anesthetics, general or local, reach the fetus in both early and late pregnancy. Fetal serum levels will usually approach maternal levels. The effects of these anesthetizing drugs on the fetus may include decreased motor activity, failure to establish spontaneous respiration, hypothermia, and a poor sucking response. Because the hepatic and renal systems are not yet mature in the newborn, excretion of the drugs by the newborn's systems will take longer. Physicians and therapists are conducting studies on the use of transcutaneous electrical nerve stimulation (TENS) during labor and delivery as an adjunct for pain relief. Most of these studies conclude that significant percentages of women find TENS helpful for pain relief during labor and delivery.[5,12,23,27,29] There are other studies that show no negative fetal effects.[2,3,7]

Studies and protocols are also available on the use of TENS for postsurgical cesarean rehabilitation.[11,22] Transcutaneous electrical nerve stimulation is used to control postsurgical pain, and is combined with a therapeutic exercise program to control flatulence and increase function within the first 36 hours of delivery. This combination also helps reduce the mother's need for pain-relieving medication which passes into the breast milk.

GYNECOLOGIC PHARMACOLOGY

Conjugated estrogens are another class of drugs therapists may encounter being used by women of all ages. They are sometimes administered to treat the symptoms of menopause. They are also used in combination with progesterone as oral contraceptives for women. In the past, estrogens in the form of diethylstilbestrol (DES) have been administered for prevention of premature labor. This drug has been shown to cause an increased incidence of vaginal adenosis in the female children of pregnant women who have taken it.[5]

It has been reported that 25% of women of reproductive age take oral contraceptives.[1] Birth control pills combine a synthetic estrogen with a progesterone component. Therapists should be aware that the increased hormonal levels in the body may contribute to ligamentous laxity, predisposing these women to joint dysfunctions. Other common and annoying side-effects may include nausea, cyclic swelling, weight gain, intermittent bleeding, and breast tenderness with increased size. Reports agree that there is a higher proportion of spontaneous abortions in women who conceive during the first 2 months after discontinuing oral contraceptive use. The most dangerous condition associated with women who take oral contraceptives is thromboembolic disease.[25] This danger appears to increase to significant levels in combination with smoking, obesity, and age over 35 years. Nevertheless, in women who do not have other risk factors, the drugs' risks do not appear to outweigh their benefits.

Estrogen of animal origin is used to treat some of the symptoms of women during and after menopause. Symptoms include vasomotor dysfunctions, atrophy of vaginal epithelia, dyspareunia, irritability, insomnia, and urinary incontinence because of atrophy of bladder epithelia. A long-term effect can be osteoporosis, or demineralization of bone. Osteoporosis is responsible for an increased frequency of bone fractures among older women, particularly fractures of the femur, the distal forearm, and the vertebral body. Disabling fractures are a major cause of death for elderly women. Many clinical studies exist to show that exogenous estrogens inhibit bone loss in these women. Weiss and coworkers report that risks of fractures are reduced by 50% to 60% when estrogen therapy is maintained for at least 6 years.[31]

However, hormone replacement therapy remains controversial. The question remains of how long to continue therapy. The signs and symptoms may reappear with the same intensity even when the therapy is withdrawn after many years. Such hormone replacement postpones natural adaptation to lower estrogen levels. Various sources discuss concerns for estrogen therapy being linked to cancer, heart disease, and gallbladder dysfunction. Certain clinical conditions, such as a history of thromboembolism, liver disease, and vascular disease, may be aggravated by estrogen therapy. Once again, a skilled authority on the matter must decide the risk/benefit ratio for the individual involved.

Alternatives do appear to exist for many women. Supplements of calcium in combination with vitamin D are likely to benefit women of postmenopausal age. Physical exercises involving weight-bearing activity will provide the stresses to the bone that are needed to decrease demineralization, increase muscle tone, and improve proprioceptive channels. Increased development of rehabilitation programs for the longer-lived population would not only improve the quality of life but may actually save lives.

CASE 1   A 32-year-old woman was pregnant with her first child. She had a job that demanded many hours on her feet. In addition, she had been taking an aerobics class for pregnant women. After class one night, she felt intense pain around her right lumbosacral area, as well as in her groin area. Walking and standing increased the pain. She began taking aspirins, knowing that they might help her painful joints. However, the pain would not cease, so she went to her obstetrician. The obstetrician sent her to an orthopedic physician, who recognized that it was unwise to give her medication. The orthopedic physician recommended that she go home to bed rest. The woman returned to the obstetrician, in despair, realizing she could not afford to leave work. The obstetrician decided to try an approach new to her, that of physical therapy. The woman went to see a therapist. After a thorough evaluation, an assessment was made indicating sacroiliac and pubic symphyseal dysfunction. The therapist taught the woman how to use ice to decrease pain and inflammation. The therapist treated the woman with mild mobilizations to bring the pelvic bones back into symmetry. A lumbopelvic support was provided to increase stability. A therapeutic home exercise program was instiued to help normalize flexibility as much as possible. Thorough posture and body mechanics education was given, with the precaution of avoiding rapid weight-bearing activities, such as jogging in place. With such an approach, this woman was able to manage her pain throughout the rest of her pregnancy, and to continue her job, drug free.

CASE 2   A 34-year-old woman was entering the hospital to deliver her second child by a scheduled cesarean section. She had had a cesarean section with her first child, and remembered having taken substantial pain medication because of postoperative pain. She decided not to breast-feed her first child because she was aware that many drugs freely enter breast milk. In addition, she was disappointed because the medication made her sleepy throughout the first 2 days after the birth of her child.

With the second cesarean section, however, she had decided to use a TENS unit postoperatively to help manage incisional pain. With a therapist's guidance, she incorporated into the first 36 hours an exercise program involving abdominal massage, breathing exercises, and leg and trunk exercises. She reported that flatulence was only a minimal problem the first 3 days, and she required less than one-third of the pain medication that was needed for her first cesarean section. Her alertness and function increased quickly. In addition, because of the low dosage and short duration of medication, she was less concerned about drugs passing into the breast milk during breast-feeding. She stopped wearing the TENS unit on the third day, and continued to progress with an exercise program.

REFERENCES

 1. Arrata WS: Oral contraceptives: General considerations. In Hafez ES (ed): Human Reproduction: Conception and Contraception, pp 509–520. New York, Harper & Row, 1980
 2. Bundsen P, Ericson K: Pain relief in labor by transcutaneous electrical nerve stimulation. Acta Obstet Gynecol Scand 61:1–5, 1982
 3. Bundsen P et al: Pain relief in labor by transcutaneous electrical nerve stimulation. Acta Obstet Gynecol Scand 60:459–68, 1981
 4. Collins TF, Welsh JJ, Black TN et al: A comprehensive study of the teratogenic potential of caffeine on rats when given by oral intubation. Report on Caffeine, FDA, September 1980
 5. Davies JR: Ineffective transcutaneous nerve stimulation following epidural anaesthesia. Anaesthesia 37:453–4, 1982
 6. Elkeles RS: Treatment of diabetes in pregnancy. In Lewis P (ed): Clinical Pharmacology in Obstetrics, pp 157–165. London, Wright PSG, 1983
 7. Erkkola R, Pikkola P, Kanto J: Transcutaneous nerve stimulation for pain relief during labour. Ann Chir Gynecol 69:273–277, 1980
 8. Fidler J, Ellis C: Analgesia in pregnancy. In Lewis P (ed): Clinical Pharmacology in Obstetrics, pp 49–57. London, Wright PSG, 1983
 9. Fofar JO, Nelson MN: Epidemiology of drugs taken by pregnant women. Clin Pharmacol Ther 14:632, 1973
10. Gallery ED: Antihypertensive treatment in pregnancy. In Lewis P (ed): Clinical Pharmacology in Obstetrics, p 88. London, Wright PSG, 1983
11. Gent D, Gottleib K: Caesarean rehabilitation. Clin Manage 5:13–19, 1985
12. Grim LC, Morey SH: Transcutaneous electrical nerve stimulation for relief of parturition pain. Phys Ther 65:337–40, 1985
13. Handbook of Nonprescription Drugs, Washington, American Pharmaceutical Association, 1980

14. Hawkins BF: Teratogenesis in humans. In Kuemmerle H (ed): Clinical Pharmacology in Pregnancy, pp 113–124. New York, Thieme-Stratton, 1984
15. Herbst AL, Ulfelder H, Poskanzer DC: Adenocarcinoma of the vagina, association of maternal stilbestrol therapy with tumor appearance in young women. N Engl J Med 284:878, 1971
16. Jones KL, Smith DW, Vileland C, Streissguth AP: Pattern of malformation in offspring of chronic alcoholic mothers. Lancet 1:1267–1271, 1973
17. Kuemmerle HP: Clinical Pharmacology in Pregnancy, p 162. New York, Thieme-Stratton, 1974
18. Lams J, Rayburn WF: Drug effects on the fetus. In Rayburn WF, Zuspan FP (eds): Drug Therapy in Obstetrics and Gynecology, p 9. Norwalk, Appleton-Century Crofts, 1982
19. Lander CM, Edwards VE et al: Plasma anticonvulsant concentrations during pregnancy. Neurology 27:128, 1977
20. Landesman-Dwyer S, Emmanuel I: Smoking during pregnancy. Teratology 19:119, 1979
21. Rayburn W, Schad RF: Iron preparations, vitamins, and antiemetics. In Rayburn WF, Zuspan FP (eds): Drug Therapy in Obstetrics and Gynecology, pp 24–28. Norwalk, Appleton-Century Crofts, 1982
22. Riley JE: The impact of transcutaneous electrical nerve stimulation on the postcaesarean patient. J Obstet Gynecol Nurs 11:325–329, 1982
23. Robson JE: Transcutaneous nerve stimulation for pain releif in labor. Anaesthesia 34:357–360, 1979
24. Speidel BD, Meadow SR: Maternal epilepsy and abnormalities of the fetus and newborn. Lancet 2:839, 1972
25. Spellacy WN: Progestagen and estrogen effects on carbohydrate metabolism. In Josimovich JB (ed): Uterine Contraction, pp 327–339. New York, John Wiley & Sons, 1973
26. Stamm H: Antiemetics. In Kuemmerle H (ed): Clinical Pharmacology in Pregnancy, pp 363–365. New York, Thieme-Stratton, 1984
27. Stewart P: Transcutaneous nerve stimulation as a method of analgesia in labour. Anaesthesia 34:361–364, 1979
28. Turner G, Collins E: Fetal effects on regular salicylate ingestion in pregnancy. Lancet 2:338–339, 1974
29. Vincenti E et al: Comparative study between patients treated with transcutaneous electrical stimulation and controls during labour. Clin Exp Obstet Gynecol 9:95–97, 1982
30. Weathersbee PS, Olsen LK, Lodge JR: Caffeine and pregnancy. Postgrad Med 62:64, 1977
31. Weiss NC, Ure CL et al: Decreased risk of fractures of the hip and lower forearm with postmenopausal use of estrogen. N Engl J Med 303:1195–1198, 1980

Pulmonary Pharmacology   5

Cynthia Coffin Zadai

The use of pharmacotherapy in the treatment of pulmonary patients relates specifically to the pathologic tissue changes and resulting pathophysiology of pulmonary disease, primarily airway obstruction and inflammation. This chapter will initially present the abnormal components of acute and chronic lung disease; identifying and defining the concepts most directly addressed by drug therapy. Medications will then be presented in groups according to their physiologic effect. Finally, the clinical use and common therapeutic combinations of drugs will be described as the chapter concludes with two case studies.

PATHOPHYSIOLOGY OF PULMONARY DISEASE

Primary pulmonary patients are most commonly grouped together under the single label of chronic obstructive pulmonary disease (COPD). Within this broad category are patients with the more specific diagnoses of emphysema, chronic bronchitis, asthma and, less commonly, broncchiectasis, and cystic fibrosis. Although the pathologic processes for each diagnosis are noticeably different, the clinical presentation, symptoms, and examination findings of these patients may be similar. In fact, it is common to find a combination of disease processes responsible for the similar complaints and problems of this patient population. *Emphysema* is characterized by "abnormal enlargement of the terminal air spaces. In part, the condition is an expression of normal senescence, a loss of elastic tissue from the lung leading to expiratory collapse of the larger air passages, difficulty in expiration and dilatation

97

of the terminal airways."[5] *Chronic bronchitis* is defined clinically as subjects who have "a chronic or recurrent productive cough on most days for a minimum of 3 months per year in not less than 2 successive years."[2] This cough is a response to an excess of secretions from hypertrophy and hyperplasia of mucous-secreting glands. Additionally, in patients with an unusually high degree of bronchospasm, airway smooth muscle may be increased and peribronchiolar fibrosis may occur. When comparing the two disease processes, emphysema initially and predominantly affects terminal airways or more peripheral tissue. It progresses centrally to larger airways to produce obstruction through airway collapse. Chronic bronchitis affects primarily the conducting airways, producing obstruction by occlusion caused by excess secretions, bronchospasm, or both.[16] Clinically, it is common to find these disease processes coexisting.

Asthma is an airway disease characterized by hyperreactivity to a variety of stimuli. Periods of illness are usually intermittent and can vary from mild to severe.[16] During remission periods, there is generally no demonstrable pulmonary function abnormality. The precipitating factors for asthma include allergens, infections, medications, exercise, emotion, and environment. The airway obstruction abnormality in this patient group is characterized by spasm of bronchial smooth muscle, edema of the mucosa and submucosa, and excessive secretion of viscous mucus.[16]

Bronchiectasis can be defined as irreversible dilatation of the bronchial tree. The abnormality includes impaction of smaller bronchi and bronchioles with thick purulent secretions accompanied commonly by cellular infiltration and swelling of the bronchial walls. All forms are accompanied by bronchial dilatation and destruction. In diffuse disease a pattern of obstruction is well recognized by pulmonary function testing.[9,16]

Cystic fibrosis, a hereditary disease transmitted by a mendelian-recessive process, is a disease of the exocrine glands. The fundamental abnormality is the secretion of thick tenacious secretions from these glands that leads to their cystic dilatation and fibrous atrophy.[16,19] Pulmonary involvement includes mucous plugging in the bronchial tree that obstructs airflow, increased susceptibility to infection and, possibly, asthma. Either chronically or during periods of infection, patients can develop atelectasis, cylindrical and cystic bronchiectasis, and abscesses.[16,19]

The common characteristics of these disease processes then includes obstructed airways and susceptibility to, or presence of, inflammation and infection. Airway obstruction occurs as a result of change in the elasticity of the tissue, smooth-muscle contraction, plugging related to secretions, or diameter reduction resulting from vascular engorgement or cellular infiltration. Inflammation and infection are seen as either precipitators or compounding factors in airway obstruction. Pharmacotherapy is directed at these abnormal process components either directly or in combination.

THEORY OF BRONCHOSPASM

Neurologic Control

Pharmacologic management of bronchospasm relates specifically to the autonomic nervous control within the pulmonary system. The available drugs promote bronchodilation by chemically stimulating or blocking specific neurons at either neuroreceptor or neuroeffector sites. A conceptual review of this system provides a basis for understanding drug management and its efficacy.

The *autonomic nervous system* is divided into the parasympathetic and sympathetic branches and is considered to be the unconscious control system of the body. These systems maintain the balance of the body's opposing effects on the smooth muscle and glands.[18] (Fig. 5-1). The *parasympathetic branch* controls the essential functions of digestion, bladder and rectum discharge, and basal secretion of bronchial mucus. The *sympathetic branch* regulates functions typically described as our fight-or-flight responses: heart rate and blood pressure, change in blood flow from periphery to muscles and heart, rise in blood sugar, and bronchial dilatation. The regulation of these responses occurs through chemical transmission of impulses at both ganglionic synapses and nerve fiber endings.[18] Pulmonary drugs either augment or inhibit the chemicals used in transmission of impulses.

Neurotransmitters and Cellular Mediators

Current research now supports the theory of a balance between the sympathetic and parasympathetic neurologic systems that maintains bronchial smooth-muscle tone. The parasympathetic system, which uses acetylcholine as its neurotransmitter, is responsible for mild constriction of bronchial smooth muscle through vagal stimulation to the bronchioles.[29] The sympathetic system uses acetylcholine as the neurotransmitter at the ganglionic junction and norepinepherine as a neurotransmitter at the neuroeffector sites.[16] The neural supply of the sympathetic system to the bronchioles is less evident and the fibers are mainly distributed to the blood vessels in the lung.[29] The sympathetic effects of bronchodilatation are then mainly gained through intracellular mechanisms. β_2-Receptors found in bronchial smooth-muscle cells are associated with the enzyme adenylate cyclase that catalyzes the conversion

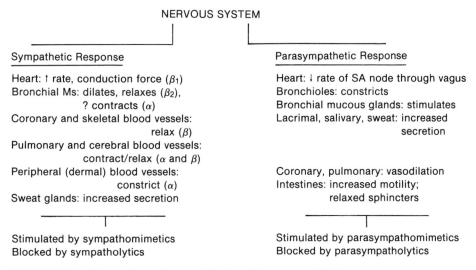

NERVOUS SYSTEM

Sympathetic Response

Heart: ↑ rate, conduction force (β_1)
Bronchial Ms: dilates, relaxes (β_2),
    ? contracts (α)
Coronary and skeletal blood vessels:
    relax (β)
Pulmonary and cerebral blood vessels:
    contract/relax (α and β)
Peripheral (dermal) blood vessels:
    constrict (α)
Sweat glands: increased secretion

Stimulated by sympathomimetics
Blocked by sympatholytics

Parasympathetic Response

Heart: ↓ rate of SA node through vagus
Bronchioles: constricts
Bronchial mucous glands: stimulates
Lacrimal, salivary, sweat: increased
    secretion

Coronary, pulmonary: vasodilation
Intestines: increased motility;
    relaxed sphincters

Stimulated by parasympathomimetics
Blocked by parasympatholytics

FIGURE 5-1. Comparison of sympathetic and parasympathetic system responses.

of adenosine triphosphate (ATP) to cyclic adenosine 3', 5'-monophosphate (cAMP).[22] Elevated concentrations of cAMP are associated with bronchodilatation through bronchial smooth muscle relaxation and the inhibition of mast cell degranulation. Mast cell degranulation releases histamine, which is a cellular mediator that also causes bronchial smooth-muscle contraction. Other cell mediators that contribute to bronchospasm include eosinophil chemotactic factor of anaphylaxis (ECF-A), which is stored in the cytoplasmic granules of mast cells; and slow-reacting substance of anaphylaxis (SRS-A) and platelet aggregation factor (PAF), which are synthesized and released during allergic response. Bronchospasm is probably produced cellularly through the effect of these mediators on bronchial smooth muscle. The synthesis and release of these mediators is inhibited through the action of cAMP promoting mast cell stability.

Other intracellular mechanisms affecting bronchial smooth-muscle tone are those reactions that accompany parasympathetic stimulation. Activation of acetylcholine receptors converts guanosine triphosphate (GTP) to cyclic guanosine 3', 5'-monophosphate (cGMP) which produces bronchoconstriction.[13,16]

It is the balance between the parasympathetic system producing bronchoconstriction and the sympathetic system producing bronchodilation that provides the concept of bronchial smooth-muscle tone (Fig. 5-2). Without parasympathetic stimulation the airways would be flaccid, without sympathetic stimulation there would be bronchoconstriction. Hence, a balanced system provides for normal function.[16]

Mediation of Bronchospasm

Bronchoconstriction is produced within the smooth muscle of the bronchial tree by either an increase in parasympathetic stimulation or by a decrease or blocking of the sympathetic receptors or effectors. This can occur by stimulating production of acetylcholine with direct-acting parasympathomimetics or cholinergic agents or by preventing the degradation of acetylcholine by agents known as indirect-acting parasympathomimetics. More commonly, bronchospasm is produced as a result of lack of cAMP production or rapid cAMP degradation. Inadequate levels of cAMP can result from blocking of β_2-receptor sites; an imbalance between cAMP and cGMP within the cell, a result of stimulation of sympathetic α-fibers; or vagal parasympathetic stimulation.[23] Bronchospasm, then, is mediated through increased stimulation of β_2-receptor sites and promotion of cAMP production; through neural stimulation by sympathomimetics that decreases degradation of cAMP; by methylxanthines that inhibit production of cGMP by anticholinergics,

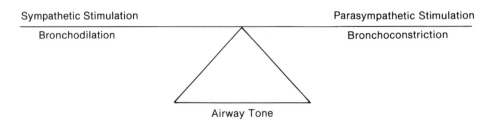

FIGURE 5-2. Maintenance of tone.

and by stabilization of the mast cell through increasing cAMP or use of cromolyn sodium (see Fig. 5-1).

PHARMACOLOGIC INTERVENTIONS

Sympathomimetics

The sympathomimetic drugs comprise the most commonly chosen group of agents for the mediation of acute bronchospasm. When originally presented for use with pulmonary patients, the main agent was epinepherine, a naturally occuring catecholamine that nonselectively stimulates the sympathetic nervous system to promote bronchodilatation. This generalized stimulation produces bronchodilatation through stimulation of β_2-receptors; however, α- and β_1-fibers of the sympathetic system are stimulated as well, creating counterproductive physiologic responses. The side-effects of epinepherine stimulation are most dramatically observed in the cardiovascular system (Fig. 5-3). Pharmacologic research has produced progressively more specific agents that act selectively to produce stimulation of only the β_2-fibers. Theoretically, the sympathomimetic agents work by stimulation of the β_2-receptors, increasing the activity of the enzyme adenylate cyclase in the cell membrane, which catalyzes the formation of cAMP. It has been postulated that adenylate cyclase, itself, may be the β_2-receptor.[23] Sympathomimetics can be grouped into nonselective and selective categories (Table 5-1).

NONSELECTIVE AGENTS

Epinepherine

Epinepherine is a drug that stimulates action at α-, β_1-, and β_2-receptors. Responses to it include vasoconstriction at the bronchial mucosa, decreased production of mucus, increased inotropic and chronotropic cardiac response, and bronchial smooth-muscle relaxation.[23] Because there are both smooth-muscle contraction produced by α-stimulation and smooth-muscle relaxation produced by β_2-stimulation, individual responses can vary. Epinepherine is rapidly assimilated

α	β_1	β_2
Bronchoconstriction		Bronchodilatation
Vasoconstriction	Inotropic and chrontropic cardiac stimulation	Vasodilatation
Sphincter contraction in GI tract and bladder		
		Skeletal muscle tremor
Increased hepatic glycogenolysis	Increased lipolysis	Increased muscle glycogenolysis

FIGURE 5-3.   Sympathetic stimulation and its physiologic effects.

TABLE 5-1
Sympathomimetics

Drug	Primary Effect	Side-Effect
NONSELECTIVE		
Epinepherine	α, β_1, β_2	Tachycardia, palpitations, increased BP, headache, nervousness, muscle tremor
Isoproterenol	β_1, β_2	Tachycardia, initial hypertension, palpitation
SELECTIVE		
Isoetharine	β_2	Tachycardia and increased BP, skeletal muscle tremor
Metaproterenol sulfate	β_2	Tachycardia or hypertension may be seen, muscle tremor
Terbutaline sulfate	β_2	Muscle tremor, less frequently tachycardia or hypertension
Albuterol	β_2	Muscle tremor, less frequently tachycardia or hypertension

by sympathetic nerve endings and metabolized by catechol-O-methyltransferase (COMT) and monoamine oxidase (MAO). Monoamine oxidase is present in the gastrointestinal tract; therefore, epinepherine is not effective when given by mouth. It is given in effective doses only subcutaneously. Delivered intravenously it can cause death from ventricular arrhythmia, cerebral hemorrhage, or sudden hypertension. Epinepherine is available in pressurized aerosol cannisters without prescription as Primatene or Bronkaid. Its use as an inhalant has been superseded by the selective β_2-medications.

Isoproterenol (Isuprel)

Isoproterenol is the most potent bronchodilator of the sympathomimetics. It has a strong relaxant effect on bronchial and gastrointestinal smooth muscle, with little or no hypertensive effect. Because of its nonselective stimulation of β_1- and β_2-receptors, it also produces potent cardiac side-effects.[12] Isoproterenol is metabolized by COMT and degraded in the liver. It is, therefore, most frequently delivered either by pressurized cannister inhaler or as a mist by air-driven compressor and nebulizer. The dose per puff, or mist content, varies with different preparations. The cardiac side-effects can be significant including tachycardia and arrhythmias. If a patient is not getting the desired bronchodilatation with isoproterenol a different drug is generally chosen, rather than increasing either the frequency or dose. During the early 1960s a significant increase in mortality from asthma in Great Britain was later traced to the over-the-counter availability of pressurized adrenergic aerosols that delivered five times more isoproterenol per puff than other preparations. Death rates dropped when these cannisters returned to prescription status.

β_2-SELECTIVE AGENTS

Selective sympathomimetics are those drugs that preferentially stimulate the β_2-receptors and have minimal α- or β_1-effects.

Isoetharine (Bronkosol)

Isoetharine is a primary β_2-stimulant with minimal α- or β_1-activity. It is far less effective on bronchial smooth muscle than isoproterenol but has 300 times less effect on the cardiovascular system.[18] It is metabolized by COMT and, therefore, is not given orally. The drug can be delivered by pressurized cannister or nebulizer through inhalation. Its peak effect is seen in 15 min to 60 min and its duration is 1-1/2 hr to 3 hr. Normal side-effects include tachycardia and blood pressure increase, as well as the most common selective sympathomimetic side-effect: skeletal muscle tremor. Skeletal muscle tremor has been documented to occur in 20% to 35% of patients receiving β_2-selective sympathomimetics.[30] There is some evidence this results from stimulation of a β_2-type receptor in skeletal muscle.

Metaproterenol Sulfate (Alupent, Metaprel)

Metaproterenol, a somewhat recently available drug, was used extensively in Europe before becoming available in the United States. It is reported to be more effective than isoetharine, yet not as effective as isoproterenol.[18] It is also primarily a β_2-stimulant with little cardiac effect. Metaproterenol is not metabolized by COMT; therefore, its duration of action is reported to be up to 4 hr, and it is available in oral preparations. Side-effects are more likely to occur with systemic than with aerosol administration and can include the previously described muscle tremor, tachycardia, and hypertension.

Terbutaline Sulfate (Bricanyl, Brethine)

Terbutaline is also a selective β_2-specific sympathomimetic, but it is somewhat different in that it is not generally administered by inhalation. It is not metabolized by COMT; therefore, it provides a longer duration (up to 4 hr subcutaneously; 4 hr to 6 hours orally) and can be taken orally. This drug is also given in small doses subcutaneously compared with the oral route and is reported to be twice as potent as metaproterenol on bronchial smooth muscle, with less cardiac stimulation.[18] Its side-effects, which vary with the mode of delivery, include tachycardia, increased blood pressure, and muscle tremor. Terbutaline has also been noted to increase the velocity of mucous transport.

Albuterol (Proventil, Ventolin)

Albuterol is not a catecholamine-structured drug. It is a β_2-stimulant with an even longer duration of up to 6 hr. It can be absorbed through inhalation or through the intestinal tract and is excreted in the urine. It appears to be approximately one-fifth as potent as isoproterenol on bronchial smooth muscle.[18] This drug is considered superior to currently approved sympathomimetics in its specificity and duration of action when administered by inhalation, but it may be inferior to metaproterenol and isoetharine when taken orally. The common sympathomimetic side-effects may occur.

Parasympatholytics

The parasympatholytic class of drugs promotes bronchodilation by two routes. The first is to block stimulation of parasympathetic receptors and production of the mediator cGMP, thereby blocking the mechanism that produces bronchial smooth-muscle contraction and airway tone. The second route interferes with the enzyme phosphodiesterase, whose role is to promote basal tone in the airways by breaking down cAMP. Phosphodiesterase interference produces muscle relaxation and bronchodilation. These drugs then block the routine parasympathetic responses of bronchoconstriction, increased mucociliary activity, decreased heart rate, and pupillary constriction.

ATROPINE

The use of atropine as a bronchodilator relates directly to the patient's level of resting vagal tone.[20] If a person has normal resting tone, the use of atropine to block stimulation of normal tone may not produce a dramatic bronchodilation. However, in persons with greater than normal-resting tone the bronchodilation might be quite dramatic. The range of response to atropine includes bronchodilation, drying of secretions, increase in heart rate, and pupillary dilatation. Consequently, the side-effects of dried and thickened secretions and tachycardia could be of importance in selected pulmonary patients. Secretion problems related to airway obstruction were discounted in 1977 by Light and George.[11] The drug is delivered by aerosol nebulizer and has a reported duration efficacy of 2 hr to 5 hr, depending on the dose.[18]

IPRATROPIUM BROMIDE (ATROVENT)

Ipratropium bromide is an anticholinergic/parasympatholytic agent that appears to prevent an increase in intracellular concentration of cGMP.[20] Physiologic effects are primarily local and site specific. The most common clinical use for this drug is in combination with a sympathomimetic bronchodilator to promote maintenance management of bronchospasm in COPD patients. It is not indicated for acute reversal of bronchospasm.

Methylxanthines

The methylxanthine class of drugs includes caffeine, theophylline, and theobromine, and the drugs are referred to as *xanthine derivatives* or methylxanthines (Table 5-2). They share in common the side effects of cerebral stimulation, skeletal muscle stimulation, bronchodilatation, pulmonary vasodilation, smooth-muscle relaxation, coronary vasodilatation, cardiac stimulation, and diuresis.[18] The primary xanthine of interest in pulmonary patients is theophylline.

THEOPHYLLINE (AMINOPHYLLINE)

Therapeutically, theophylline exerts its primary effects through decreased airway resistance (bronchodilatation), decreased pulmonary vascular resistance (vasodilatation), and stimulated ventilation. The mechanism of theophylline action is not

TABLE 5-2
Methylxanthines

Generic Drug	Trade Name	Delivery Form
Theophylline	Theo-Dur	Tablet
	Slo-Phyllin	Tablet/capsule
	Elixophyllin	Capsule/elixir
	Aerolate	Capsule
	Fleet Theophylline	Retention enema
Aminophylline	Aminodur Dura-Tabs	Tablet
	Aminophylline suppositories	Suppository
	Aminophylline ampule	Intravenous solution
Oxtriphylline	Choledyl	Tablet/elixir

ADVERSE SIDE EFFECTS

Cardiovascular: tachycardia, palpitations, arrhythmia/hypertension, headache/hypotension, shock

Gastrointestinal: nausea, anorexia, abdominal pain, indigestion, vomiting, hematemesis, diarrhea, melena

Nervous system: anxiety, irritability, agitation, insomnia, tremulousness, twitching, dizziness, fainting, seizures

---

well or fully understood. It is presented here as a parasympatholytic because a portion of its action relates to the inhibition of phosphodiesterase, thereby increasing cellular levels of cAMP. However, there is not equal inhibition of the phosphodiesterase enzymes, and the concentration of theophylline required to inhibit phosphodiesterase would be toxic in vivo.[18,26] Additionally, there is some evidence in rats that theophylline acts as a prostaglandin antagonist, and intracellular effects on calcium have been described.[4,8] Theophylline, then, causes bronchodilatation, possibly through a variety of mechanisms but most significantly in a different mode from the sympathomimetics. Therefore, these drugs are commonly seen together therapeutically, and their effect is synergistic.[24]

The bronchodilator effect of theophylline is approximately proportional to the logarithm of serum concentrations within the 5–20 mg/ml range.[10,14] This effect has also been demonstrated for exercise-induced bronchospasm.[17] Serum concentrations above 10 mg/ml effectively inhibited bronchospasm during treadmill exercise testing. Frequency and severity of symptoms in chronic asthma are most effectively decreased when serum levels are maintained on a continuous around-the-clock basis between the 10 mg/ml and 20 mg/ml range.[25]

Conversely, the side-effects of theophylline can also be monitored by serum levels. Common problems include nausea, vomiting, headache, diarrhea, irritability, and insomnia. These effects are associated with serum levels higher than 20 mg/ml. At the higher levels, side-effects have included seizure, cardiac arrhythmias, and death.[27]

Theophylline is administered intravenously, orally, and rectally. It is quickly absorbed and distributed through extracellular and, to a smaller extent, intracellular water.[28] It is eliminated in several forms: unchanged through the kidneys or metabolized in the liver.

The method of delivery depends on the clinical situation. Long-term users rely on oral forms that produce slow, constant absorption over 12 hr to maintain stable blood levels. This can be accomplished through commercial preparations such as Theodur, Slo-Phyllin, or Sustaire. When rapid increase in serum levels is necessary for acute, unresponsive bronchospasm, the medication is delivered intravenously.

Anti-Inflammatory Agents

Inflammatory response is one of the commonalities among pulmonary patients. It is part of the disease process in asthma, bronchitis, bronchiectasis, pneumonia, and even possibly emphysema.[7] As previously described in this chapter, inflammation produces swelling, vascular engorgement, hypersecretion of mucus, and bronchoconstriction in the pulmonary system. There are several drugs used that attempt to either prevent or reverse that process.

CROMOLYN SODIUM (INTAL)

Cromolyn sodium is not technically an anti-inflammatory drug or a bronchodilator. It is presented here because its primary action is to prevent an inflammatory response in patients with allergic bronchospasm. This action is thought to occur through stabilization of the mast cell membrane, thereby preventing release of the chemical mediators that cause bronchoconstriction.[24] This drug, then, can be used only prophylactically.

Cromolyn is delivered by either an aerosol inhaler or by capsule in a spinhaler device. The capsule containing a dry powder is placed inside the device and punctured. A propeller inside the device is spun to allow the inhalation of the air-suspended powder particles. Side-effects of drug delivery include bronchospasm in response to the irritating powder. Inhalation of a sympathomimetic 10 min to 15 min before the cromolyn dose may allow more effective entry. Positive response to this drug may take at least 3 to 5 days and, possibly, up to a month. It is, therefore, recommended for use only in severe perennial asthma.[3]

CORTICOSTEROIDS: Dexamethasone Sodium Phosphate (Decadron); Beclomethasone Dipropionate (Vanceril or Beclovent); Prednisone; Prednisolone; Hydrocortisone (Cortef); Methylprednisolone (Medrol); Triamcinolone Acetonide (Azmacort)*

The major indication for use of corticosteroids with pulmonary patients is for their anti-inflammatory effects including bronchodilation, decreased secretion production, and reduced mucosal edema.[18] There are several hypotheses for the mechanisms behind these physiologic effects that include

- Stimulation of specific corticosteroid receptors in the cytoplasm of target tissues to influence protein synthesis in the cells responsible for inflammatory response

*Aerosol delivery of triamcinolone acetonide (Azmacort) has been accomplished within the last year.

- Cell and lysosomal membrane stabilization preventing release of inflammatory mediators
- Adenylate cyclase activation, promoting production of cAMP

Most probably, the effects are mediated through more than one mechanism. The physiologic effects produced include vasoconstriction and reduced capillary permeability in the bronchial microvasculature, relaxation of bronchial smooth muscle, and reduced mucosal edema.[24] The additional benefits may include restored responsiveness to adrenergic bronchodilators.

Corticosteroids can be given by mouth, inhaled as an aerosol, or intravenously. Their route of delivery and dose depend on the patient and the acuteness of their condition (Table 5-3). The greatest drawbacks in using steroids are the serious side-effects seen with long-term administration. Side-effects can include weight gain with cushingoid facies, osteoporosis, edema, echymoses from capillary fragility, cataracts, steroid diabetes, muscle wasting and weakness, stress ulcers, emotional problems, and interference with response to infection.[24]

Because these substances are normally produced by the body and there is a feedback mechanism to control their level, the normal production is decreased over time when their levels are artificially increased. Steroid therapy, then, is a careful balance to provide adequate amounts of drug, prevent major side-effects, and not produce a steroid-dependent patient. This balancing act was aided by the

TABLE 5-3
Corticosteroids

Drug	Delivery/Action Length	Advantage/Disadvantage
Hydrocortisone (cortisol)	Intravenous/short	Effective in status asthmaticus/can cause electrolyte disturbance
Prednisone	Oral/intermediate	Inexpensive, effective/not as effect in patients with liver disease
Prednisolone	Oral/intermediate	Quickly effective p.o./more expensive than prednisone
Methylprednisolone	IM, oral/intermediate	Rapidly effective, minimal side-effects/more expensive
Betamethasone	IM, oral/long aerosol	More potent than dexamethasone/less potent than beclomethasone/can develop candidiasis with aerosol use
Dexamethasone	Oral, IM, IV,/long	Variety of forms available/efficacy questioned in asthma
Beclomethasone	Aerosol/variable	Minimal side-effects/hoarseness and candidiasis
Triamcinolone acetonide	Aerosol/variable	Minimal side-effects/hoarseness and candidiasis

TABLE 5-4
Antibiotics

Drug Category	Delivery	Action
Penicillins	Oral, IM, IV	Bactericidal
Cephalosporins	IV, IM	Bactericidal
Aminoglycosides	Parenteral	Bactericidal
Tetracyclines	Oral	Bacteriostatic
Erythromycin	Oral, IV	Bacteriostatic

development of aerosolized steroids that provide high levels of topical activity with minimal systemic absorption, thereby decreasing side-effects.[18]

Antibiotics

Antibiotics have proved to be some of the most useful drugs developed to treat pulmonary disease because of their ability to significantly decrease morbidity and mortality related to infection. Their primary action is to kill or inhibit the microorganisms responsible for producing infection. These agents can be classified as bactericidal or bacteriostatic and operate in one of the following ways: (1) inhibition of cell wall synthesis, (2) inhibition of cell membrane function, (3) inhibition of protein synthesis, (4) inhibition of nucleic acid synthesis[18] (Table 5-4). Antibiotics are further classified as broad-spectrum, which are useful against both gram-positive and gram-negative bacteria, or narrow-spectrum, which are effective against only a few organisms. This classification is most important clinically because these drugs can be effective only if used with organisms that are sensitive to their mode of action. Use of an agent that is ineffective for any given infecting organism will simply complicate the infection by killing competing organisms and promoting growth of the resistant infecting colony.

PENICILLINS (Penicillin G, Penicillin V, Oxacillin, Cloxacillin, Methicillin, Ampicillin, Amoxicillin, Carbenicillin)

The mode of action for penicillin is to inhibit cell wall synthesis. It can be delivered either orally or parenterally and is used to treat infections with staphylococci, *Haemophilus influenzae*, gonococci, and syphilis-causing organisms. Penicillin allergy is a major side-effect that produces responses that can include various skin rashes, urticaria, and anaphylactic shock.[18]

CEPHALOSPORINS: Cephalexin (Keflex); Cephalothin (Keflin); Cephaloridine (Loridine); Cephradine (Velosef); Cephaloglycin (Kafocin)

The cephalosporins' mode of action is bactericidal, inhibiting bacterial cell wall synthesis. The drug is administered IV, which can cause thrombophlebitis, or IM, which can be painful. It is a broad-spectrum agent that is effective against many common gram-positive cocci, some gram-negative organisms, particularly, *Klebsiella* sp. The worst side-effects of cephalosporin administration can be nephrotoxicity, including acute tubular necrosis.[18]

AMINOGLYCOSIDES (Streptomycin, Gentamicin, Tobramycin, Kanamycin, Amikacin, Neomycin)

Aminoglycosides have a bactericidal action that interferes with the bacteria's protein synthesis. These drugs are poorly absorbed through the gastrointestinal tract, thus they are given parenterally. Their efficacy is somewhat drug-specific, for example, streptomycin is used with tuberculosis, gentamicin with pneumonia caused by aerobic gram-negative bacteria, and tobramycin with pneumonias caused by *Pseudomonas aeruginosa*. These drugs are associated with a significant amount of toxicity including ototoxicity, neuromuscular impairment, and renal tubular damage.[18]

TETRACYCLINES (Tetracycline, Oxytetracycline, Chlortetracycline, Methacycline, Doxycycline)

The tetracycline class of antibiotics can be either bacteriostatic or bactericidal by interfering with the bacteria's protein synthesis. These drugs are administered orally and should be taken with an empty stomach to promote absorption. They are effective with atypical pneumonias including those caused by mycoplasmata. Side-effects include gastrointestinal irritation with nausea, vomiting, and diarrhea, as well as bone marrow depression and allergic responses such as skin rashes or anaphylactic shock.

CLINICAL MANAGEMENT

Patient Assessment

Clinical assessment of the patient with pulmonary disease requires both subjective observation and objective measures. The patients with chronic pulmonary disease, described initially in this chapter, may be stabilized on a given drug regimen; however, they are continually susceptible to disease exacerbation, allergic responses, or acute infection. Consequently, obtaining baseline data in this population provides an objective measure to assess decline or improvement in clinical status, whereas subjective assessment can indicate the need for repeat measurement and change in the therapeutic program. Commonly useful clinical assessment measures are vital signs, thoracic physical examination findings, pulmonary function test values, arterial blood gas or oxygen saturation levels, chest x-ray findings, sputum culture results, exercise test results, and blood values. These clinical findings and values, in combination, can document the presence of infection with an increase in bronchoconstriction; stabilization of bronchospasm with therapeutically safe medication blood levels; colonization of the patient with a new infecting organism that has produced an acute lung infiltrate; or stabilization of airway reactivity in response to exercise.

Typically, the pharmacologic management can be grouped into categories of immediate and long-term therapy. Many of the patients can fall into either category at any given point.

Immediate Therapy

Acute pulmonary symptoms refer primarily to the presence of bronchospasm. This can be documented by change in the forced expiratory volume in 1 sec (FEV_1). Initial changes in expiratory flow are most commonly treated with β_2-selective sympathomimetics by inhalation.[10] Care must be taken to instruct the patient about the most efficacious method for delivery. The patient exhales to begin. Two-thirds of the way through a slow, deep inhalation, the patient should activate the cannister and deliver the drug without stopping inhalation. At maximum inhalation the patient holds his breath for 10 sec, then exhales.[15] If the drug used in this manner is not effective and the bronchospasm increases, the patient will require additional medication. The second level of therapeutics would typically be methylxanthine, delivered intravenously. Objective monitoring of vital signs, blood levels, oxygenation, and pulmonary function continues. Patients are also continued on a regimen of inhaled sympathomimetics; however, with increasing bronchospasm, the method of delivery may change to a nebulized form of the drug. This can be effectively delivered by a therapist who is assisting the patient. The techniques of positioning and breathing patterning are used to facilitate efficacious use of ventilatory musculature and maximize ventilation/perfusion ratios. Attention must also be given to the breathing pattern to achieve maximum drug delivery.

If signs and symptoms of bronchospasm continue for 1 to 2 hours after the initiation of therapy, corticosteroids are generally used. They are delivered by IV in loading doses appropriate for the individual patient. Often supportive measures include adequate hydration, oxygenation, and institution of mechanical ventilation if respiratory failure ensues.[10] Additionally, patients are assessed for precipitating or accompanying infection.

Long-Term Therapy

Pharmacologic therapy for chronic bronchospasm is most effectively and safely managed with theophylline in doses that achieve and maintain effective serum levels. In individuals with primarily extrinsic asthma, this can be accomplished, albeit more expensively, with cromolyn sodium. Additional therapy for minor flare-ups can be managed with inhaled sympathomimetics. For patients with intractable bronchospasm that cannot be managed by the preceding medications, corticosteroids are used. The major goal of steroid therapy is to use short courses that permit continued adrenal function and produce minimal side-effects. Patients that require long-term steroid therapy can decrease their side-effects by alternating daily dosages. In levels less than 20 mg q.o.d.; however, this technique has not been found effective.[26] The risks of long-term corticosteroid therapy can be minimized by the use of prednisone, prednisolone and methylprednisolone, or by the use of inhaled rather than systemic corticosteroids.[1,6] For most effective oral therapy the drug is administered as a single dose in the morning.

Management of infection in the chronically ill also relates to clinical assessment and objective documentation. Extended antibiotic use is not considered useful in COPD patients because they may acquire infections with resistant strains of bacteria.[18] Antibiotic therapy is generally started at the first clinical sign of infection. It is useful to know with which strains of organisms the patient is chronically colonized. Sputum specimen evaluation for Gram stain, culture, and antibiotic sensitivity can aid the specificity of drug management.

Pharmacologic management of pulmonary patients is a complex process that many times requires trial and error to determine what combination of drugs most effectively resolves the patient's problems. Professionals working with this population require a background familiarity with available agents, in a constantly changing drug environment, as well as the clinical skills to assess their patients who require these complex drug regimens. Subjective and objective observations of baseline function and functional performance can greatly contribute to the determination of the most effective therapy combinations.

CASE 1 **History of Present Illness**

This is the first hospital admission at this facility for a 33-year-old white woman with a long history of asthma and three previous admissions to another facility for acute exacerbations. She reports that she had been doing well until about 1 week ago, when she developed a chest cold with cough, initially nonproductive, but over the past 2 days productive of greenish sputum. She relates this to other family members who have had upper respiratory infections. Sunday, her chest began to feel tight, and the patient developed shortness of breath with wheezing. She tried to treat this at home with regular medications (aminophylline, 200 mg, five times a day; albuterol, 4 mg, four times a day, Alupent Inhaler two puffs four times a day), and added ampicillin 250 mg times three or four doses on the day before admission, with no improvement. She denies chills, diaphoresis, chest pain. Oral temperature was 99° at home.

The patient had asthma as a young child, from about the ages of 6 to 10, that was essentially unmedicated and not problematic. This was associated with eczema. She then developed more severe asthma at aged 21, and was hospitalized twice during 1982 and 1983. The patient was hospitalized with her most serious episode at which time she was, by her own report, nearly intubated in the ICU in 1985. Since that time she has been on a continuous dosage of prednisone, between 2.5 and 50 mg q.d. (typical dosage 50 mg q.d.), which was recently tapered and stopped upon conversion to Vanceril. Vanceril was subsequently stopped in June. She reports an excellent response to steroids but stopped them because of her desire to conceive. Her condition has been subjectively deteriorating since the termination of her medications. She reports asthma typically exacerbated by upper respiratory infection. She develops some wheezing with exercise that is relieved with an inhaler. She denies allergies, household pets, occupational exposures, nasal polyps, aspirin use, exacerbation by cold or hot air. She does have a significant family history, with mother and maternal grandmother with asthma.

Available past laboratory results are significant for a peripheral eosinophil count of 25% with a white blood cell count of 7.2, and negative sputum fungal cultures. There are no previous pulmonary function tests available.

Past Medical History

Medical illnesses: (1) Asthma, as in HPI. (2) hypertension — thought to be secondary to steroids:

Surgical illnesses: None.

Obstetrical/gynecologic history: (1) P1, G1; (2) birth control pills times 3 years continuously, discontinued 3 months ago; (3) Last menstrual period 8/15/88. The patient began her period again on the first day of admission.

Allergies

None

Tobacco use: None

Alcohol use: About one drink per day

History of blood transfusions: None

Medications on Admission

*   Aminophylline 200 mg five times per day
*   Alupent two puffs four times a day
*   Albuterol 400 mg p.o. four times a day
*   Hydrochlorothiazide 50 mg q.d.
*   Potassium supplements

Family History

Mother and maternal grandmother with asthma. Father died of an MI in his 60s. Grandmother with thyroid carcinoma. Otherwise negative.

Social History

Married, works as homemaker, with a 3-year-old child.

Review of Systems

Positive for some blood-streaked sputum. Negative for change in weight, sleep, TB, PD, hepatitis, nausea, vomiting, diarrhea, dysuria, anemia, diabetes, thyroid disease.

Physical Examination

General appearance: pleasant white female, slightly SOB,? cushingoid face

Vital signs: T, 99.6°; pulse, 88; BP 120/90; RR, 16
HEENT: WNL, PERRLA
Mouth: w/o oral mucosal lesions or exudate
Neck: w/o adenopathy or thyromegaly
Skin: warm, dry, w/o lesions
Lungs: BS throughout, diffuse end expiratory wheezes
CV: PMI, 5th (L)ICS, regular rate w/o murmur, S_3, S_4, or JVD
Abdomen: WNL
Extremities: w/o cyanosis, clubbing, edema or calf tenderness
Neuologic: WNL

Laboratory Data

Theophylline level equaled 5.6
Hematocrit 47.7 with a white cell count of 6.8
Differential significant for 28% eosinophils
Sodium 134, potassium 4.4, chloride 101, total CO_2 26, BUN 9,
   creatinine 0.9, glucose 87
Sputum revealed numerous PMNs, gram-positive cocci in groups.
   Culture grew out *Haemophilus hemolyticus* and *Neisseria* sp
FEV_1 prebronchodilator 1.2, postbronchodilator 2.0
FVC prebronchodilator 0.8, postbronchodilator 1.5.

Hospital Course

Problem 1: Asthma. The patient was bolused in the emergency
   room with Solu-Medrol 125 mg IV, and aminophylline 200
   mg IV, followed by maintenance doses of Solu-Medrol 125
   mg t.i.d. and aminophylline 30 mg/hr IV. The patient received
   Alupent nebulizer treatments g. 1 hr in the emergency room
   and q. 2 hr while on the floor. The patient responded quite
   well and Alupent treatments were decreased to q. 2–4 hr and
   to q. 4 hr on the day after admission. Aminophylline was increased to 50 mg per hour IV on day 2 secondary to subtherapeutic theophylline levels. The patient was also bolused with
   an additional 300 mg of aminophylline in two separate doses.
   On 9/14, theophylline level was 10.0. Despite subtherapeutic theophylline levels, the patient was doing extremely well,
   with clear lungs and no subjective complaints of shortness
   of breath. The patient was switched to prednisone 60 mg p.o.
   q.d. on day 2, and aminophylline 200 mg p.o. five times per
   day on day 3, and to Alupent Inhaler q. 4 hr on day 3. The patient continued to do quite well and was discharged on day 5
   with a theophylline level pending (theophylline level on 9/15
   equaled 6.6). Because of subtherapeutic theophylline levels,
   aminophylline was increased to 1400 mg/day in five divided
   doses. The patient was to get a theophylline level checked 2
   to 3 days after discharge.
Problem 2: Hypertension. During the hospitalization, the patient's
   blood pressure remained in the range of 120–130/70–90 off

of hydrochlorothiazide. It was decided to discharge the patient off her hypertensive medications and to have her physician follow this.

Medications on Discharge

- Aminophylline 1400 mg p.o. in five divided doses daily
- Prednisone 30 mg p.o. q.d. in a tapering dose
- Alupent Inhaler two puffs q.i.d.
- Vanceril Inhaler three puffs following Alupent Inhaler when the oral prednisone dose is down to 20 mg q.o.d

Follow-Up

1. The patient is to have theophylline level drawn on the 18th or 19th of September.
2. Appointment with physician on 9/25/88.
3. Refer to physical therapy outpatient clinic.

Discharge Diagnoses

1. Asthma, acute exacerbation
2. Hypertension, probably steroid-induced

Condition on Discharge

Ambulating

Discussion

Pharmacotherapeutic management of this patient is typical of that described in the clinical management section of this chapter. This patient had irreversible bronchospasm that required hospitalization and a combination of intravenous steroid, intravenous methylxanthine, and inhaled sympathomimetic drugs. As the patient improved, her medications were altered to accommodate outpatient management of chronic hyperreactive airways. The patient was discharged on oral therapy, tapering to inhaled steroid and oral methylxanthine drugs with continuation of the aerosol sympathomimetic. She was referred to physical therapy for outpatient management of bronchopulmonary hygiene and an exercise-conditioning program. Throughout a 12-week period the patient progressed from her discharge medications, q.o.d. bronchopulmonary hygiene and low level walking program, to elimination of bronchopulmonary hygiene, methylxanthines, and steroids, with progression to a four-times a week jogging program that required only an aerosol sympathomimetic before exercise.

CASE 2   **Chief Complaint**

The patient is a 64-year-old man with chronic obstructive pulmonary disease, diabetes mellitus, coronary artery disease, and ischemic cardiomyopathy managed with milrinone (experimental vasodilator that increases inotropy), admitted with chest pain.

History of the Present Illness

The patient's cardiac history dates to a myocardial infarction in 1970. In December 1985, he developed symptoms of congestive heart failure. Cardiac catheterization in April 1986 showed an occluded right coronary artery with 50% stenosis in the left anterior descending and left circumflex marginal coronary arteries. The pulmonary capillary wedge pressure was 15 mmHg, left ventricular ejection fraction was 17%.

In May 1986, he began an amrinone regimen, which was discontinued after 2 to 3 weeks, because he developed fever, chills, and nausea. He was admitted to the hospital in October 1986, and a radionuclide ventriculogram showed a left ventricular ejection fraction of 19%, with right ventricular ejection fraction of 55%, diffuse hypokinesis, and apical akinesis, and severe septal hypokinesis. On 10/14/86, he underwent cardiac catheterization again; pulmonary capillary wedge pressure was 15 mm Hg, increasing to 32 mm Hg with modest exercise. With intravenous milrinone, cardiac index increased to 2.8 and pulmonary capillary wedge pressure decreased to 10 mm Hg. He did moderately well thereafter, with evident improvement in his left ventricular function — repeat radionuclide ventriculogram on 1/17/87 showed a left ventricular ejection fraction of 27%.

In July 1988, the patient reported a dramatic increase in angina, with decreasing exercise tolerance. His weight had increased 3 lb at that time. He was told to double his furosemide (Lasix) dose (see medications on admission, below) and take prophylactic sublingual nitroglycerin before exercise. At home, his weight increased further. In the week before his admission, metolazone was added to his regimen for 2 days. This therapeutic intervention resulted in a 5 to 6 lb weight loss, but on the day before admission, the patient still felt poorly.

On the morning of admission, the patient awoke with burning substernal chest pain which radiated to the throat, jaw, and left arm. This was unrelieved by three sublingual nitroglycerin. The patient also noted palpitations. He was given Nitrol Paste and intravenous morphine at the local hospital emergency room and was transferred to the city hospital. The patient denies orthopnea, paroxysmal nocturnal dyspnea, peripheral edema, or a change in his chronic nocturia.

Past Medical History

1. Chronic obstructive pulmonary disease – a 40 pack-year tobacco smoking history. March 6, 1987, FEV 1.58 liter (43% of predicted); FVC 4.36 liter (82% of predicted). DLCO 6.5 (23% of predicted.
2. Diabetes mellitus, type II.

Allergies

Tetanus toxoid

Medications on Admission

- Milrinone 5 mg, p.o., five times per day
- Digoxin, o.125 mg, q.d.
- Aldactone, 25 mg, b.i.d.
- Lasix, 120 mg, b.i.d.
- Glyburide, 2.5 mg, q.d.
- Lopressor, 50 mg., b.i.d.
- Metolazone,, 2.5 mg, b.i.d.
- Potassium chloride, 60 mEq/day
- Albuterol, 2 puffs, q.i.d.
- Vanceril inhaler, 4 puffs, q.i.d.
- aspirin, 1000 mg/day

Physical Examination

General appearance: considerably obese, middle-aged, white man
  in mild distress
Vital signs: HR 122, BP 130/100 sitting, 130/80 supine, RR 20,
  afebrile
Skin: cool and moist
PERRL, EOM intact
Neck, supple without thyromegaly or lymphadenopathy
Breath sounds: clear to auscultation and percussion
Heart: JVP $\geq$ 5 cm H_2O, PMI not appreciated, distant heart sounds
  with intermittent gallop, carotid pulses full
Extremities: pedal pulses unpalpable, trace edema at ankles

Laboratory Data

Blood: Hct 54.3%; Hgb 18.0; WBC 15.2; PT and PTT WNL; Plt 205K
UA: 0-1 WBC; 0 RBC
Chemistries: Na, 130; K, 3.3; Cl, 95; HCO_3, 26; BUN, 29; Creat, 1.6;
  Glu, 238; CPK, 88; LDH, 199
Digoxin level: less than 0.5
SGPT, 75 (40 is maximum normal)
Cholesterol, 160; HDL cholesterol, 18
Chest x-ray: cardiomegaly, hyperinflation consistent with COPD,
  no pulmonary edema, infiltrate, or diffusions
ECG: sinus tachycardia rate 104, normal intervals, axis 40°, in-
  verted T waves in leads II, III, AVF, with downsloping S-T
  segments, poor R wave progression, nonspecific S-T and T
  wave abnormalities consistent with digoxin, PVCs

Hospital Course

Problem 1: Coronary artery disease. The possibility of a myocardial infarction to explain this episode of the patient's chest
  pain was ruled out by serial enzymes and electrocardio-

grams. The patient had one episode of chest pain in the coronary care unit, terminated with reduction in heart rate from approximately 120 to the 90s with intravenous metoprolol. The patient underwent cardiac catheterization on 7/23/88 with the following results: coronary artery pressures 40/26, mean 32; pulmonary capillary wedge mean 10; cardiac index 1.6; left ventricular ejection fraction 38% (probably an overestimate because of postextrasystolic potentiation); global hypokinesis; coronary artery anatomy not significantly changed from April 1986. Diltiazem was added to the patient's anti-ischemic regimen.

Problem 2: Ventricular ectopy. Upon admission to the Coronary Care Unit, the patient had frequent ventricular premature beats which were reduced in number as his hypokalemia was corrected. For multifocal and unifocal couplets, the patient was treated with lidocaine for 4 days. Off lidocaine, the patient had one or two sets of multifocal premature ventricular contractions per day, monitored.

Problem 3: Chronic obstructive pulmonary disease. It was never clear how much of the patient's severe shortness of breath was attributable to his chronic obstructive pulmonary disease. His therapy of albuterol inhaler and Vanceril inhaler was not changed.

Condition on Discharge

Ambulatory, feeling somewhat fatigued

Medications on Discharge

- Aspirin, 325 mg, q.d.
- Diltiazem, 30 mg, p.o., q.i.d. (calcium channel blocker)
- Isordil, 10 mg, p.o., q.i.d. (vasodilator)
- Metoprolol, 75 mg, b.i.d. (selective β-blocker)
- Digoxin, 0.125 mg, q.d. (cardiac glycoside)
- Milrinone, 5 mg, p.o., five *i.d.* (vasodilator)
- Aldactone, 25 mg, b.i.d. (antihypertensive)
- Lasix, 120 mg, b.i.d. (antihypertensive)
- Slow-K, 3 tablets, q.i.d.
- Glyburide, 2.5 mg, q.d. (decreases blood sugar; effective with type II diabetics)
- Albuterol inhaler, 2 puffs, q.i.d. (selective sympathomimetic)
- Vanceril inhaler, 2 to 4 puffs, q.i.d. (steroid)

Discharge Diagnoses

1. Coronary artery disease
2. Congestive heart failure, cardiomyopathy
3. Ventricular ectopy
4. Presumed viral syndrome

Discussion

This patient is typical of the complex individual with cardiopulmonary medication. He requires cardiac drugs that block his β-receptors to decrease cardiac sympathetic response. However, blocking the β_2-receptors promotes bronchoconstriction in this patient with chronic obstructive pulmonary disease. He requires stimulation of his β_2-receptors to promote bronchodilation. Consequently, his β-blocking cardiac drug is a β_1-selective drug and his pulmonary β-stimulating drug (sympathomimetic) is a β_2-specific drug.

REFERENCES

1. Ackerman GL, Nolan CM: Adrenocortical responsiveness after alternate day corticosteroid therapy. N Engl J Med 278:405, 1968
2. American Thoracic Society: Chronic bronchitis, asthma and pulmonary emphysema. Am Rev Respir Dis 85:762, 1962
3. Bergner RK, Bergner A: Rational asthma therapy for the outpatient. JAMA 232:1243, 1975
4. Brisson GR, Malaisse-Lagie F, Molaisse WJ: The stimulus-secretion coupling of glucose-induced insulin release VII. A proposed site of action for adenosine 3'5'-cyclic monophosphate. J Clin Invest 52:232, 1972
5. Cumming G, Semple SG: Disorders of the Respiratory System. Oxford, Blackwell Scientific Publications, 1973
6. Harter JG, and Novitch AM: Evaluation of steroid analogues in terms of suitability for alternate day steroid therapy. J Allergy 37:108, 1966
7. Hoidal JR, Niewoehner DE: Pathogenesis of emphysema. Chest 4:679, 1983
8. Horrobin DF, Manku MS, Franks DJ et al: Methylxanthine phosphodiesterase inhibitors behave as prostaglandin antagonists in a perfused rat mesenteric artery preparation. Prostaglandins 13:33, 1977
9. Landau LI, Phelan PD, Williams HE: Ventilatory mechanics in patients with bronchiectasis starting in childhood. Thorax 29:304, 1974
10. Levy G, Koysooko R: Pharmacokinetic analysis of the effect of theophylline on pulmonary function in asthmatic children. J Pediatr 86:789, 1975
11. Light RW, George RB: Oral atropine in the treatment of chronic asthma. Ann Allergy 38:58, 1977
12. Lockett MF: Dangerous effects of isoprenaline in myocardial failure. Lancet 2:104, 1965
13. Mathewson HS: Promising new bronchodilator drugs. Respir Ther 1:47, 1982
14. Mittenko PA, Ogilvie RI: Pharmacokinetics of intravenous theophylline. Clin Pharmacol Ther 14:509, 1973
15. Newman SP, Pavia D, Clarke SW: How should a pressurized β-adrenergic bronchodilator be inhaled? Eur J Respir Dis 62:3, 1981
16. Pare JAP, Fraser RG: *Synopsis of Diseases of the Chest.* Philadelphia, WB Saunders, 1983
17. Pollock J, Kiechel F, Cooper D et al: Relationship of serum theophylline concentration to inhibition of exercise-induced bronchospasm and comparison and cromolyn. Pediatrics 60:840, 1977
18. Rau JL: *Respiratory Therapy Pharmacology,* 2nd ed. Chicago, Year Book Medical, 1984
19. Robbins SL, Cotran RS, Kumar V: *Pathologic Basis of Disease, 3rd ed.* Philadelphia, WB Saunders, 1984
20. Simonsson BG, Jonson B, Strom B: Bronchodilatory and circulatory effects of inhaling increasing doses of an anticholinergic drug, ipratropium bromide (SCH 1000). Scand J Respir Dis 56:138, 1975
21. Stolley PD: Asthma mortality: Why the United States was spared an epidemic of deaths due to asthma. Am Rev Respir Dis 105:883, 1972

22. Sutherland EW, Robison GA: The role of cyclic 3':5' AMP in responses to catecholamines and other hormones. Pharmacol Rev 18:145, 1966
23. Webb-Johnson DC, Andrews JL: Bronchodilator therapy (first of two parts). N Engl J Med 297:476, 1977
24. Webb-Johnson DC, Andrews JL: Bronchodilator therapy (second of two parts). N Engl J Med 297:758, 1977
25. Weinberger M: Theophylline for treatment of asthma. J Pediatr 92:1, 1978
26. Weinberger M, Hendeles L, Ahrens R: Pharmacologic management of reversible obstructive airways disease. Med Clin 65:579, 1980
27. Weinberger M, Hendeles L: Commentary: Role of dialysis in the management of theophylline toxicity. Dev Pharmacol Ther 1:26, 1980
28. Weinberger M, Hendeles L, Ahrens R: Clinical pharmacology of drugs used for asthma. Pediatr Clin N Am 28:47, 1981
29. Widdecome JG, Sterling GM: The autonomic nervous system and breathing. Arch Intern Med 126:311, 1970
30. Ziment I: Respiratory Pharmacology and Therapeutics. Philadelphia, WB Saunders, 1978

Rheumatology 6

Judy Feinberg
Rebecca Barton
Marlene A. Aldo-Benson

More than 36 million Americans have some form of arthritis.[2] Although many of these people do not require specialized medical care, many others require management by a rheumatologist and a team of rehabilitation professionals. The purpose of this chapter is to provide an overview of the more common rheumatic diseases and their management, with emphasis on drug therapy and the implications of these drugs in the overall management of the patient.

OVERVIEW OF THE RHEUMATIC DISEASES

Osteoarthritis

Osteoarthritis, another name for degenerative joint disease, is the most common of the rheumatic diseases. It is estimated that 16 million people in the United States have osteoarthritis severe enough to cause pain or limitations in activity.[2] Clinically this disorder is characterized by slowly developing joint pain, stiffness, and limitation of motion, during which radiographically progressive deteriorization of the joint and loss of articular cartilage is noted. There is, however, no correlation between symptoms and radiologic findings. The most symptomatic patient may have no abnormalities shown on an x-ray film, whereas the asymptomatic patient may show advanced changes.

There are two broad categories of osteoarthritis. Primary osteoarthritis occurs more frequently in women and, although the specific cause is unknown, there is a definite genetic predisposition. Etiologic factors have been identified in secondary osteoarthritis. They include occupational stress, trauma, structural abnormalities, and other systemic diseases that can effect cartilage metabolism.

The hips, knees, and spine are the most commonly involved joints. In the upper extremity the carpometacarpal joint at the base of the thumb is often involved in primary osteoarthritis. Heberden's and Bouchard's nodes are characteristic osteophytes located at the distal interphalangeal and proximal interphalangeal joints of fingers. The prevalence of osteoarthritis increases with age, and changes are seen on x-ray films as early as the third decade. There are no laboratory tests that identify the disease, and the diagnosis is based primarily on history, physical examination, and x-ray findings. Pain usually occurs after using affected joints and is relieved by rest early in the disease but may be persistent in the later stages. Crepitus and pain on passive motion are frequent findings. A secondary synovitis is common.

The prognosis depends somewhat on the joints involved and the required activities of the patient. Treatment involves the use of analgesic drugs, such as acetaminophen; thermal modalities to decrease pain; isometric exercises; and instruction in joint protection principles. Anti-inflammatory drugs may be helpful in the treatment of osteoarthritis, especially when secondary synovitis is present. Analgesics are also useful adjuncts.

Rheumatoid Arthritis

Rheumatoid arthritis is chronic, systemic, inflammatory disease characterized by exacerbations and remissions. It is estimated that over 7 million people in the United States have rheumatoid arthritis.[2] The course of this disease cannot be predicted at the onset, but spontaneous remission, if it occurs, will occur within the first 2 years. Disease that is intermittent at first may then become more sustained with time. Approximately 35% of people with rheumatoid arthritis have a monocyclic course, 50% are polycylic, and 15% are progressive. The onset of rheumatoid arthritis occurs most often between the ages of 20 and 60, with peaks at 35 and 45 years. The overall female/male incidence of rheumatoid arthritis is 3:1. With onset under the age of 60 there is a 5:1 female/male ratio, and with onset over the age of 60 the ratio is about equal. All racial and ethnic groups are represented. A genetic predisposition is now strongly suspected.[19]

The cause of rheumatoid arthritis is unknown, but the disease is perpetuated by a continual, poorly defined immune reaction in synovial tissue that leads to synovial inflammation, hypertrophy of the synovium, weakening of the capsules, tendons, and ligaments and, occasionally, destruction of cartilage and bone.[11] Diagnostic criteria include symmetric joint swelling of at least 6-weeks duration, morning stiffness, pain on motion, or tenderness. The American Rheumatism Association (ARA) criteria for classification of rheumatoid arthritis lists 11 features of the disease. A diagnosis of rheumatoid arthritis requires the presence of seven of these features. The presence of five of these features is considered definite rheumatoid arthritis, and the presence of three is consistent with probable rheumatoid arthritis. A diagnosis of possible rheumatoid arthritis is made with the presence of only two features, if joint symptoms have been present for 3 months. There are 20 exclusion criteria to assist with differential diagnosis.[14] The small joints of the hands and feet are most frequently involved, followed in descending order of frequency by the wrists, ankles, knees, hips, elbows, and shoulders; however any joint with articular cartilage may be involved including the sternoclavicular and temporomandibular joints. Joint involvement is manifest clinically by heat, swelling, erythema, and pain. Morning stiffness, malaise, fatigue, fever, and anorexia are the more common systemic manifestations of rheumatoid arthritis. Extraarticular manifestation may involve inflammation of the lungs, heart, blood vessels, and eyes.

Although the diagnosis of rheumatoid arthritis is made primarily from history and physical examination, there are laboratory tests that may assist in determining diagnosis as well as prognosis. The rheumatoid factor test, which identifies an autoantibody directed against the patient's own immunoglobulin, is found in about 40% to 50% of patients in the early stages and 80% to 90% of patients later. It also occurs in 2% to 4% of the normal population under 65 years of age and in 10% to 20% of people over age 65. Reaction of the rheumatoid factor test may also be positive in systemic lupus erythematosus and other diseases. A high titer of rheumatoid factor, the presence of erosion as seen by x-ray films, the presence of subcutaneous nodules, and a positive antinuclear antibody (ANA) reaction also assist in making a diagnosis. If reactions to these test results are positive, there is increased likelihood of more severe, destructive disease. An acute onset of the arthritis and onset of disease later in age tend to be more favorable prognostic signs. The ARA, in addition to having criteria for the diagnosis of rheumatoid arthritis, have functional classification and stage classification that are based on x-ray findings. Studies of the natural history of the disease reveal that after 10 to 15 years a few patients will be in remission, but the majority will be functional.[18] Approximately 15% of rheumatoids are in class I (remission or ability to perform normal activities); 40% are in class II (moderate restriction, adequate for normal activities); 30% are in class III (marked restrictions, inability to perform most duties of usual occupation of self-care), and only 15% are in class IV (incapacitation, confinement to bed or wheelchair).

The goals of management of rheumatoid arthritis include relief of pain and inflammation, maintenance of optimal function, and education of the patient. Relief of inflammation is accomplished primarily by drugs, with the other goals addressed by various rehabilitation professionals who bring to bear numerous modalities. Aspirin or other nonsteroidal drugs are the drugs of choice in the management of the inflammation in rheumatoid arthritis. Other drugs are added in a stepwise fashion depending upon the severity of the symptoms and may include gold or hydroxychloroquine (Plaquenil), which may induce remission in otherwise insufficiently controlled disease. Systemic glucocorticoids and immunosuppressive drugs should be reserved for patients exhibiting severe, systemic involvement.

Juvenile Rheumatoid Arthritis

Juvenile rheumatoid arthritis (JRA) is characterized by chronic synovial inflammation of unknown cause. It affects 200,000 children in the United States. There are three subtypes of juvenile rheumatoid arthritis — systemic, polyarticular, and pauciarticular. About 20% of children with JRA have the *systemic type* of disease, which is characterized by high intermittent fevers, erythematous papular evanescent rash, lymphadenopathy, hepatosplenomegaly, and anemia. The musculoskeletal manifestations may initially appear as arthralgias and myalgias only, and a chronic polyarthritis may develop months or years later. *Polyarticular* and *pauciarticular* subsets each represent 40% of children with JRA. Juvenile rheumatoid arthritis may begin at any age but is rare before the age of 6 months, and has two peaks between ages 1 and 3 and 8 and 12 years. In general, girls are affected more often than boys; however, sex and age ratios differ in different subgroups. There is no clear evidence of genetic predisposition for juvenile rheumatoid arthritis except in late-childhood pauciarticular disease, which may be associated with the HLA-B27 antigen and familial spondylarthropathy.

Diagnosis of juvenile rheumatoid arthritis, like that of rheumatoid arthritis, is primarily based on history and physical examination. There are no diagnostic laboratory tests for JRA, and the reaction to the rheumatoid factor test is generally negative. The ANA test reaction is frequently positive in patients with pauciarticular disease. Young children frequently do not complain of severe joint pain or pain at rest, but these children tend to limit any motion that results in pain and, therefore, stiffness is common. Older children do complain of more pain. Juvenile rheumatoid arthritis can affect growth because of a generalized growth retardation associated with chronic childhood illness or from the localized effects of inflammation on epiphyseal growth, which can result in bony overgrowth or undergrowth around the affected joints. Iridocyclitis may occur in JRA patients with few associated signs and symptoms and, therefore, can lead to blindness.[16] This is most likely to occur in young patients with pauciarticular disease and positive reactions to the ANA tests. Routine slit-lamp examinations are recommended for children with JRA to avoid this potentially disastrous complication.

The prognosis for most children is good. At least 75% enter into long remissions, with little or no residual effects. The few patients with consistently positive rheumatoid factor reactions are more likely to develop severe chronic arthritis and, therefore, have a worse prognosis than those who have rheumatoid–factor-negative reactions.[13] The major goals of therapy are relief of symptoms and maintenance of joint function, motion, and strength. Drug therapy includes the use of aspirin or nonsteroidal agents. If these are not effective, gold therapy is generally considered. Systemic glucocorticoids are contraindicated, except in the most severe cases of systemic JRA.

Systemic Lupus Erythematosus

Systemic lupus erythematosus (SLE) is a systemic, inflammatory, multisystem disease in which autoantibodies play a major role. The autoantibodies may be directed against cells themselves (e.g., erythrocytes, platelets) and, therefore, damage the cells, or they may form antigen–antibody complexes that deposit in various tissues and, thus, cause inflammation in these tissues (e.g., kidney, blood vessels, synovium). There is apparently some hereditary predisposition to the disease, but it is not directly inherited. Four of five cases occur in females, primarily in the adolescent and young adult, but it can occur at any age. The incidence is higher in black women than in Caucasian women.

Systemic lupus erythematosus presents a diverse clinical picture, depending upon the organ system involved. The onset may be insidious and begins with a fever, fatigue, weakness, or weight loss. Other common presenting symptoms may be rash or polyarthritis, myositis, anemia, pneumonitis, thrombocytopenia, alopecia, and renal, cardiac, or neurologic problems may also be present. The clinical diagnosis is made on the basis of multiorgan involvement. A characteristic facial rash (called a "butterfly" rash because of the symmetric cheek involvement) is a most frequent feature. Polyarthritis or arthralgia is seen in over 90% of patients. Glomerulonephritis occurs in only about 45% and central nervous system involvement in 25%. Laboratory tests that assist in the diagnosis are a positive reaction to the ANA test, and positive results from an LE preparation and kidney or skin biopsy.

The prognosis is variable and depends on organ involvement. Renal, neurologic, or myocardial damage represent poorer prognosis, and nephritis accounts for 50% of all fatalities. The arthritis is generally not deforming, but deforming arthritis without x-ray evidence of erosion occurs in 15% of patients after 4 years of disease. Aseptic necrosis (usually of the hip) occurs in 5% to 8% of SLE patients treated for at least 5 years, especially those who received large-dose steroid therapy, even for a short time.[13] Treatment of SLE is aimed at decreasing the inflammation, and drug therapy depends on the organs involved. Arthritis symptoms are treated with modalities and drugs similar to those used for rheumatoid arthritis. Nonsteroidal anti-inflammatory drugs are used in the treatment of SLE, but if these are not sufficient to control inflammation, antimalarial drugs such as hydroxychloroquine may be added. Steroid therapy is often used in higher doses in acute vasculitis, renal, or central nervous system involvement, and may be used in low doses for skin or joint involvement.

Progressive Systemic Sclerosis

Progressive systemic sclerosis (PSS) is a generalized disorder of the connective tissue involving the skin, synovium, and small arteries of the esophagus, intestinal tract, lungs, heart, and kidney. *Scleroderma* is a frequent label describing the fibrotic and degenerative changes involving only the skin and the synovium. The cause of PSS is unknown; however, recent studies suggest that an immunologic factor may be important in its pathogenesis. The disorder can affect any age group, sex, or race; however, it is most common in women in the age group of 30 to 50. It has also been noted frequently in coal miners, and because of this, silicosis has been suggested as a predisposing factor. Diagnosis of PSS is made by physical examination and history, with the most notable finding being the characteristic skin tightening. The blood count is usually normal; however, anemia may occur later, secondary to visceral involvement. Mild hypergammaglobulinemia (IgG) is often found and 25% to 35% of patients have positive reactions for rheumatoid factor.[13] The course of the disease is variable, but it is often slowly progressive and may become disabling secondary to the characteristic skin tightening. Visceral involvement may lead to life-threatening conditions.

The skin involvement often begins with an edematous phase in which swelling of the hands, forearms, feet, and legs occurs. This finger swelling is often referred to as being "sausagelike." Polyarthritis and joint stiffness may occur along with muscle weakness. This is then replaced by an indurative phase characterized by thickening, tightening, and hardening of the skin. The skin becomes taut and shiny, losing the normal wrinkle and skin folds. Range-of-motion may become limited in the affected areas, most notably in the fingers but also involving the face, neck, shoulders, trunk, elbows, knees, and feet. Hyperpigmentation may occur as well as subcutaneous calcification, bony resorption, and atrophy of the soft tissue.

Progressive systemic sclerosis with *diffuse scleroderma* is a classification in which there is symmetric, diffuse involvement of the skin affecting the trunk and extremities. Relatively early appearance of visceral involvement occurs. The *CREST syndrome* is a classification in which there is relatively limited involvement of the skin, primarily the fingers and face. The five identifiable features of CREST are calcinosis, Raynaud's phenomenon, esophageal dysmotility, sclerodactyly, and telangectasia. Calcinosis or calcification of the soft tissue may be localized to a fingertip or may be diffuse, contributing to severe joint contractures. *Raynaud's phenomenon* is a paroxysmal interruption of the blood flow to the fingers and occurs in 98% of patients with PSS.[13] Vasospasm results in blanching, erythema, and cyanosis of the hands, with associated burning pain, numbness, or aching. Cold exposure, trauma, or stress may induce this vasospasm. Esophageal dysfunction is characterized by difficulty with swallowing and esophageal reflux. *Sclerodactyly* refers to the sclerotic skin changes and tapering of the digits. *Telangectasias* are small reddish spots in the skin that are a result of chronic dilation of the capillaries and arterial branches. The most common internal involvement is esophageal dysfunction. Decreased peristaltic activity may contribute to symptoms of reflux and difficulty in swallowing. The rest of the gastrointestinal tract is less frequently involved but may result in malabsorption problems. Pulmonary function may become impaired by interstitial and alveolar fibrosis. Dyspnea upon exertion is the most frequent symptom. The earliest physiologic abnormality is a subnormal diffusing capacity, with later development of obstructive disease. Cardiac disease is characterized by myocardial fibrosis. The severity of symptoms depends on the degree of cardiac fibrosis and presence or absence of concurrent lung fibrosis. Renal disease is a major cause of death in PSS.[13] Malignant arterial hypertension can abruptly develop and is associated with rapidly progressive and irreversible renal insufficiency. Nearly all patients eventually show evidence of visceral involvement, with the prognosis significantly worse if the kidney, heart, or lung are involved.

Treatment of the disease is symptomatic. No single drug or combination of drugs have proved valuable, and efficacy has been difficult to assess because of the slowly progressive nature of PSS. Drug agents such as D-penicillamine and colchicine are used to inhibit the overgrowth of collagenous connective tissue. Corticosteroids are generally ineffective and are used only with inflammatory complications such as myositis. Immunosuppressive therapy is currently being studied. Other drugs may be used in the treatment of the specific symptoms, such as antihypertensive drugs in the presence of renal disease or vasodilating drugs for the treatment of Raynaud's phenomenon.

Polymyositis/Dermatomyositis

Polymyositis is a disease characterized by diffuse inflammation of the striated muscles. Polymyositis accompanied by a characteristic skin rash is referred to as *dermatomyositis*. The disease is characterized by a gradual onset of weakness that is usually symmetric and proximal. The cause is unknown, and myositis is often associated with other collagen vascular diseases. In older patients with polymyositis, there may be an increased prevalence of malignant neoplasms. Polymyositis can occur at any age; however, it is found more frequently in females. Symptoms may include proximal muscle weakness (shoulder and pelvic girdle musculature), arthralgias and myalgias, Raynaud's phenomenon, and dysphagia. The prime clinical manifestation of muscle weakness is the patient's initial complaint of not being able to perform activities requiring proximal muscle strength such as lifting the arms to comb hair or getting on or off of a low surface such as a chair. This muscular weakness may also involve the neck muscles, pharyngeal musculature, and muscles of respiration. The cardiac muscle is unaffected because it is nonstriated; however, myocarditis and conduction abnormalities can occur.[13] A small percentage of patients develop intestinal disturbances.

Diagnosis of polymyositis/dermatomyositis is based upon the presence of proximal muscle weakness, elevation of serum muscle enzyme levels, characteristic muscle biopsy, and an electromyogram, with no neurologic findings, and occasional heliotropic rash of the eyelids.[15] The course of the disease is characterized by exacerbation and remission and is dependent upon the severity of the symptoms. Prognosis is generally better when the disease is slowly progressive and occurs at a younger age.

Management of polymyositis is based upon reducing the inflammation occurring in the muscles. Corticosteroids are frequently used with the dosage tapered as the symptoms improve. Immunosuppressive and cytotoxic agents have also been used in some cases, with improvement noted. Supportive measures must also be used. The dysphagia must be treated to prevent aspiration, and pulmonary function must be monitored to prevent respiratory distress. Prevention of contractures through proper positioning and nonresistive, range-of-motion exercises are important during the inflammatory phase, with therapy becoming more aggressive as the inflammation decreases.

Gout

Gout is a disease that has been described for centuries. It is characterized by an acute attack of monoarticular inflammation that may subside on its own within 2 weeks. Gout usually occurs in men, especially in the 40 to 50 age group. The lower extremity joints are typically involved, especially the great toe. The acute attack leaves the joint extremely painful, red, and swollen and is sometimes mistaken for cellulitis. If untreated, gout will recur with an increase in the frequency of the attacks and an increase in the number of joints involved.

Gout is associated with hyperuricemia, caused by either increased production of uric acid, decreased excretion of uric acid, or a combination of both. Uric acid and its salts have only limited solubility in biologic fluids; crystals can, therefore, deposit in the joints, the kidneys, or other tissue. In the joints, this deposition may precipitate the attacks of inflammatory arthritis. The uric acid deposits, or crystals, are known as *tophi*. Untreated, the tophi can erode the joints and bones and create functional impairment as in other forms of destructive, erosive arthritis.

Diagnosis of gout depends on history, physical examination, the presence of uric acid in the joint, elevated serum uric acid levels, and therapeutic response to colchicine. Treatment of gout is twofold; treating the acute attack and treating the hyperuricimia. One should treat the latter after the initial attack has been treated and has subsided. Colchicine is the traditional initial treatment. The nonsteroidal anti-inflammatory drugs (NSAIDs) may be used instead of colchicine, with phenylbutazone and indomethacin frequently being the chosen drugs. The patient then continues with the baseline dose of colchicine indefinitely. After the patient has been symptom-free for 1 month, the hyperuricemia should be treated. Suggested drugs for this are probenecid, sulfinpyrazone, and allopurinol.

Vasculitis and Arteritis

Inflammation of the blood vessels characterize vasculitis and arteritis. They occur as a primary entity or with a rheumatic disease. The symptoms depend upon the vessel involved. The following classifications may be helpful in understanding the different conditions existing within the rheumatic disease population.

Leukocytoclastic vasculitis may occur in SLE and rheumatoid arthritis, but also it may be a primary disease. Symptoms may include purpura, hematuria, abdominal pain, and arthralgia. Primary leukocytoclastic angitis may be due to drug reaction and is usually self-limited; however, it can be fatal if there is renal involvement. Treatment with steroids is usually effective.

Wegener's granulomatosis is characterized by formation of necrotizing granulomata in the lungs or upper respiratory tract and glomerulonephritis. Symptoms usually are rhinorrhea, sinusitis, arthralgia, cough or dyspnea, and evidence of renal disease. Diagnosis is made upon biopsy of the lesion. Corticosteroid treatment alone is not effective, but the disease is responsive to cyclophosphamide (Cytoxan) therapy.

Polyarteritis nodusa involves inflammation of the medium-sized arteries. Its cause is unknown, but it often affects older men and often resembles SLE because of its multiple organ involvement. Nonspecific symptoms, such as malaise, fever, and fatigue, are often present, but there are frequently symptoms specific to the organ system involved. Polyarteritis may also manifest itself as a nervous system disease, affecting both the peripheral and central nervous systems. Symptoms would depend on the system involved. For example, peripheral neuropathy of the radial nerve might be exhibited clinically by wristdrop. Severe headaches or changes in consciousness may be representative of central nervous system involvement. Diagnosis is made by biopsy and the presence of eosinophilia in the blood count. The disease is often fatal, but steroids can provide symptomatic relief. Often cyclophosphamide is necessary in treating this disease.

Giant cell arteritis is a form of vasculitis that can be a complication of polymyalgia rheumatica (PMR) or can occur independently. *Polymyalgia rheumatica* is a clinical syndrome found in the population who are over 50 years of age, and it is characterized by severe aching and stiffness in the neck/shoulder girdle and pelvic girdle. Systemic symptoms may also be present. Giant cell arteritis is inflammation of the temporal and cranial arteries, usually affecting women in the 50 to 80 age group. Complications secondary to this can include sudden blindness or a cerebrovascular accident. Again, steriods are usually the treatment of choice.

All forms of vasculitis are serious and potentially life-threatening. Treatment is essential, most often with steroids. Treatment of the secondary symptoms, such as arthritis and neuropathy, may be supplemented by intervention provided by the allied health personnel, depending on the symptoms exhibited.

Rheumatoid Variants: Ankylosing Spondylitis, Psoriatic Arthritis and Reiter's Syndrome

The rheumatoid variants are similar to rheumatoid arthritis in that they first appear as a chronic inflammatory arthritis and other systemic features such as fatigue, malaise, weight loss, and fever. However, peripheral joint involvement tends to be asymmetric, with common involvement of the sacroiliac joints. Iritis may be present, and there is a common presence of the HLA-B27 antigen.

Ankylosing spondylitis (AS) is characterized by low-back pain with inflammation of the sacroiliac, spinal apophyseal, and sternal joints. Peripheral large-joint involvement may also be present. Prolonged morning stiffness and pain are typical symptoms. This disorder usually occurs in young males, and there does appear to be a genetic predisposition to the disease because the majority of AS patients exhibit the presence of the HLA-B27 on their lymphocytes. Diagnosis is made by history of low-back pain with limited lumbar spine mobility and typical changes, seen on x-ray films, in the sacroiliac joints or, in advanced cases, ankylosis of the spine. The disease can be slowly progressive with resultant disabling limitations such as decreased chest wall expansion and limited spinal mobility and bony ankylosis, or it can stop at any stage, with only resultant pain-free deformity. Treatment includes NSAIDs or aspirin to reduce inflammation. An extremely important aspect of therapy is patient education in proper exercise, good body mechanics, and compensatory methods to increase independence, if a deformity is present.

Psoriatic arthritis is an inflammatory arthritis associated with the presence of psoriatic skin lesions. In some cases, it closely resembles rheumatoid arthritis, although it usually causes less disability. It classically involves the distal interphalangeal joints but, frequently, the other peripheral joints are involved as in rheumatoid arthritis. Involvement is often asymmetric and swelling is characteristically sausagelike in appearance. Nail lesions of psoriasis are frequently seen. In some cases, the changes seen on x-ray films in psoriatic arthritis, such as the marked osteolysis seen in arthritis mutilans, can distinguish it from rheumatoid arthritis. Laboratory test results are nonspecific for psoriatic arthritis. Treatment is usually administration of NSAIDs or aspirin. Large doses of steroid can provide temporary relief in the skin and joints but are infrequently used because of their side-effects. Immunosuppressive drugs are also very effective but, again, are used only in the most severe cases because of their toxicity. Gold is also used similarly to its use in rheumatoid arthritis. Physical intervention through therapy is similar to that described for rheumatoid arthritis.

Reiter's syndrome is a rheumatoid variant characterized by urethritis, conjunctivitis, and arthritis. It is primarily a disease of young males, with a high percentage having the HLA-B27 antigen. The arthritis that occurs is usually an acute asymmetric polyarthritis commonly affecting the weight-bearing joints. Recurrence is common, and a chronic arthritis can develop with joint damage. Other symptoms may be more systemic, such as fever and weight loss. Onset may be associated with venereal exposure after sexual contact or following infectious diarrhea (e.g., with salmonellae or schigellae). Treatment is symptomatic, with the use of NSAIDs to reduce inflammation and pain. Physical and occupational therapy may be effective in the physical management of chronic arthritis.

TEAM MANAGEMENT OF RHEUMATIC DISEASE

Many of the rheumatic diseases impact sufficiently on the individual that the expertise of a variety of physician specialists is required, as well as ancillary rehabilitation specialists. Drug therapy, which will be the focus of the next section of this chapter, is only one aspect of the total management program. This section will briefly introduce the reader to the specialists involved in the management of patients with rheumatic diseases and describe the roles of each.

The *rheumatologist* is an internist who specializes in the diagnosis and management of rheumatic diseases and is generally the person who makes referrals to other specialists and oversees the comprehensive management plan. The *orthopaedic surgeon* may provide surgical interventions, such as synovectomy early in a disease process or a total arthroplasty in the latter stages. The *physiatrist* may be involved in directing the rehabilitation, for example, of an advanced rheumatoid arthritis patient.

The various rehabilitation professions have a great deal to offer patients with rheumatic diseases. The multidisciplinary care is best provided in a comprehensive, coordinated, and integrated manner as described by Gross and associates.[6] The involvement of rehabilitation professionals with a particular patient depends on the needs of the patient as well as the availability of the health professional.

The *nurse educator* provides education to the patients and their families about their illness and its treatment and also acts as a liaison between the physician, the patient, and the rehabilitation team. The *occupational therapist* (OT) assesses upper-extremity range-of-motion and strength as well as the patient's ability to perform activities of daily living. Treatment provided by the OT includes splinting to reduce inflammation and pain and to maintain optimal positioning, instructing patients in principles of joint protection and work simplification, and providing adaptive devices to assist with daily-living activities. The *physical therapist* (PT) assesses joint range-of-motion, functional strength, posture, and gait. Treatment by the PT includes instructing patients in an exercise program, and in the use of home heat, and also makes provisions for ambulation aids. The *social worker* assesses the emotional and social needs of the patients and their families and makes referrals to community agencies as indicated. Consultation with a *dietitian* may be important for a weight-loss program or other special dietary needs related to a patient's specific illness. A *rehabilitation psychologist* may provide a pain-management program by use of biofeedback or relaxation techniques.

All of these disciplines combine together to offer patients with rheumatic disease a comprehensive care plan. Because most rheumatic diseases are chronic, periodic reevaluation and reinforcement of the prescribed treatment plans are necessary. Good patient rapport is necessary to gain and maintain compliance over months or years of a medical regimen. An integrated team of rehabilitation professionals working with patients and their families can best enhance compliance by reducing obstacles.

COMMONLY USED DRUGS AND THEIR SIDE-EFFECTS

Drug therapy is extremely important in the management of patients with rheumatic diseases. Usually, there is no one drug of choice. Selection of the best medication is a complex procedure. A drug that works well for one patient may not be effective for another with a seemingly similar disease. It is not uncommon for a patient to require a combination of drugs to manage some of the rheumatic diseases or to require periodic changes in their medication regimen. For rheumatoid arthritis and some of the spondyloarthropathies, the rule-of-thumb for physicians prescribing antirheumatic drugs is to start with a first-line drug, such as aspirin or another nonsteroidal anti-inflammatory drug (NSAID), and to add or substitute higher-level drugs in a stepwise or pyramid fashion (Fig. 6-1). The lower items of the pyramid are more generally applicable to the treatment of rheumatoid arthritis and are used in virtually all patients, whereas the higher-ranked ones are relevant only in certain patients. The higher-level drugs have more anti-inflammatory properties but, also, have potential for more serious side-effects. In addition, their usefulness in arthritis is not as well established.[9] It is imperative that patients taking these antirheumatic drugs adhere closely to their physicians orders because each patient's regimen is designed specifically for that patient and because changes in one aspect of the regimen may affect the entire regimen.

The following section will describe the most commonly used drugs for the management of rheumatic disease, their potential side-effects, and any information relevant to the rehabilitation professional. There are numerous drugs available for the treatment of rheumatic diseases, and new drugs are frequently being introduced. This discussion of drugs will focus primarily on the families or types of drugs used and is not mean to be exhaustive.

Aspirin

Aspirin is a salicylate that, when used in large doses, is effective as an anti-inflammatory agent. A dosage of 12 to 20 tablets per day would be considered anti-inflammatory, whereas fewer than 9 tablets per day would provide only an analgesic response. Aspirin is the oldest and most-widely used form of arthritis therapy and is still the treatment of choice for rheumatoid arthritis as well as for most other inflammatory arthritides. Aspirin is generally effective within the first 2 to 4 weeks. If no improvement is seen within 2 to 4 weeks, then another NSAID should be tried.

The most common side-effect of aspirin therapy is gastrointestinal symptoms such as nausea and heartburn. These side-effects can be prevented or diminished by making sure that patients take aspirin with food and never take it on an empty stomach, that is, not before or after a meal but during it. Buffered or enteric-coated aspirin will also help prevent these common side-effects. Toxicity from aspirin is

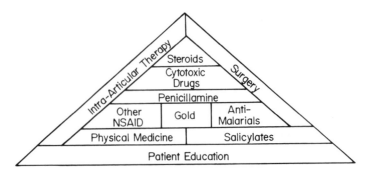

FIGURE 6-1. The therapeutic pyramid of drug administration. (McCarty DJ: Arthritis and Allied Conditions—A Textbook of Rheumatology, p 668. Philadelphia, Lea & Febiger, 1985, reprinted by permission)

characterized by tinnitus (ringing or buzzing in the ears). Reducing the dosage will reverse this symptom, and normal hearing will return. Physicians will sometimes use tinnitus as a guideline to determine therapeutic levels of aspirin.

A therapeutic anti-inflammatory level of salicylates is approximately 25 mg/dl. This may be tested by a simple laboratory test of the blood. Some patients may not be able to reach therapeutic levels because of improper absorption, or they may develop side-effects that require discontinuation of the drug before a therapeutic level can be achieved. Because of the short half-life of aspirin it must be taken regularly at 4-hr intervals to maintain therapeutic levels. Some patients may require a time-release aspirin at night to avoid an increase in symptomatology in the morning.

Advantages of aspirin therapy are that it is inexpensive, is effective, and has few serious side-effects. Disadvantages are that some patients find it difficult or impossible to take so many pills so often, and others may feel that, because aspirin is nonprescription, it is not "real" medicine and, therefore, they may not comply with their physician's recommendations.

It is important to educate patients about their salicylate regimen, including providing them with a list of other nonprescription products (e.g., cold and cough preparations, analgesics, and sleep aids) that contain aspirin. Additional aspirin ingestion may cause toxicity; therefore, both the patient and physician need to be aware of other sources of aspirin.

Nonsteroidal Anti-Inflammatory Drugs

There are several of these drugs that are used alone or in combination with aspirin to control inflammation through inhibition of prostaglandin synthesis. When given as a single dose, they may have an analgesic effect. Regular use with a sufficient dosage may result in decreased stiffness, pain, and swelling. The drugs are similar in their use and effect, but they differ in terms of their side-effects.

PHENYLBUTAZONE AND OXYPHENBUTAZONE

Phenylbutazone (Butazolidin) and oxyphenbutazone (Oxalid) are potent anti-inflammatory agents and are chemically related. Phenylbutazone was first introduced into the United States in 1952. It was the first alternative to aspirin as a NSAID. It has a potentially fatal toxic effect and most generally is now reserved for a particular indication or a short period of treatment, such as in gout. Long-term use has been found effective in difficult cases of ankylosing spondylitis. The dosage of these drugs is usually 100 mg to 300 mg daily.[5] One should establish a minimum maintenance dosage as soon as possible. The most common side-effect is gastric intolerance, which can be avoided or reduced if the drug is taken with meals or if enteric-coated tablets are used. Other side-effects may include rash, fluid retention, allergic reactions, thyroid inhibition, and renal damage. The most severe side-effect is bone marrow depression, with decrease in platelet and blood cell production.[5] The patient should be advised of these side-effects, and regular blood counts and urine analyses performed every month. This drug should not be used with gold, antimalarials, anticoagulants, or steroids, nor should it be used in patients who have congestive heart failure or edema.[5]

INDOMETHACIN

Indomethacin (Indocin) has been used in the treatment of rheumatic disorders for over 15 years and has analgesic and anti-inflammatory actions. Indomethacin generally should not be used in conjunction with other NSAIDs, including aspirin. Side-effects include gastrointestinal irritation with peptic ulcer formation, dizziness, headaches, edema, and weight gain.[15] It is more generally used in the treatment of ankylosing spondylitis, gout, osteoarthritis, rheumatoid arthritis, and acute musculoskeletal disorders (eg, bursitis and tendonitis). Dosage ranges from 25 mg/day to a maximum of 200 mg/day, with the usual dosage being 25 mg two or three times a day.[12]

IBUPROFEN

Ibuprofen (Motrin) is a relative new drug, introduced in 1969. It is said to have analgesic, anti-inflammatory, and antipyretic properties, with its main mode of action being based on inhibition of prostaglandin biosynthesis. It has been used clinically in the management of rheumatoid arthritis, juvenile rheumatoid arthritis, osteoarthritis, nonarticular rheumatoid conditions, and soft-tissue injuries, as well as dysmenorrhea. Side-effects are few, but its toxicity potential is still being studied. Fewer gastrointestinal complaints have been noted, but occcasional nausea, dyspepsia, heartburn, and peptic ulceration may occur. Its use is contraindicated in patients with active peptic ulcers, bronchospasm, or allergic sensitivity to aspirin. Dosage is usually 400 mg to 600 mg given four times a day, up to a total of 2400 mg. It can be used in conjunction with corticosteroids. Use with aspirin is controversial, with some sources noting it is of little value and others feeling it may have a synergistic effect.[1,15]

NAPROXEN

Naproxen (Naprosyn) is known for its analgesic, anti-inflammatory, antipyretic, and uterine-relaxant activities. Therefore, it is widely used with a variety of rheumatic diseases, such as rheumatoid arthritis, osteoarthritis, ankylosing spondylitis, and acute gout, as well as for dysmenorrhea. Side-effects are few with rare adverse reactions. Gastrointestinal complaints, such as heartburn, nausea, and dyspepsia, are reported. Rare reactions may include impairment of renal function, thrombocytopenia, bone marrow depression, and jaundice. Its long half-life allows it to be given in a twice-a-day dosage of 250 mg to 500 mg each dose.

FENOPROFEN CALCIUM

Fenoprofen calcium (Nalfon) has been found to be effective for the treatment of mild to moderate pain in rheumatoid arthritis or osteoarthritis. Some relief in arthritic symptoms may occur in a few days, but optimal results may take up to 4 to 6 weeks. Side-effects are similar to the other NSAIDs including dyspepsia, nausea, anorexia, headache, and dizziness. There have been reports of nephrotic syndrome, thrombocytopenia, bone marrow depression, and anemia. These may be reversible if the drug is withdrawn early.[3] Typical dosage is 300 mg to 600 mg three to four times a day.

TOLMETIN SODIUM

Tolmetin sodium (Tolectin) has been used in the treatment of rheumatoid arthritis, osteoarthritis, juvenile rheumatoid arthritis, ankylosing spondylitis, and soft-tissue diseases. It has been found to be effective in the control of chronic inflammation. Therapeutic response usually occurs within 1 week. Gastrointestinal complaints are the most common side-effects. Headache and dizziness may also occur. Skin rash, edema, and hypertension are other occasional side-effects. Dosage is usually 400 mg, three times a day with the total dose not to exceed 2000 mg.

SULINDAC

Sulindac (Clinoril), a new NSAID, has been found effective in the relief of pain and inflammation in osteoarthritis, rheumatoid arthritis, ankylosing spondylitis, periarticular diseases, and acute gout. It is usually well tolerated with side-effects reducible through a reduction in dosage. Common side-effects are gastrointestinal complaints, rash, dizziness, headache, tinnitus, and edema. The usual dosage is 150 mg to 200 mg, twice a day.

The preceding review is certainly not exhaustive, but it is representative of the commonly used NSAIDs. Many patients tolerate NSAIDs better than aspirin, and often patient compliance is improved. Physicians find these drugs to be a valuable way to conservatively treat a variety of rheumatic conditions. The primary disadvantage is their cost.

Drugs Used Only for Gout

COLCHICINE/ALLOPURINOL

Colchicine, in some form, has been used for centuries in the treatment of gouty arthritis. Today, it is used in a high dose for treatment during the acute gouty flare. Colchicine should be administered as soon as possible after the onset of the acute attack, otherwise its success diminishes. The initial dosage is one 0.6 mg tablet each hour. This continues until the pain is relieved or the patient begins to feel the effects of its diuretic properties, as evidenced by diarrhea or other gastrointestinal complaints. However, because sudden death may occur with high doses, no more than 6 mg/day should be used. The dosage is then tapered to a daily dose of 0.6 mg, if the arthritis was mild, or 1.2 mg, if the patient has moderate or severe chronic tophaceous gout. Daily ingestion of colchicine as a prophylactive drug does not increase side-effects nor make the drug intolerable in the patient. This prophylactic dosage may be tapered even more, or discontinued, if the patient remains symptom-free for a period (e.g., 1–2 years in mild arthritis).

Allopurinol is a drug that influences uric acid metabolism and, therefore, is used to control uric acid production in patients with gout. Allopurinol causes a reduction in urate synthesis. This drug is recommended for use during the hyperuricemia after the acute gout attack has been treated. Side-effects include gastrointestinal intolerance, skin rash, alopecia, bone marrow depression, and vasculitis. Decreasing the dosage may eliminate these side-effects. Starting doses for allopurinol should be 100 mg. The average dosage is 300 mg, but it may be increased to 400 mg to 600 mg daily in more severe cases.

Second-Line Drugs Used to Treat Rheumatoid Arthritis

Second-line drugs are often added to the treatment regimen in patients with rheumatoid arthritis whose disease has not responded well enough to aspirin or NSAIDs. It is felt that these drugs may inhibit joint damage in some patients and, in some cases, they may induce remissions; however, their side-effects are also more severe.

GOLD

Gold sodium thiomalate (Myochrysine) and aurothioglucose (Solganal) are injectable compounds used in the treatment of rheumatoid arthritis. Gold sodium thiomalate is a water-soluble compound that is easier to administer than the oil-based aurothioglucose, but aurothioglucose has a lower frequency of adverse reactions. Gold therapy is indicated for patients with rheumatoid arthritis and, less frequently, for psoriatic arthritis, when aspirin and NSAIDs have been insufficient to control inflammation or when patients develop erosive disease as shown by x-ray studies made during NSAID therapy. Because gold is a slow-acting antirheumatic drug, it is necessary to continue analgesic and other anti-inflammatory therapy. About 70% of patients treated early in the course of their disease experience good or excellent results with gold therapy.

Gold therapy should be started with a small test dose (10 mg) to identify any idiosyncratic reaction, then weekly injections of 25 mg to 50 mg should be administered for approximately 20 weeks. Larger doses do not increase efficacy but do increase toxicity. Responses are not generally seen until after 3 to 4 months of treatment. If a patient does not respond to gold therapy in 6 months, gold should be stopped and another drug initiated. If effective, the interval between injections is then increased to 2 weeks, 3 weeks, and eventually 4 weeks, over the next several months. If gold therapy helps, then the patient should be maintained on this regimen for life. If administration of the gold is stopped, an exacerbation of the disease will result, and patients seldom respond to the second course of gold therapy.[15]

Toxicity with gold therapy is high. During a standard course (20 injections of 50 mg) approximately 35% of patients experience toxic side-effects, and these are severe enough to require discontinuance of the drug in about 14%.[17] The most common side-effect is a rash, which is seen in 30% of patients treated with gold. Other side-effects include stomatitis, proteinuria, leukopenia, and thrombocytopenia. Because of the potential for these serious side-effects, a complete blood count and urinalysis should be done each week prior to each injection. If the reaction is minor, the gold may be temporarily discontinued and then resumed with a 10-mg dose, followed by a 25 mg dose, and then a return to a full dose. Bone marrow depression and renal damage require permanent discontinuation of gold. These side-effects may be managed early by discontinuing the gold, but other drug treatment may be required to treat gold-induced problems.

Oral gold (Auranofin) has just recently been approved for use in rheumatoid arthritis. Trials of this drug, to date, suggest that oral gold is slightly less effective than injected gold but has fewer side-effects.[13]

Advantages of gold are that gold has the potential to induce remission of the disease and patients do not have to take many pills per day. Disadvantages include the need to go to a physician's office weekly for the injection, blood, and urine tests, and toxicity with the use of this drug is high. Compliance, therefore, is based on whether or not the patient comes in for the injections regularly, rather than on how many pills he takes at home between appointments.

It is very important that patients understand about gold therapy before beginning treatment. The patient's cooperation in making the weekly appointments is integral for success of this regimen. The patient must also understand the potential side-effects of this treatment and the nature of the drug, that is, that it is slow acting and no response will be seen for 3 to 4 months.

HYDROXYCHLOROQUINE

Hydroxychloroquine sulfate (Plaquenil) is an antimalarial drug used in the treatment of rheumatoid arthritis and SLE. It is felt to have an action similar to gold, although it has not been shown to alter the radiographic progression of the disease. It is also a slow-acting drug. Effects are not seen for at least 4 weeks and, usually, it takes 3 to 6 months before significant benefits are observed. It is used in combination with salicylates or NSAIDs because of its slow action.

The side-effects of hydroxychloroquine include nausea, diarrhea, skin rash, ototoxicity, and hemolytic anemia. Retinal toxicity can occur, and once symptoms of impaired vision have occurred, the defect is considered irreversible and may even progress.[13] Light exposure accelerates ocular toxicity, and patients should be advised to wear sunglasses when in bright sunlight to minimize this effect.[9] Retinal toxicity can be detected early by performing a test of red vision with a tangential screen and 2-mm red disk. Discontinuation of the drug at first sign of an abnormal test can prevent significant loss of vision. Therefore, eye examination is recommended every 6 months while taking this drug.

Advantages of this drug are that it is generally well-tolerated and potential side-effects can be avoided. A disadvantage is that it is slow acting. Patient education is similar to that required with patients considering initiation of gold therapy.

PENICILLAMINE

Penicillamine is a derivative of penicillin and is found in three forms; D, DL, L. D-Penicillamine is the form used in clinical practice to treat rheumatoid arthritis. This drug is used in place of gold and, although its action is slow (6 weeks to 3 months), it may restrain the progression of the disease. Penicillamine does not cure rheumatoid arthritis, but studies have shown a reduction of rheumatoid symptoms, an improvement in articular indices, a decrease in the need for anti-inflammatory drugs, and a decrease in erosive activity.[10] Indication for its use is in active, progressive rheumatoid arthritis that has previously been uncontrolled by small doses of steroids, anti-inflammatory agents, or gold.

The potential toxicity of this drug is serious, and the patient considering its use should be made aware of this. The following list contains potential adverse reactions: skin rash, oral ulcerations, poor wound healing, gastrointestinal disturbances, proteinuria with development of nephrotic syndrome, leukopenia, thrombocytopenia, bone marrow depression, autoimmune diseases, and loss of taste. The following tests are performed every 2 weeks during use of the drug: a complete blood count, a platelet count, and an urinalysis. Because of this necessarily frequent monitoring, some patients are not able to consider use of the drug because it may be inconvenient and expensive. The initial dosage of the drug is usually 250 mg/day, increasing the dose 250 mg every 2 to 4 weeks until there is an effect or a maintenance dose of 1500 mg is achieved. Many patients are unable to tolerate this high of a maintenance dose. Dosage is slowly reduced if side-effects occur or with remission of the disease. Penicillamine is taken with water between meals or at bedtime. There has been no evidence of interaction between penicillamine and NSAIDs; however, it is customary to avoid coprescribing drugs of the phenylbutazone group with penicillamine.[10]

Glucocorticoids

ORALLY ADMINISTERED

Cortisone, hydrocortisone, and prednisone are examples of glucocorticoids, a class of naturally occurring adrenal hormones with characteristic effects on the intermediary metabolism of glucose. They are used in the treatment of rheumatic diseases because of their potent anti-inflammatory properties. Glucocorticoids have numerous serious side-effects and, therefore, clinical use requires careful assessment of the benefits to be gained versus the risks involved. The physician must consider the severity of the disease and be aware of any predisposition of the patient to steroid complications. In general, the incidence and severity of side-effects parallel increasing doses and duration of treatment; therefore, steroids should be prescribed in the smallest dose for the shortest time to accomplish the desired effect. For most rheumatic diseases, the drug is not curative but it is palliative. It is probable that it does not alter the course of rheumatoid arthritis as a disease. Rather, it may even permit or hasten its progression because the patient may avoid rest and overuse damaged joints.[15] Nonetheless, there are indications for steroid use in certain patients with rheumatic diseases, such as rheumatoid arthritis, SLE, polymyositis, polyarteritis, and polymyalgia rheumatica.

There are numerous side-effects of steroid therapy that include obesity; cataracts; osteoporosis; aseptic necrosis; myopathy; hypertension; peptic ulcers; edema, secondary to sodium and water retention; behavioral disturbances; impaired wound healing, secondary to thin, fragile skin; and increased risk of infection.[4] Large doses and long-term steroid use may produce symptoms that mimic the disease being treated, for example, steroids may include myalgia, arthralgia, hypertension, and edema. Therefore, the physician may be faced with determining whether to increase or to decrease steroid dosage because of an apparent increase of disease symptoms that may be caused by a flare of the disease, or they may be side-effects of the drug therapy. Because of the natural rhythm of the pituitary adrenal axis, steroids are less likely to cause side-effects if administered only once a day, preferably in the morning, because this least disturbs the normal rhythm of the axis. Pituitary adrenal function is suppressed with steroid use and may remain suppressed for up to a year after prolonged use. Steroid therapy must be gradually tapered. Abrupt withdrawal of steroids can lead to adrenal insufficiency and death.[15]

The advantage of a short course of steroid therapy is that it can provide a dramatic decrease in inflammation in a seriously ill patient. The disadvantage is the numerous side-effects that can occur even with short-term steroid therapy. Patients being considered for steroid therapy should be apprised of the benefits, the risks, and the alternatives. Because of the dramatic and immediate improvement obtained with steroids, the short-sighted patient may request steroid therapy without an awareness of the risks of such treatment.

Once a patient is on high-dose steroid regimen, they may display a state of euphoria or false sense of well-being. Patient education at that time is difficult because the patient may not perceive the need for education or for instruction. Hence, it is recommended that any verbal instructions given to a patient on a high-dose steroid regimen be reinforced with written instructions for later reference by the patient or his family.[11]

ADMINISTERED BY INJECTION

Intra-articular injection of corticosteroids may give good local symptomatic relief with few side-effects. Although not a cure for joint inflammation, hydrocortisone injection can produce a decrease in joint temperature, tenderness, pain, and swelling within 24 hr. This symptomatic relief lasts from a few days to several weeks. In addition to intra-articular injections, tendonitis and tenosynovitis may be effectively treated by local injection.

Potential side-effects include infection and postinjection flare. About 1% of people experience an exacerbation of the inflammation immediately after injection. Joint instability from osteonecrosis and weakened capsular ligaments occur in repeatedly injected areas; therefore, the frequency of steroid injections should be limited to no more than once every 4 to 6 months and no more than three injections within 1 year to avoid changes. It is unknown whether the damage occurs because of the steroid or because the relief from pain allows overuse of the damaged joint.

In general, indications for intra-articular corticosteroid injection include

1. When only one or a few joints are involved (after infection is ruled out)
2. When a few joints have active inflammation, even in the presence of a more generalized low-grade involvement
3. In rheumatoid arthritis as an adjunct to systemic drug therapy, especially for "resistant" joints
4. When systemic therapy is contraindicated
5. To assist in rehabilitation and prevent joint deformity

Contraindications include

1. Presence of infection in or near a joint
2. Multiple severe joint involvement
3. Severe joint destruction
4. Arthritis in joints with no synovial space
5. When previous injections have produced little or no benefit[7]

Patients should be informed of the potential for a postinjection flare and should be cautioned not to overuse the injected part for several days after the injection.

Immunosuppressives

The immunosuppressive drugs were originally used in the treatment of cancer patients. Their use in the treatment of rheumatoid arthritis began with the concept of rheumatoid arthritis being a disease of hyperimmunity. The use of these potent drugs is reserved for treating severe disease that has previously been resistive to therapy with more traditional drugs. A discussion of some of the more commonly used immunosuppressive drugs follows.

METHOTREXATE

Methotrexate is given orally or intramuscularly in a dosage of 7.5 mg to 15 mg once a week, and it has been used in psoriatic arthritis, dermatomyositis and rheumatoid arthritis. Approval by the FDA has been received for its use in psoriatic arthritis.[15] Methotrexate interferes with folic acid metabolism, thereby reducing all metabolism. Side-effects include hair loss, oral ulcers, and severe liver disease.

AZATHIOPRINE (IMURAN)

Azathioprine has been used with rheumatoid arthritis, psoriatic arthritis, and SLE. Studies have found that this drug has provided symptomatic relief as well as prevention of new erosions in rheumatoid arthritis.[8] Azathioprine interferes with DNA synthesis and destroys rapidly dividing cells. Side-effects include bone marrow suppression, gastrointestinal intolerance, liver damage, and infections. The dosage is 2 mg/kg per day.

CYCLOPHOSPHAMIDE (CYTOXAN)

Cyclophosphamide is also an alkylating agent that kills cells and has been found effective in treating rheumatoid arthritis. In some instances, it may decrease bony erosions and induce remission of the disease. It is more useful in treating life-threatening vasculitic disease. It has a high toxicity, however, and can produce alopecia, nonreversible hemorrhagic cystitis, and suppression of gonadal function.[15] Dosage is generally 100 mg to 150 mg daily, with this dose producing the necessary leukopenia.

The preceding drugs are extremely toxic and need to be carefully monitored through monthly or weekly blood counts. Yearly liver biopsies are recommended with methotrexate treatment. The potential for increased malignancies after many years has not been ruled out and should limit the use of these drugs to patients with severe disease, in whom other therapy has failed, or to potentially life-threatening disease.

IMPLICATIONS FOR REHABILITATION PROFESSIONALS

Because most of the rheumatoid diseases are chronic, one of the most important aspects of the treatment program is patient education. The health professionals provide assessment and make treatment recommendations, but the ongoing management becomes the responsibility of the patient. The rehabilitation professional can play an important role in clarifying and reinforcing the proper treatment program with individual patients. It is imperative that the rehabilitation professional work closely with the referring physician and know and understand the physician's philosophy of treatment before discussing these issues with patients. Often the rehabilitation professional is faced with questions about medications from patients with rheumatic diseases. By providing the patient with correct information the rehabilitation professional not only increases or reinforces the patient's education but also tends to improve rapport with the patient. By demonstrating a general knowledge about the patient's disease and its management, the rehabilitation professional conveys the concept of a coordinated, integrated approach in the care of the patient. The rehabilitation professional who recognizes signs of drug toxicity or side-effects and refers the patient back to his physician provides a potentially invaluable service to the patient who may not be aware of the problem or who, for some reason, is reluctant to contact the physician before his next scheduled appointment. Reduction of the incongruities in the complex treatment programs that many patients with rheumatic diseases have (e.g., drug, exercise, and splinting regimens) and demonstration of a consistency in approach can help to reduce obstacles to compliance and enhance the disease outcomes.

Evaluation results can be affected by relatively fast-acting drugs such as aspirin and other NSAIDs. Joint range-of-motion and grip strength, for example, can be objectively affected in as little as 30 min after ingestion of a fast-acting anti-inflammatory medication; therefore, rehabilitation professionals need to be aware of the time of serial evaluations relative to the patient's medication regimen. The observed improvements may be a result of medication rather than rehabilitation efforts; therefore, the rehabilitation professional should be consistent in the time selected for reassessment of certain physical measures.

Complex medication regimens can involve many rehabilitation professionals. The rehabilitation nurse should make sure that patients not only understand and know when to take their medications, but she should also make sure that the patient is able to take all doses prescribed at the prescribed times. For example, she should make sure a factory worker can take a break to take his aspirin every 4 hr while on the job. The social worker should discuss with the patient whether or not he can afford to buy the required amounts of medications. And the occupational therapist should assess whether or not the patient can open the medication containers and take his medicine independently. If any of these problems cannot be resolved, then alternative arrangements need to be made. Sometimes this means recommending to the physician that he consider use of another similar drug. For example, if the factory worker cannot take a break to take his aspirin, then he will not be able to maintain the therapeutic blood levels of salicylate required to appropriately treat his disease. However, changing his drug therapy to a drug taken only twice a day would eliminate the problem of taking medication at work and allow the patient to achieve therapeutic doses of the medication. Patients requiring medication for pain in addition to anti-inflammatory medications may respond to techniques such as transcutaneous nerve stimulation (TENS), biofeedback, or various relaxation procedures for managing pain. These techniques may allow a decrease in, or elimination of, pain medication and, therefore, a decrease in the potential for interaction of side-effects of medication. Again, this team approach helps to reduce obstacles to compliance that may otherwise go unnoticed.

Side-effects of some of the most potent anti-inflammatory drugs have implications for rehabilitation professionals as well. The physical therapist needs to take precautions with patients on long-term steroid therapy because these patients may develop osteoporosis and, thereby, suffer fractures more easily. Their fragile skin also bruises more easily. Therapists should discuss with their referring physician precautions or limitations to be observed following steroid injections. Although physicians may differ in their opinions, most feel that patients should be protected from overuse of the injected area for some period after injection of steroids into a joint or bursa. Patients taking immunosuppressive drugs or steroids are also at risk of infection; therefore, therapists should be aware of potential danger to these patients when scheduling, for example, location of treatment. Steroid therapy may also induce a sense of euphoria in some patients. This can make patient education by any rehabilitation professional difficult because these patients will not perceive a need, for example, of learning joint protection principles. Provision of small amounts of education materials with written reinforcement for later reference, as well as review of materials at a later date, may improve effectiveness. Involving the family or significant others may also be helpful in patient education and ultimately in enhancing compliance with the treatment regimen.

The case studies that follow present information illustrating why rehabilitation health professionals need to be knowledgeable about drug management in the arthritis patient. Although the therapist may not be directly involved in the drug education of the patient or in the prescription of drugs, it is helpful and sometimes crucial that the rehabilitation professional be able to recognize drug side-effects and be aware of dose and effect. These case studies will illustrate how the allied health professional can be instrumental in assisting with patient understanding and compliance with their drug regimen.

CASE 1   Mrs. Brown, a 56-year-old woman, with a 5-year history of rheumatoid arthritis, has multiple joint involvement including the hands, wrists, knees, and shoulders. Several hours of morning stiffness and quite severe pain are often present with persistent swelling. A high-dose aspirin regimen was tested, but this was discontinued secondary to gastric disturbance. Several other NSAIDs have been used, but none has controlled her symptoms, and function continues to decrease. She is unable to perform household chores adequately and frequently needs assistance with self-care tasks, such as bathing and dressing. A month ago, a regimen of gold injections was instituted because use of NSAID agents failed to adequately control her symptoms and because examination of her x-ray films revealed erosive changes at the wrists and knees.

Mrs. Brown came to clinic today for her fourth gold injection and was also referred to physical therapy for evaluation and instruction in exercise and use of heat. Physical therapy evaluation revealed deficits in range-of-motion at the shoulders and knees, and the patient demonstrated poor understanding of joint protection principles and appropriate exercise techniques. She was somewhat receptive to the instructions received in physical therapy but questioned the validity of performing them when the "gold is not having any effect on my symptoms anyway." Mrs. Brown was noticeably discouraged with her lack of improvement physically when she had had high expectations for improvement when placed on the gold therapy. This discouragement was also reflected in the patient's reluctance to totally accept the prescribed physical therapy program.

The physical therapist acknowledged Mrs. Brown's frustration with her lack of improvement but reinforced the importance of compliance with both the prescribed drug regimen as well as with the exercise to prevent loss of motion. Mrs. Brown was reminded that improvement in symptoms and functions is slow with gold therapy, sometimes taking up to 3 to 4 months. Maintaining physical function and movement during this time was stressed. Mrs. Brown was able to express her dissatisfactions during this period, and some misunderstandings were clarified. Ultimately, compliance with her drug regimen was enhanced as well. The rehabilitation professional also shared this information with the physician, who, because of increased awareness of the patient's concerns and level of understanding, was able to reinforce the encouragement given by the therapist, and reassure the patient.

CASE 2   Mrs. Jones is a 34-year-old black woman, with a 7-year history of SLE. Her disease was initially manifested as a polyarthritis involving the hands and feet with systemic features of fatigue, anorexia, and fever. A characteristic butterfly rash was present, and the patient gave a history of photosensitivity. The patient recently developed increasing proteinuria, with subsequent discovery of renal involvement. Before this, the patient had been treated with various NSAIDs to control the symptoms of polyarthritis. With the development of renal involvement, she was placed on a steroid regimen. Several weeks later, it was noted that the patient began exhibiting a flattened affect, impaired short-term memory, and other behavioral disturbances. Mrs. Jones was hospitalized with the intent of observing her symptoms, further evaluation for possible central nervous involvement, and regulation of her steroid therapy. Occupational therapy was requested for perceptual, motor, and cognitive assessment to establish a baseline of behavior. The patient was well known to this therapist from previous clinic visits for treatment of arthritis symptoms. The physician requested that occupational therapist follow this patient and aid the physicians as they altered her steroid doses. The occupational therapist gave daily input on the patient's cognition and behavior to help ascertain whether the symptoms exhibited were related to her drug therapy or to the disease process. This input aided the physician in regulating drug dosage.

CASE 3   Mr. Smith has a 5-year history of polymyositis that first evidenced as proximal muscle weakness involving the shoulder and pelvic girdles. Initial symptoms were weakness during self-care activities and inability to climb stairs or get on or off a chair. The patient's disease has been characterized by exacerbations and remissions. Exacerbations have been controlled with high doses of steroids which were eventually tapered to a lower maintenance dose. Mr. Smith was admitted to the hospital for increasing respiratory involvement and exacerbation of muscle weakness. He was referred to occupational therapy, physical therapy, and respiratory therapy. All three services must be aware of Mr. Smith's long history of steroid therapy for several reasons. Osteoporosis is a frequent side-effect of steroid therapy; therefore, one must be careful to avoid aggressive manual muscle testing in a patient such as this and to use caution during transferring, passive range-of-motion, or percussion therapy. Steroid myopathy, which is another side-effect of steroid therapy, may decrease muscle strength and may present problems in a patient's general functional ability. Finally, general care of the patient's skin through proper positioning must be addressed because of his thin skin, and because of a tendency for poor wound healing and an increased risk of infection if pressure sores result.

REFERENCES

1. Adams SS, Buckler JW: Ibuprofen and flurbiprofen. In Huskisson EC (ed): Anti Rheumatic Drugs, pp 243–264. New York, Praeger Publishers, 1983
2. Arthritis Foundation: Basic Facts. Answers to Your Questions. Atlanta, Arthritis Foundation, 1983
3. Burt RA, Gruber CM, Irons MR: Fenoprofen Calcium: A review. In Huskisson EC (ed): Anti Rheumatic Drugs, pp 233–242. New York, Praeger Publishers, 1983
4. Castles JJ: Glucocorticoids. In McCarty DJ (ed): Arthritis and Allied Conditions, 10th ed, pp 512–524. Philadelphia, Lea & Febiger, 1985
5. Fowler PD: Phenylbutazone. In Huskisson EC (ed): Anti Rheumatic Drugs, pp 353–370. New York, Praeger Publishers, 1983
6. Gross M, Brandt K, Feinberg J et al: Team Care for patients with chronic rheumatic disease. Allied Health 11:239–247, 1982
7. Hollander JL: Arthrocentesis techniques and intrasynovial therapy. In McCarty DJ (ed): Arthritis and Allied Conditions, 10th ed, pp 514–553. Philadelphia, Lea & Febiger, 1985
8. Huskisson EC: Azathioprine. In Huskisson EC (ed): Anti Rheumatic Drugs, pp 597–604. New York, Praeger Publishers, 1983
9. Lightfoot RW: Treatment of rheumatoid arthritis. In McCarty DJ (ed): Arthritis and Allied Conditions, 10th ed, pp 668–676. Philadelphia, Lea & Febiger, 1985
10. Lyle WH: Penicillamine. In Huskisson EC (ed): Anti Rheumatic Drugs, pp 521–554. New York, Praeger Publishers, 1983
11. Melvin JL: Rheumatic Disease: Occupational Therapy and Rehabilitation, 2nd ed. Philadelphia, FA Davis, 1982
12. Rhymer AR, Gengos DC: Indomethacin. In Huskisson EC (ed): Anti Rheumatic Drugs, pp 265–278. New York, Praeger Publishers, 1983
13. Rodnan GP, Schumacher HR: Primer on the Rheumatic Diseases, 8th ed. Atlanta, Arthritis Foundation, 1983
14. Ropes MW, Bennett GA, Caleb S et al: 1958 Revision of diagnostic criteria for rheumatoid arthritis. Bull Rheum Dis 9:175–176, 1958
15. Rosenbaum EE: Rheumatology: New Directions in Therapy. Garden City, Medical Examination Publishing, 1979
16. Schaller JG: Treatment of juvenile rheumatoid arthritis. In McCarty DJ (ed): Arthritis and Allied Conditions, 10th ed, pp 811–818. Philadelphia, Lea & Febiger, 1985

17. Skosey JL: Gold compounds. In McCarty DJ (ed): Arthritis and Allied Conditions, 10th ed, pp 487–496. Philadelphia, Lee & Febiger, 1985
18. Steinbrocker O, Traeger, CH, Batterman RC: Therapeutic criteria in rheumatoid arthritis. JAME 140: 659–662, 1949
19. Williams RC, McCarty DJ: Clinical picture of rheumatoid arthritis. In McCarty DJ (ed): Arthritis and Allied Conditions, 10th ed, pp 650–619. Philadelphia, Lea & Febiger, 1985

The Older Patient and the Effects of Drugs on Rehabilitation

7

Diane M. White
Carole Bernstein Lewis

The older person is the largest consumer of drugs.[42] Hence, when a rehabilitation professional is treating a functional disability, the interplay of the drugs the patient is taking is more than likely to impact upon the patient's performance. This chapter will discuss some of the major concepts of the older patient and the effects of drugs on rehabilitation. The chapter Appendix lists many of the more commonly used drugs and their trade names.

WHAT MAKES THE ELDERLY UNIQUE?

In 1890, 3% of the United States population was over the age of 65.[50] Today the over-65 population is about 10.8%.[50] With the aging of the baby boomers some demographers speculate that the segment of the United States population over 65 years of age could reach 20% to 25%.[50]

In the current 65-and-older population, some interesting health statistics become evident. Older persons (over 65 years old) visit the doctor 43% more often than younger persons. They have twice as many hospital stays, for twice as long. Of this group 75% have a chronic disability.[50] The three leading chronic disabilities for this age group are heart conditions, visual impairment, and arthritis.[50]

Despite the large percentage of older persons with chronic conditions, 87% had no limitation of their mobility.[50] (i.e., they do not have to use a cane, crutch, wheelchair, or walker).

The statistics for drug use in the elderly are not as well established or as clear as the general health information. In long-term care facilities, one study showed that older persons received at least eight different drugs for their first 10 days in the facility.[42] In addition, a study made in 1976 showed that one-third of the residents in a long-stay institution received between 8 and 16 drugs daily. The class of drugs most frequently used by the older consumer is cathartics, followed by analgesics, tranquilizers, and diuretics. A final concern over drug use of the older patient is the high consumption of over-the-counter (OTC) medications. A study done by Lamy in 1982 showed that 60% of the well elderly consumed some type of OTC drug.

Beyond statistical information affecting drug use of older persons and the rehabilitative outcomes, there are some rehabilitative concepts. The first of these concepts that is singular to older patients is the multiplicity of their problems. In contrast to younger patients, elderly patients often have more than one disability. There are two ways that this can impact upon rehabilitation. First, the disease itself can cause changes in the older person's performance. Second, the drugs used in treating the mixture of disorders can affect the person's functional level. Therapists must be cognizant of both of these intervening variables when working with older patients.

This concept of multiple functional abnormalities leads us to the next concern, that of differentiating normal age changes from pathologic age changes. In the realm of rehabilitation it is important to be aware of changes that occur in the body systems as a result of the aging process versus those changes that are a result of a disease. For example, presbycusis, hearing loss, is a normal change with age. Tinnitus, on the other had, is a disease. Rehabilitation professionals can help both problems by designing functional adaptions to the environment. Tinnitus and its symptoms can be further helped, to some extent, with surgery and sedatives. Rehabilitation professionals need not attribute all changes seen in elderly patients to normal aging. Sometimes the changes may be due to disease. When this is the case, different interventions must be considered and goals must be reexamined.

Another concept affecting rehabilitative outcomes is that of variability. Variability has been proved in only a few cases; however, its ramifications for rehabilitation are significant. Basically, the concept of variability states that some functional determinations in older persons are more variable than those of younger persons. For example, reaction time generally slows as one ages, but it can also be more variable. Therefore, an older person's reaction time scans a broader response time than a younger person's. This concept also can affect our treatment programs and goals. We cannot always expect similar responses to exercise or drug regimens in our older patients.

The fourth concept that can impact upon rehabilitative outcomes as well as on drug interactions is hypokinetics. *Hypokinetics* is decreased activity. Many changes attributed to aging may well be the effects of hypokinetics.[54] Decreased bowel mobility, increased bone demineralization, and increased muscular atrophy are but some results of hypokinetics that are oftentimes confused with normal aging. An older person's decreased activity level may substantially affect their rehabilitative potential as well as their ability to tolerate various drugs. In addition, various drugs may contribute to an older person's decreased activity level. Hence, rehabilitation professionals need to be aware of the effects of hypokinetics on older persons.

The final concept that impacts upon rehabilitation is optimal health. Figure 7-1 schematically outlines the Rogers Health Status Scale.[40] This scale outlines the var-

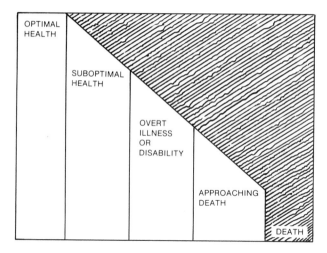

FIGURE 7-1. A schematic representation of the Health Status Scale. (Adapted from Rogers ES: Human Ecology and Health. New York, Macmillan, 1960).

ious areas of health. Optimal health is the area of complete physical, psychologic and social well-being. The next area is suboptimal health. Most people are in this category. The area of overt illness or disability is where most rehabilitation professionals see their patients. Intervening at this phase was appropriate when our health care system revolved around the critical care model of health care delivery. Today, however, we are more concerned with chronic conditions that most often respond to interventions in the area of suboptimal health. The older person can be visualized as being on a skateboard. When this person is in optimal health it is a balanced situation. However, once he or she starts down the slope, it can be a quick trip to approaching death. Our job as rehabilitation professionals is to push the older person into optimal health. One means of doing this in the realm of rehabilitation is to be aware of, and sensitive to, the effects of various drugs on an older person's independent functioning. This is the purpose of this chapter. It is hoped that sharing of the ideas that have already been presented and those to come, can better equip the therapist to understand the sensitive nature of the health care picture of the older adult.

Age Changes That Affect Drug-Taking Behavior

Sensory and mental status changes can affect drug-taking behavior of older persons. All five senses tend to decline with age.[33] The sense of hearing can affect drug-taking behavior in the older person. If the ability to hear declines, all of the important information necessary to properly take the drug may be lost or cause confusion. In addition, verbal reminders may also be lost if an older person is hard of hearing.

The sense of vision also decreases as one ages. This loss of vision is called presbyopia. Some changes with presbyopia that can affect drug-taking behavior are the ability to discriminate between pastels or very dark colors. Most pills are pastel and may be easily confused by an older person. Color coding is a good idea for proper pill use, but only if the colors look different. Remember, pastels all look similar, as do all dark colors. Labeling may also be difficult to distinguish, and instructions may be misinterpreted. Large, clear print is helpful for a vision-impaired older person.

Taste and smell decrease with age. Because an older person cannot taste or smell food as well, they may not eat properly, and various drugs may affect them differently.

Finally, the sense of touch does decrease with age. However, no real impediments to drug use have been shown. The symptomology of arthritis, however, may make it more difficult for older persons to handle various drugs or drug containers. Encouragement and assistance may help alleviate this impediment.

Changes in mental status can also affect drug-taking behavior. Blazer reports that as many as 50% of the elderly are depressed.[3] One of the signs of depression is loss of interest and self-esteem.[3] These people, therefore, may be less motivated to take care of themselves. In addition, depressed people tend to have more negative self-reports. This may make it more difficult for rehabilitation professionals to accurately assess these patients' outcomes. It must be emphasized that these mental status changes are not normal signs of aging. They can be due to disease, social concerns, or even be caused by patient's medication regimen itself, as will be discussed later.

Pathologic changes in mental status that can affect drug-taking behaviors of older persons relate to the various types of brain syndromes. The symptoms of brain syndromes are judgment impairments, memory loss, and fluctuating levels of cognition. These may contribute to erratic and undependable drug-taking behavior. Older persons with a brain syndrome may be helped with a written schedule and frequent reminders from family members or support personnel.

Again, it cannot be emphasized enough that all of these factors presented interplay with one another to make the older patient unique. Each person must be considered individually when determining goal objectives and possible rehabilitative processes. Remember that throughout an evaluation of a patient drug therapy can be an "obstacle to successful rehabilitation as well as a help."[1]

Physiologic and Pharmacokinetic Changes in the Older Patient

Introductory information about the elderly and some changes with age that affect drug-taking behavior have just been discussed. Aside from the physiologic changes that have been presented, there are certain other physical changes that individuals undergo as they age that cause what are considered pharmacokinetic changes. These changes alter the way in which a drug is handled by the older patient.

Pharmacokinetics describes the processes by which the body absorbs, distributes, metabolizes, and excretes a drug. The study of pharmacokinetics is important in helping to determine the expected drug response of an individual patient to a given drug regimen. The ultimate concern of pharmacokinetic factors is the drug's tissue concentration—how much drug actually gets to the site of action to exert its drug effect and how does the patient respond to this amount of drug. Too much drug can lead to drug toxicity; too little drug means that the therapeutic

objectives are inadequate. It has been shown and cited in several important publications that pharmacokinetic changes with age are significant.[22,23,28,39,45,53] Figure
7-2 shows the factors affecting the concentration of the drug at its site of action.

ABSORPTION

Absorption is the passage of drugs from the gastrointestinal tract into the blood-
stream. There are a number of changes in the gastrointestinal tract of the elderly
that might be expected to alter drug absorption.[46] These include:

1. An increase in the gastric pH, which might alter the solubility and ionization of
    drugs. This, in turn, might affect the degree and rate of absorption.
2. A decrease in intestinal blood flow, which might reduce or delay absorption.
3. A decrease in rate of gastric emptying and gastric mobility.
4. A decrease in the mucosal cell absorbing area.

A review of the literature on drug absorption and aging reveals that, in many
instances, aging has little effect on the rate and intent of drug absorption, despite
what might be anticipated.[22,28,53] When there does seem to be age-related changes
in drug absorption, studies indicate that it is not the aging, as such, that affects
the absorption adversely. Acetaminophen, aspirin, and indomethacin are just a
few of the drugs absorbed from the gastrointestinal system by passive diffusion.
Their absorption in the elderly appears to be unaffected by aging as does that of
many other drugs absorbed in this manner. Digoxin and levodopa, on the other
hand, are drugs that seem to be absorbed less rapidly or to a smaller extent in
the older population.[31,45,47] These findings are possibly a result of other factors
influencing the absorptive process, rather than of aging itself. Such factors may
include drug interactions that decrease or increase absorption or delay or increase
gastric emptying; first-pass effect of the liver, which can either increase or decrease
the bioavailability of the drug; impaired metabolism of a drug; decreased renal
excretion of the drug; altered volume of distribution, protein binding, and disease
states, which can alter the course of absorption. The only drug for which there
is evidence of a decreased extent of absorption is prazosin. Its bioavailability is
60% that of a younger subject.[31,45] It is evident that future studies on absorption
processes in the elderly will reveal more than is currently known.

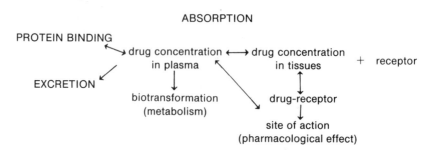

FIGURE 7-2. Factors affecting the concentration of drug at its site of action
(adapted from Refs. 22 and 7)

DISTRIBUTION

The drug distribution in the body determines its concentration at the target site of action. In the normal distribution process, a drug first enters the portal circulation and passes through the liver, where it may be changed by enzymes. The drug then enters the systemic circulation, where it may bind to proteins in the blood or in cells, be dispersed in body water, or accumulate in certain organs. With this in mind, it is easy to see that distribution is affected by how well an organ is perfused (cardiac output), by the drugs preferential protein binding, by solubility of a drug into and out of a target site, and by total volume of a particular compartment (total body water, lean cell mass).

Because with aging, there is decreased lean body mass, decreased total body water, increased body fat, and a decrease in plasma albumin (affects protein binding of drugs), there should be age-related changes in drug distribution among the elderly. This is indeed true, although alterations do not occur in a predictable fashion. In elderly patients there is a decrease in total body water (51% to 53%) and an increase in total body lipids (4% to 30%).[53] This results in a decreased volume of distribution for some hydrophilic drugs (quinine, ethanol, antipyrine) as well as an increase in the volume of distribution of some lipophilic drugs (chlordiazepoxide, diazepam).[22,46,47] A drug's *volume of distribution* is the volume of fluid into which the drug appears to distribute with a concentration equal to that in the plasma. This apparent volume of distribution is a function of the lipid versus water solubilities and of the plasma and tissue protein-binding properties of the drug. Volumes of distribution that are larger than the plasma compartment (greater than 3 liters) indicate that the drug is also present in tissues or fluids outside that compartment. When there are factors present that tend to keep the drug in plasma (low lipid solubility, binding to plasma protein, or decreased tissue binding), the apparent volume of distribution is reduced. On the other hand, when factors decreasing the plasma concentration (decreased plasma protein binding, increased tissue binding, increased lipid solubility) exist, the volume of distribution is increased. With an increase in the volume of distribution of lipid-soluble drugs there is the potential for prolongation of drug action because of the increase in fatty tissue found with the older patient (drug is in the tissue instead of the plasma). The volume of distribution of the hydrophilic drugs decreases because the total body water decreases, resulting in an extended half-life (drug remains in the plasma longer). There is considerable variation between drugs in their patterns of distribution to different tissues and compartments of the body, and the age-related changes seen in the elderly make the situation even more unpredictable. This results in the elderly being more susceptible to a drug's side-effects or toxic effects. Protein binding of drugs to serum proteins, such as albumin, is also an important factor in determining the volume of distribution of a drug. In the plasma a drug is transported in two forms, either "free" drug or "bound" drug. The "free" drug in the plasma is that fraction which is available to diffuse into the tissues and also is subject to renal excretion and to enzymatic degradation. The result of lower serum albumin levels, whether occurring in healthy old age or as a consequence of disease, is a reduction in the number of drug binding sites. The higher level of free drug available, then, leads to an enhanced therapeutic effect. Again, the potential for side-effects and toxic effects exists. In addition to the reduced binding sites associated with lower serum albumin levels, there is the concern of competition for those sites when two or more highly protein-bound drugs are administered. For example, phenytoin, warfarin, salicylates, sulfonamides, and benzodiazepines are all more than 90% bound to serum proteins.[53] A decrease in serum protein binding of these drugs can occur either because of the decrease in the actual number of sites associated with aging or because of an interaction with other bound drugs that bind with more affinity to the sites. Regardless of the cause, the results are the same—more free drug, resulting in exaggerated and adverse effects.

Biotransformation is the process of metabolism of a drug either to active metabolites (having a drug effect) or to inactive metabolites that are then excreted by the kidneys. It is one route by which drugs are removed from the body. Since the rate of elimination of a drug influences the duration of its effect, factors that alter this rate of elimination will more than likely change the length of time that the drug stays in the body. Age-related changes in drug hepatic metabolism result in decreased metabolism of some drugs (though not all) and a decrease in the first-pass effect. These findings, quite naturally, have significant consequences for some drugs.

Some of the factors involved in bringing about these changes include

1. A possible decrease in the size of the liver with aging.[31,45]
2. A decrease in the hepatic blood flow with aging[22,31,45]
3. A decrease in the hepatic enzyme activity resulting in decrease rate of hepatic metabolism[22,23,45]

Changes in the hepatic metabolism of drugs with aging are highly variable and unpredictable. The elderly probably have a diminished capacity to metabolize drugs. This together with a decrease in the hepatic blood flow make the elderly susceptible to reduced elimination of such drugs as chlormethiazole, labetalol, lidocaine, and possibly propranolol.[45] Several other drugs that are affected by changed hepatic enzymatic activity include acetaminophen, chlordiazepoxide, diazepam, phenylbutazone, phenytoin, theophylline, and warfarin.[22]

Hepatic enzyme activity may also be enhanced or inhibited by concurrently administered drugs. Stimulation of enzyme activities (enzyme induction) can occur as a result of a number of chemical compounds. The antihistamines, barbiturates, doxycycline, ethanol, phenytoin, prednisone, and cortisone all induce enzymes, thus bringing about not only their own metabolism but, also, the metabolism of other compounds.[22,41] This will be shown later to be an important factor in drug interactions.

RENAL EXCRETION

Renal excretion is another method by which the body removes or eliminates the drug. The effects of age on renal function exert a profound influence on the elimination of a number of drugs. The physiologic changes that take place with aging include decreased renal blood flow (probably secondary to reduced cardiac output), decreased glomerular filtration, and decreased tubular excretion. These changes result in a decrease in the renal elimination of many drugs.[45]

Digoxin and aminoglycoside antibiotics are excreted by glomerular filtration.[28] Because the glomerular filtration rate can decrease by as much as 40% to 50% with age, the rates of elimination of these two drugs are reduced with age, resulting in possible increased accumulations and increased drug toxicities. Also, because tubular function deteriorates with age, penicillin and procainamide elimination is reduced (these drugs are actively secreted by the renal tubules). One other important factor is that in addition to the physiologic and pathophysiologic effects exerted on the renal status of an elderly patient, one must consider the effects that therapeutically prescribed drugs have on the kidneys. Many medications that are prescribed for the elderly may cause disturbances in the fluid and electrolyte balance of the body. Some can be toxic to the kidneys. Others can further decrease the rate of elimination of certain drugs because of a direct effect on the kidneys to cause urinary retention (anticholinergics, decongestants). Declining renal function, whether it be a drug effect, disease effect, or age effect, is probably the most important factor responsible for adverse drug effects in the elderly.[22]

ALTERED TISSUE SENSITIVITY

In addition to absorption, distribution, metabolism, and excretion, there are two other factors to which the elderly are susceptible that alter the way in which they respond to a drug. The first is a change in the receptor density or sensitivity to a drug. The second is impairment of homeostatic mechanisms (those mechanisms that stablize the normal physiologic state of the individual).

Changes in the sensitivity to drugs have been reported in the elderly without any pharmacokinetic explanation for the altered response. For example, elderly patients would seem to be more sensitive to warfarin than younger subjects because they show an increased anticoagulant effect from the drug.[28] Similarly, studies indicate that altered or increased sensitivity seems to affect the aged brain in particular, with the elderly patient being more confused and disoriented after administration of barbiturates, hypnotics, anticholinergics, and dopaminergic drugs that would be well tolerated by younger adults.[28,39] Other drugs involved include nitrazepam (increased impairment of performance) and propranolol (larger dose needed to have proper effect; may be related to decreased receptors that handle the drug).

Impairment of normal homeostatic mechanisms is the other factor resulting in altered responsiveness to drugs. It includes several things.

1. Drug sensitivity may be altered by the presence of disease, either directly or through the pathologic processes themselves or as a complication of the disease. Many of the elderly are exposed to multiple disease processes that play a profound role in how the body reacts to a drug. For example, the increased risk of hemorrhagic complications of anticoagulants in the elderly is, in part at least, due to degenerative vascular disease diminishing the homeostatic response.
2. Drug-induced postural hypotension is particularly evident in this aged group. The resultant effects of this response—dizziness, confusion, agitation, and weakness—might not be seen in younger patients who have more efficient homeostatic mechanisms.
3. The elderly have impaired thermoregulatory capacity. Several psychoactive drugs can cause hypothermia in the elderly not only the result of the pharmacologic effect of the drug but also as a result of a reduction in physical activity.
4. The regulation of blood sugars and the neurologic control of bowel and bladder functions may also be less efficient in old age. This may result in increased sensitivity to the adverse effects of some drugs.

Summary

The effects of aging on drug handling are complex, and are further complicated by the effects of disease and multiple drug use. Changes in physiologic functions with aging lead to changes in the way drugs affect the body. These changes do not occur at the same rate for everyone. Therefore, it is important to treat each patient individually.

With the exception of drug absorption, which is not significantly altered, age changes in pharmacokinetics lead to clinical concerns of prolonged drug action or an increase in untoward effects of drugs (because more drug is available). Of the pharmacokinetic changes, decreased renal elimination and a reduced first-pass effect are particularly important. Hepatic enzymatic activity changes and renal elimination changes are important factors in making the elderly, who are already susceptible, even more "sensitive" to medications. Unfortunately, because of all the factors involved, the effect that a drug will exert on an older patient is difficult to determine.

DRUG THERAPY OF COMMON MEDICAL PROBLEMS

Cardiovascular Disease

CORONARY ARTERY DISEASE

Coronary artery disease is the single most frequent cause of death in the elderly.[36] Many persons, especially older persons, have no obvious symptoms. The narrowing of their vital coronary vessels may progress for many years before any adverse effects are evident. Indeed, in many instances a heart attack is the first sign of the disease. However, half or more of the victims of coronary artery disease will experience a warning, usually in the form of *angina pectoris*—chest pain caused by a temporary shortage of oxygen to the heart muscle. Coronary artery disease may appear as angina pectoris, myocardial infarction, rhythm disturbances, or cardiac failure.

ANGINA PECTORIS

Angina pectoris is often absent in elderly patients who have coronary artery disease. Factors causing this include an increase in the threshold for deep pain sensation, restriction of mobility by locomotor or neurologic disorders, and angina present earlier in life causing collateral coronary circulation to develop. Other subtle signs of coronary artery disease need to be recognized when angina is not present (dyspnea, epigastric discomfort, shortness of breath, arrhythmia, unusual giddiness, or new onset of confusion). Drugs of three pharmacologic classes are used prophylactically to treat angina—nitrates, β-blockers, and calcium channel blockers.

Sublingual nitroglycerin and the longer-acting oral or transdermal forms of nitroglycerin are the first choices for treatment of angina, even in the elderly patient. Isosorbide dinitrate (5 to 20 mg four times a day) may be effective for as long as 4 hr. It is also occasionally given as a sublingual dose that works in 3 to 5 min, but it is rapidly metabolized by the liver. Transdermal patches of nitroglycerin (Nitrodisc, Nitrodur, Transderm) are placed on the skin from which absorption of the drug occurs over a 24-hr period. A new patch should be applied if the product loosens. As a rule, nitroglycerin products should all be stored in their original containers because of the tendency to vaporize onto other materials. (This, of course, does not apply to the patches applied to the skin.) Side-effects of nitroglycerin include postural hypotension, headache, flushing due to cutaneous vasodilation, and dizziness. Care should be taken in the elderly who already are sensitive to hypotensive effects.

β-blockers are also useful for angina. This class of drugs include propranolol, atenolol, and nadolol. The longer-acting preparations (atenolol and nadolol) have the added advantage of a reduced dosage frequency, thereby, improving compliance in the elderly.[30] The β-blockers appear to exert their antianginal effect by reducing the oxygen requirement of the heart through catecholamine blockade. They are carefully prescribed for patients, especially the elderly, who suffer cardiac failure, asthma, lung disease, or insulin-dependent diabetes.[15,30] Unusually slow pulse rate (bradycardia), dizziness, light-headedness, mental confusion, or depression may all be side-effects. Hypoglycemia may go undiagnosed with the use of these drugs because β-blockade masks the clinical signs.

The use of calcium channel blockers (also called calcium antagonists and slow channel inhibitors) has broadened the therapeutic choices in the treatment of angina as well as other cardiovascular disorders. Verapamil, nifedipine, and diltiazem can be used in place of β-blockers as initial therapy, or as an alternative when β-blockers are contraindicated. Most of the adverse effects are associated with the vasodilator effects of the drugs (dizziness, light-headedness, peripheral edema, hypotension). Nifedipine, a direct vasodilator, is highly bound to protein. Verapamil is completely absorbed and metabolized rapidly in the liver through the first-pass phenomenon. On the basis of pharmacokinetic changes, both effects are important for the elderly. Dosage of all of the antianginal agents may need to be altered for the elderly.

MYOCARDIAL INFARCTION

Because in old age myocardial infarction is manifested by atypical symptoms, such as confusion, syncope, hemiparesis or dizziness, its diagnosis is sometimes difficult. Fifty percent of infarctions in elderly patients have other than classic presentations (silent infarction and noncardiac presentations).[36] In general, however, treatment of these patients is essentially the same as that of their younger counterparts. Opiates may be prescribed for pain. Lower doses in the elderly are required because of increased tissue sensitivity to the drug, increased half-life of the drug in old age and, therefore, the potential for increased side-effects. Other measures can be taken to symptomatically treat the patient.

CONGESTIVE HEART FAILURE

Congestive heart failure (CHF) is extremely common in old age, accounting for the fact that in those over 75, 18% are taking diuretics and 17% are taking digoxin.[28] Management of this disease in the elderly is not unlike that in younger patients—correction of underlying disease states, such as hypertension; bed rest; a sodium-restricted diet; and the administration of digitalis glycosides, diuretics, and vasodilators. Physical changes of decreased kidney function, decreased body size, and electrolyte abnormalities among the elderly, though, may make the elderly more susceptible to the side-effects of these drugs. Extreme attention should be given to monitoring these medications.

Digoxin is the most widely used of the digitalis preparations. Dosages of the drug range from 0.125 mg to 0.25 mg given daily. It has a low therapeutic index in and of itself but, the margin of safety with its use is probably even lower in the elderly. Several factors predispose the elderly to the drug's toxic effects. They include

1. The volume of distribution of digoxin is apparently reduced in the elderly.[15] This results in higher levels of the drug if doses are not lowered.
2. Renal function declines in the elderly. Because most patients excrete 85% of the digoxin as unchanged drug in the kidneys,[15] significant renal impairment will result in elevated levels of the drug.
3. The decrease in the glomerular filtration rate with advancing age results in higher levels of the drug.[15,28]
4. A decrease in the lean body mass[15,30] results in lower dose requirements to avoid toxicity.
5. Drug interactions with other drugs are not infrequent with the use of digoxin. Some drugs, for example diphenoxylate, may increase the absorption of digoxin, whereas others (metoclopramide) may decrease the drug's absorption. Quinidine is another example of a drug that causes an increase in the serum digoxin level by interfering with the clearance of the drug.[15,30]
6. Electrolyte imbalances may alter the reaction to the drug. Hypokalemia, which may or may not result from other drug therapy, sensitizes the heart to digitalis toxicity.[15,28] Hypercalcemia may lead to increased cardiac excitability and arrhythmia.[15]

It is not difficult to see why proper digoxin therapy is so critical. Individualized doses, good compliance, and continual monitoring of effects, all are important. Because toxic manifestations of the drug are variably related to overdose,[26] clinical symptoms relating to too much drug should immediately result in a dose reduction. The anorexia and vomiting normally seen in the younger patients as a sign of overdose may not be seen in the elderly.[15,28,30] Other toxic effects do occur, however, and can include virtually any arrhythmia (reflected in altered pulse rate and rhythm), lassitude and general weakness, severe mental depression (sometimes labeled as dementia), headache, dizziness, acute confusional states, abdominal pain, weight loss, and vision changes.[15,26,28,30] All health professionals play an important role in monitoring the toxic effects of this drug. The recognition that these signs and symptoms may be caused by drug therapy as well as the physical condition of the patient is a start in avoiding undesirable situations.

Diuretic therapy is used both as first-line drug treatment and as adjuncts to digoxin therapy in the treatment of CHF. Because toxic effects also increase in the elderly, the use of these drugs must be monitored carefully. Hydrochlorothiazide, chlorthalidone, and furosemide are just a few of the diuretics used in treating CHF. Elderly patients are sensitive to diuretics. Indeed, several studies have shown that diuretics (also being used for hypertension) are among the most widely used drugs[9,52] and that they most frequently cause unwanted side-effects in the elderly. Hyponatremia and hypovolemia, for an example, while uncommon, do occur and can result in hypotension, anxiety, vertigo, mental confusion, or drowsiness.[1,27] Other untoward effects relate to hypokalemia, decreased carbohydrate metabolism, and hyperuricemia. Side-effects of diarrhea and vomiting, muscle disorders, and an increase in gouty attacks (uric acid), therefore, should be understandable. These potential risks of side-effects are quite important in the older patient; hence, the use of diuretic therapy in the aged must be monitored closely.

Vasodilators have also been helpful in treating CHF that is refractory to digoxin and diuretic therapy. Nitrates, hydralazine, and captopril have been used for this purpose. These vasoactive drugs can similarly cause hypotension and diminished organ perfusion, so judicial use in the elderly is again needed.

In some instances, cholesterol or lipid-reducing agents are prescribed for the elderly patient with coronary artery disease (CAD). Although it is true that elevated cholesterol and triglyceride levels are a risk in the CAD, many older patients have been treated with agents such as clofibrate when the need is not really warranted. In general, if cholesterol levels are not excessively high, the elderly patient need not be treated.[30]

HYPERTENSION

Hypertension is an independent risk factor for coronary artery disease, ischemic cerebrovascular disease, congestive heart failure, and peripheral vascular disease. Unfortunately, its prevalence rises with age.[15,21] Because this disease comes with such a high risk of morbidity as well as mortality, reduction of blood pressure (diastolic below 90 mm Hg, systolic below 160 mm Hg) is necessary and is likely to reduce the incidence of the secondary complications.

Drug therapy for hypertension is usually organized in a stepwise program with the intent of administering the most effective therapy with the least number of side-effects. This is especially important for the elderly. The first step is treatment with diuretics alone. Diuretics used to treat hypertension include hydrochloro-thiazide and other thiazides, bumetanide, furosemide, amiloride, spironolactone, and triameterene. It must be remembered that the pharmacokinetics of antihypertensive drugs may be changed by the altered physiologic functions of the elderly patient (i.e., decreased kidney function, decreased liver function). In addition, it must be kept in mind that drug interactions between antihypertensive medications and other drugs can lead to harmful consequences for the patient, especially if they lead to additive hypotensive effects.

The second step is to treat the patient with diuretic therapy as well as adre-nergic inhibiting drugs (clonidine, methyldopa, guanabenz, prazosin, β-blockers, and reserpine).[15] In the elderly, concomitant diseases determine the use of one drug over another. Depression can be a side-effect of many of these medications, but it is especially seen with reserpine. Sedation is also a side-effect. Transient adverse effects of headache, orthostatic hypotension, and weakness, all can occur. Prazosin is an interesting choice for the geriatric patient. Although there can be a first-dose effect of syncope, which occurs 30 to 90 min after this first dose is given, the reduced frequency of other side-effects makes this drug useful in geriatric therapy. Guanabenz also can be useful in the elderly, causing a smaller degree of orthostatis, as long as the elderly patient can tolerate the dry mouth and sedation it may cause. The β-blockers that are used can include metaprolol, nadolol, propranolol, antenolol, pindolol, and timolol.

The third step of antihypertensive therapy involves treatment with a diuretic, plus an adrenergic inhibiting drug, plus hydralazine.[15] Although such combination therapy is warranted, this therapy for the elderly patient causes concern. The risk of drug interactions increases as the number of drugs given increases. In addition, side-effects become more prevalent especially when additive effects occur.

The fourth line of drug therapy, the potent drugs—guanethidine, minoxidil, and captopril—are added to the patient's regimen when all else fails. Because these drugs are potent and can cause serious side-effects in the elderly, especially troublesome orthostatic hypotension, they must be used with great caution.

ARRHYTHMIAS

Arrhythmias are frequent in the elderly.[30] The treatment of cardiac arrhythmias in the elderly is similar in most ways to that of the younger patient, the differences being largely in the doses employed.[15] Drugs utilized as antiarrhythmic agents include bretylium, propranolol, disopyramide, procainamide, quinidine, lidocaine, phenytoin, and verapamil. The physiologic changes of aging (renal function and liver function decline, hepatic metabolism decline, etc.) once again alter the levels of drug in the blood of the elderly patient. Doses of these drugs needs to be reduced for the elderly.

Other situations of health concern to the elderly patient that relate to cardiovascular system include *clotting disorders* and *peripheral vascular disease*. The anticoagulant, warfarin (Coumadin), occasionally may be used to treat clotting disorders. The elderly are more sensitive to the orally administered anticoagulants for several reasons.

1. These drugs are almost completely protein-bound.
2. The potential for drug interactions is great.
3. The drugs are metabolized by the mucosal enzymes of the liver.

This is one class of drugs where the pharmacokinetic changes seen with aging make a major difference. Of special concern to the physical therapist, or any other health professional, for that matter, is the most often seen side-effect of this drug, hemorrhaging. Any activity that could cause bleeding, internally or externally (even situations that usually only bruise), can be a risk for patients receiving anticoagulant therapy. Therefore, caution must be exercised to avoid potentially dangerous activities.

The drugs one might see being used to treat peripheral vascular disease are nylidrin, cyclandelate, dihydrogenated ergot alkaloids, papaverine, nicotinic acid, and isoxsuprine. Although many patients are still receiving many of these medications, their use for the purpose of improving circulation remains controversial.

Eye and Ear Diseases

GLAUCOMA

Glaucoma, primarily a disease of the elderly, affects 1 million patients in the United States.[2] It is a major cause of vision loss and, unfortunately, like hypertension, its effects are not seen until too late. Pilocarpine is usually used first by itself or in combination with epinephrine. Timolol maleate has proved to be effective, but because it is a β-blocker, some elderly patients may be sensitive to its side-effects. Acetazolamide may lower introcular pressure by decreasing the amount of aqueous humor produced, but its use is limited because of the side-effects of acidosis, lethargy, numbness and tingling in the extremities, and potassium loss.

CATARACTS, RETINAL DETACHMENT, AND EYE INFECTIONS

The treatment of cataracts, retinal detachment, and eye infections in the elderly is essentially the same as that of the younger population.

OTOLOGIC PROBLEMS

Otologic problems that occur in the elderly, such as presbycusis (hearing loss), tinnitus, and vestibular disorders, are not necessarily treated with therapeutic intervention. In fact, in some situations because of other disease conditions or multiple-drug therapy, medication use is not beneficial. Instead, an understanding explanation and recognition of the problem with ways of working around it is the best approach.

Gastrointestinal Disorders

Well over half of the older population are likely to have a *hiatal hernia*.[28] Many patients over the age of 60 have complaints of diarrhea, *constipation*, indigestion, and hemorrhoids. *Peptic ulcer disease*, although not always widely recognized as clinically significant in the geriatric population, can be a concern for patients themselves. In fact, 80% of all ulcer deaths occur in the elderly.[8] In addition *diverticulitis* occurs with increasing frequency in old age.[19] Although therapy for these concerns may not be different from that in the young, there are a few important points to be made.

Antacids are the primary choice in treating hiatal hernias, dietary indiscretion, as well as peptic ulcer disease. They appear to work by relieving pain and accelerating ulcer healing. Their use in the elderly are of special concern for several reasons. It is true that antacids are not prescription medications, but this does not mean that they are without problems. The elderly, particularly those with altered bowel function, severe organ system disease, or renal impairment, are generally susceptible to the complications of antacids.[13] These may include constipation, diarrhea, dehydration, hypercalcemia, hypermagnesemia, sodium retention, electrolyte imbalances, and possibly, neuromuscular and neurologic dysfunction.[13] Because underlying disease and multiple-drug therapy already predispose the elderly to these effects, and others, it is easy to see why self-administration of antacids should be avoided.

The four primary neutralizing ingredients found in preparations are sodium bicarbonate, calcium carbonate, aluminum salts, and magnesium salts. All generate their own individual concerns. Use of one product over the other depends on palatability, side-effects, and whether or not the patient can tolerate the preparation. Aside from the potential for side-effects, antacids also have the potential for drug-to-drug interactions. These interactions vary in intensity and significance.[13] They may affect both the absorption and the excretion of other drugs. When it is realized that the elderly patients may treat themselves with antacids for various reasons without informing the physician, this fact becomes extremely important. For example, when digoxin is not being absorbed properly because of antacid use and, therefore, is not being effective, serious complications for the patient can result. The physician may increase the dose of the drug when the need for that is not warranted. Again, it cannot be emphasized enough that antacid therapy is not innocuous, especially for the elderly.

Cimetidine and ranitidine are histamine-receptor antagonists. They act to suppress gastric acid secretion. Unfortunately, mental confusion and agranulocytosis can be complications of therapy with these drugs in the elderly.[9,19] Cimetidine-associated mental confusion can occur as belligerence or develop as slurring of speech. These effects can occur even at normal adult doses because the bioavailability of cimetidine increases with age.[15] Cimetidine-related adverse drug interactions have also been noted, especially with warfarin, diazepam, phenytoin, theophylline, and propranolol. Because of its effects on hepatic blood flow and hepatic enzyme systems, cimetidine can also interact with many other drugs. Ranitidine has not been in use as long as cimetidine and, therefore, further investigation will be needed before it can be routinely prescribed without concern for the elderly.

Anticholinergics are sometimes used in gastrointestinal disorders. However, their use in the elderly is best avoided because of their serious side-effects. Side-effects of anticholinergics (dicyclomine and the combination drug Donnatal) can include tachycardia, urinary retention, flushing, constipation, and mental confusion. The side-effects of these agents are further increased when other drugs with similar actions are also administered together (for example, antipsychotic agents).

Laxative use or "abuse" in the elderly is a real concern. Surveys indicate that the elderly are prolific users of laxatives.[5] Unfortunately, the professional guidance that is so critical in choosing a laxative is often not available or is not utilized by the elderly. When a laxative is necessary, the elderly patient who is receiving other medications should be referred to their physician for proper care. Prescription medications may be causing the constipation, in which case, the physician may alter therapy. Lack of dietary fiber may also be a cause, as may an underlying disease. When a laxative is needed, the bulk-forming laxatives or stool softeners are usually recommended with the instruction to increase fluid intake if possible.

Hormonal Disorders

DIABETES MELLITUS

Diabetes mellitus is one of the most common diseases among older people, affecting 17% of those over 65 years and 26% of those over 85.[28] Glucose tolerance, itself, is progressively impaired with advancing age,[28,43] and aging causes a decreased tissue sensitivity to insulin.[43] Therapy principles are similar to those for younger diabetic patients. Patients can be treated with diet alone, oral hypoglycemics (tolbutamide, acetohexamide, tolazamide, chlorpropamide, glipizide) and diet, or insulin. Both oral hypoglycemics and insulin, when they cause a hypoglycemic response, can place the elderly at risk for complications. If the response is severe enough, it can result in hypoglycemic coma. Other treatment measures for diabetics revolve around controlling or caring for the long-term complications of the disease, namely, retinopathy, peripheral vascular disease, and renal disease.

THYROID DYSFUNCTION

Alterations in thyroid function are responsible for a significant amount of morbidity and mortality among the elderly.[47] It is estimated that up to 30% to 35% of all cases of *hyperthyroidism* occur in patients older than 60.[44] Therapy for the disease in the elderly generally is the same as for younger patients except that the elderly are often sicker because of their chronic debilitation and associated cardiovascular problems.[44] *Hypothyroidism* also occurs in the elderly but often goes unnoticed. Therapy involves thyroid hormone replacement (L-thyroxine). Care must be taken in initiating doses in the elderly because they are particularly sensitive to the drug's effects. Angina pectoris and cardiac arrhythmias may occur because of the increase in heart rate and contractility seen with the drug.

DISORDERS OF BONE METABOLISM

Osteoporosis means decreased bone mass, but the bone remains normally mineralized. *Osteomalacia* refers to poor bone mineralization, related basically to poor calcium absorption.[35] Both quite commonly coexist to cause pain and complications for the elderly patient. Appropriate therapeutic measures are still being studied and can include estrogen therapy, calcium therapy, exercise, and fluoride therapy. They are mentioned here because of their relationship to hormone balance, especially in the female population. Side-effects of estrogen therapy are numerous.

Neurologic Disorders

CEREBROVASCULAR DISEASE

Cerebrovascular disease (CVD; stroke) is a disturbance in cerebral circulation. Its causes are many, including atherosclerosis, embolism, hypertension, intracerebral hemorrhage, and ruptured aneurysms. Hypertension, cardiac disease, elevated blood cholesterol levels, diabetes mellitus, and peripheral vascular disease are just a few of the associated medical problems that can accompany the stroke.[37] The incidence of strokes in persons over 65 is about 60: 1000; in persons over 75 the incidence is 95:1000 persons. Over 80% of the patients who suffer stroke are older than 65 years.[48] Because the disease itself includes a number of syndromes (transient ischemic attacks, thrombosis, embolism) management depends upon the type and severity of the problem. Preventative therapy is of utmost importance because once the brain tissue has infarcted, there is no means of regenerating it.

Current treatment of CVD remains to be identified. Underlying disease should be treated if that is what is causing the stroke. Vasoactive drugs, such as isoxsuprine, cyclandelate, and papaverine, have been given to patients in the hope of decreasing the frequency of stroke. Their use still remains controversial.

Anticoagulation with heparin or warfarin (Coumadin) has been used and has been useful in preventing recurrence of disease. Unfortunately, in the elderly, even close monitoring does not eliminate complications of therapy, especially hemorrhage. Finally, antiplatelet drugs (aspirin, dipyridamole, and sulfinpyrazone) may also play a useful role in preventing recurrences.

Recovery of function after a stroke is dependent primarily on physical rehabilitation of the patient. Drugs may be used to relieve muscle spasms (diazepam, baclofen, dantrolene), pain (analgesics), or depression (doxepin) associated with stroke. Psychologic support and reassurance is extremely beneficial to patients, especially for the elderly who may feel they are losing control of their lives.

EXTRAPYRAMIDAL DISORDERS

Parkinsonism is a group of neurologic disorders marked by hypokinesia, tremor, and muscular rigidity. Parkinson's disease usually begins insidiously in patients who are older than 50 years and has its onset after age 60 in about 20% of the cases.[49] It is primarily due to deficiency of dopamine in the brain.[16] Therapy, therefore, lies with replacing dopamine as much as possible to receptor sites and improving anticholinergic responses that are necessary for the functional balance between the two neurotransmitters (dopamine and acetylcholine). When treatment is needed, benztropine, an anticholinergic drug, can be used initially. The side-effects are usually minor, even in the elderly, although acute glaucoma, bladder retention, blurred vision, and confusion can occur. L-Dopa in combination with carbidopa is the most effective and most important therapy for treatment of parkinsonism. The use of carbidopa allows the administration of larger doses of L-dopa by reducing (although not eliminating) L-dopa's peripheral side-effects. The major concern with L-dopa therapy in the elderly is a drug-induced confusional state or acute psychotic reaction.[16] Other side-effects include involuntary movements, orthostatic hypotension, and vomiting. Occasionally, a patient will develop an on-off syndrome associated with long-term drug use, which results in sudden fluctuations of performance.[16] A reduction in the dosage intervals helps in some instances but, in other instances, a longer-acting drug may be prescribed. Bromocriptine, a dopamine agonist, has been used for this purpose. Its use in the elderly, however, causes concern because of its side-effects. Amantadine hydrochloride is also sometimes useful. Although it is an antiviral agent, its ability to prevent neuronal uptake of dopamine permits it to be used alone or as an adjunct to L-dopa therapy.

Other extrapyramidal disorders of the nervous system can occur and can result, unfortunately, from drug therapy. Phenothiazines, for example, have long been associated with the production of a typical parkinsonian-type syndrome. They also may be responsible for the appearance of tardive dyskinesia, or other severe dystonic movements. Some of these side-effects can be treated by removal of the drug, lowering the dose of the drug, or addition of another agent. Other side-effects are irreversible. Lower doses of any agent should be tried initially in the elderly, especially to curtail these serious side-effects.

EPILEPSY

Epilepsy, another neurologic disorder, is not infrequent in the elderly.[16] Treatment depends greatly on the type of seizure involved. Only one drug should be used, when at all possible. Phenytoin is widely used and is effective in several seizure disorders. Because it is metabolized in the liver, elderly patients require careful monitoring. It can cause ataxia, dizziness, drowsiness, or lethargy, especially in the elderly, predisposing them to falls. Other side-effects also occur. Phenobarbital is another drug used an an anticonvulsant. It, too, has side-effects harmful to the elderly, especially drowsiness and confusion. Primidone is metabolized to phenobarbital in the body and, therefore, its effects are similar to those of phenobarbital itself. Carbamazepine is not as widely used as some of the other agents, but it is still a valid choice for anticonvulsant therapy. Other drugs include valproic acid and ethosuximide. Again, therapy for the elderly patient means treatment to achieve the desired effect with as few drugs as possible. Anticonvulsant therapy, especially because of its tendency to decrease mental alertness and cause trauma resulting from falls, is no different: monitoring is necessary.

Mental Disorders

INSOMNIA

Hypnotics have been prescribed quite frequently for insomnia in the elderly. One result is that 39% of all hypnotics prescribed in the United States in 1977 were for patients over 60 years of age.[17] Unfortunately, insomnia is not concretely defined for and by the elderly. Its causes are many. Bodily discomfort associated with pain and underlying disease, overstimulation with caffeine-containing products, acute confusion, and dementia can all coexist to cause the problem. When drugs are used in the elderly, they should be used with caution, watching for the oversedation that can result. The hypnotics used for this purpose are flurazepam, clorazepate, temazepam, triazolam, and meprobamate. Barbituates, glutethimide, and chloral hydrate are also used, but they are not really recommended for the elderly.

ANXIETY

Anxiety in the elderly usually presents itself differently from anxiety at younger ages. Therapy, however, is generally similar for both aged groups. The benzodiazepines are the major class of anxiolytic agents used for all ages. The longer-acting ones are diazepam, flurazepam, chlordiazepoxide, prazepam, and nitrazepam. Increased receptor sensitivity has been demonstrated for some of these agents,[17] and, therefore, the short-acting benzodiazepines (oxazepam, lorazepam, temazepam) might be preferred in the elderly. All of the benzodiazepines may impair psychomotor performance and coordination, so their use, especially in the elderly who might already have a compromised system, must be with caution. In addition, overall central nervous system sedation with its resulting effects on the lungs and heart must be kept to a minimum. Some elderly patients respond to the benzodiazepines with an opposite response of agitation, excitability, and confusion. All of the untoward effects of these drugs can be avoided or reduced by lower doses of the drug.

DEPRESSION

Depression is common in the elderly and continues to rise with increasing age.[47] It may result from many causes, including from drugs themselves (reserpine, methyldopa, hydralazine, propranolol, levodopa, estrogen). Fortunately for the patient, the problem of depression is treatable. Tricyclic antidepressants are the most effective and the most widely prescribed agents for this purpose. They include such compounds as imipramine, desimipramine, amitriptyline, nortriptyline, protriptyline, and doxepine. Despite their effectiveness they do cause frequent problems for the elderly (urinary retention, constipation, posture hypotension, blurred vision, confusion). In addition, they are involved in many drug interactions that pose a threat to the geriatric patient who is receiving multiple-drug therapy. First-pass metabolism is extensive for these agents, and plasma protein-binding is high. The choice of one agent over the other depends on the nature of the depression as well as potential for side-effects.

The monoamine oxidase inhibitors (phenelzine, for example) are generally less effective and more hazardous than the tricyclic drugs. Their use, especially in the elderly, is not recommended. Lithium carbonate is an alternative. It should be administered in lower doses to the elderly and to debilitated or sensitive individuals because signs of toxicity can result even at normal adult doses. Toxicity includes diarrhea, vomiting, tremors, mild ataxia, drowsiness, or muscular weakness.

CONFUSION

Confusion is a symptom of a disease rather than a disorder in itself. It is a common finding that sometimes has to be treated in the elderly. The tranquilizers used for this purpose are

1. The phenothiazines—chlorpromazine, thioridazine, fluphenazine, perphenazine, prochlorperazine, and trifluoperazine
2. The thioxanthenes—thiothixine
3. The butyrophenones—haloperidol

Side-effects that are troublesome include sedation, agitation, increased confusion, parkinsonism, postural hypotension, constipation, urinary retention, and hypothermia. In general, the elderly are more susceptible to these effects and, therefore, special care is given with their administration.

DEMENTIA

Dementia, or organic brain syndrome, is the organic loss of intellectual function. It causes are numerous. Perhaps one in ten persons aged 65 and over have some degree of dementia, and its prevalence increases steeply with age, exceeding 20% in those aged 80 and over.[18] It is an extremely difficult diagnosis for the physician who must differentiate between dementia and other mental disorders, especially confusion. When the problem of dementia results in aggressive and unacceptable behavior patterns, drug therapy is frequently implemented.

Sedatives may be the first line of defense. The shorter-acting benzodiazepines (oxazepam, lorazepam) again are preferred. Occasionally, higher doses may be required to totally sedate the patient. For patients with mild dementia who develop a depressed affect, a tricyclic antidepressant (desipramine) may help. When the sedative drugs are not effective and the patient remains a management problem from the perspective of behavior, the neuroleptic agents are necessary (haloperidol, thioridazine, chlorpromazine). They are very effective against problem behavior. Their side-effects, as previously described, make them a last-choice medication. Hence, they are never just routinely prescribed across the board for everyone who has slight bothersome behavior disturbances. Patience and compassion are frequently required to serve the patient.

Respiratory and Allergic Disorders

Elderly patients are subject to the entire spectrum of respiratory diseases, and secondary factors related to the aging process with coexisting disorders make this population even more susceptible to respiratory disorders.[41] Although treatment of the elderly patients with respiratory disorders is not unlike that of younger patients, some changes have to made when secondary underlying disease or altered physiologic function coexists. Appropriate dose adjustments have to be made to minimize the potential for drug-induced toxicities.

OBSTRUCTIVE AIRWAY DISEASE

Obstructive airway disease includes asthma, bronchitis, and emphysema. Primarily, therapy with antibiotics, bronchodilators, or corticosteroids is used to treat these conditions. Antibiotic therapy will not be discussed in this chapter. The bronchodilators include theophylline, and its derivatives, as well as several sympathomimetic drugs (epinephrine, isoproterenol, metaproterenol, terbutaline, albuterol). Corticosteroid therapy with prednisone, beclomethasone, methylprednisolone, and dexamethasone can be very valuable to the patient who is in acute distress, but long-term therapy, especially for the elderly, produces a wide range of serious side-effects and, therefore, is usually avoided.

Side-effects of these drugs are numerous. Toxic effects can result quickly, especially with theophylline. The pharmacokinetic changes with aging are very important for establishing proper theophylline doses. In addition, many pathologic conditions and drugs can alter the clearance of this drug and, thereby, the half-life of the drug. Side-effects associated with theophylline toxicity include nausea, vomiting and diarrhea; nervousness, insomnia, and headache. Patients with cardiovascular disease, hyperthyroidism, and diabetes are more prone to side-effects which can include tachycardia, palpitations, hand tremor which may or may not go away, nervousness, headache, insomnia, giddiness, changes in blood glucose levels, and fall in serum potassium levels.[41] The list of adverse effects of the corticosteroids is long and well known. It will suffice to say that the elderly are also more susceptible to these effects.[41]

ALLERGIES

Allergic reactions to a wide variety of antigens occur in all age groups. Because drug-induced allergic reactions are not uncommon, a brief discussion follows. Nearly any drug can cause an allergic reaction in one or more individuals. When the offending agent can be stopped without compromise to the patient, then this is the action of choice. If the drug is necessary, however, then the patient must either live with the allergic response or appropriate antihistamines can be prescribed. Diphenhydramine and cyproheptadine are just two examples. Although these drugs do not cause real concern in the general population, their use in the elderly patient may bring too much sedation to warrant their routine use. Caution, again, is thus especially necessary for the older patient.

Treatment of Painful Conditions

THE ARTHRITIDES

Osteoarthritis, rheumatoid arthritis, and *ankylosing spondylitis* are very debilitating diseases, especially for the elderly patient. The incidence of osteoarthritis (degenerative joint disease) is age-related. Eighty-five to one hundred percent of people over 70 years old develop this type of arthritis.[12] Although rheumatoid arthritis develops for the first time in only about 10% of the cases,[53] the frequency of long-term effects is actually much higher among the elderly. It is these long-term effects that pose a problem for the health care providers concerned with the patient.

Arthritic therapies require interprofessional involvement because supportive care is especially important. Aside from the medicinal measures than can help relieve the pain and inflammation associated with the disease, there are physical and occupational therpeutic modalities that can improve a patient's situation tremendously. In many patients, the intervention of physical therapy (rest, exercise, splinting) maintains or restores joint function, preventing deformities of the joint and, thereby, controlling the progression of the debilitation. In other patients, however, little or no improvement is seen, even with medical intervention.

The role of medicinal therapy for all of these diseases is symptomatic relief of pain and inflammation. Therapy must always be individualized, especially for the elderly patient. Concomitant disease should be considered in drug selection to avoid exacerbation with the antirheumatic drugs (i.e., ulcer disease, renal failure, hypertension).[12] In addition, the less toxic drugs should be used first in the hopes of minimizing side-effects. Treatment for the various arthritic diseases is similar. More aggressive therapy may be needed in rheumatoid arthritis, but that is not always true. The elderly, because of multiple diseases, aging, and pharmacokinetic changes, can respond to drug therapy in a manner different from that of younger adults.[12] Despite this fact therapy for both aged groups is very similar. A list of the major drugs used to treat arthritis can be seen in Table 7-1.

Simple analgesics, such as acetaminophen and aspirin in small doses, can be initially used to relieve pain. The salicylates remain the principal anti-inflammatory and analgesic agents used. Buffered aspirin (600 mg to 1200 mg four times a day) taken with food is very effective and quite often used. The high doses necessary, however, may put the elderly at risk for salicylate toxicity. If ataxia, tinnitus, confusion, and deafness occur, drug overdose should not be ruled out. Side-effects from salicylates are not that much different from other anti-inflammatory medications. They include gastrointestinal distress and gastrointestinal bleeding. This is of special importance to patients taking blood thinners. Aspirin and other nonsteroidal anti-inflammatory medications should not be used in patients receiving warfarin. Choline magnesium trisalicylate may be tried instead. Other salicylate products include salsalate and diflunisal.

The nonsteroidal anti-inflammatory drugs (NSAIDs) are the next choice for inflammatory control. The propionic acid compounds (fenoprofen, ibuprofen, naproxen) are usually prescribed initially when the inflammation is not marked.[6,12] Other agents similar to these drugs in terms of anti-inflammatory effects are meclofenamate, sulindac, and mefenamic acid. For conditions in which the inflammation is prominent, such as acute conditions of rheumatoid arthritis, more potent NSAIDs are utilized. Indomethacin falls into this category. Unfortunately, this drug is poorly tolerated by the elderly, causing dizziness, disorientation, and severe headaches. Tolmetin also has been used. Piroxicam is newer anti-inflammatory agent that can be given once daily to patients with compliance problems.

Most patients usually respond similarly to all NSAIDs, but one patient can respond quite differently to one category of drugs versus another one (i.e., aspirin, versus ibuprofen, versus sulindac).[12] Because this can occur, a patient is often switched from one drug to the next in an effort to attain the maximum benefits from therapy. Side-effects of the NSAIDs, as a class, can include symptoms of gastrointestinal

TABLE 7-1
Drugs Used to Treat Osteoarthritis and Rheumatoid Arthritis

Drug Class	Generic Name	Trade Name(s)
Simple analgesics (relief of pain only)	Acetaminophen	Tylenol
	Aspirin (in low doses)	
	Codeine	
Salicylates	Aspirin/buffered aspirin	
	Choline magnesium salicylate	Trilisate
	Salsalate	Disalcid
	Diflunisal	Dolobid
Nonsteroidal anti-inflammatory drugs	Fenoprofen	Nalfon
	Ibuprofen	Motrin, Rufen
	Naproxen	Naprosyn, Anaprox
	Indomethacin	Indocin
	Tolmetin	Tolectin
	Sulindac	Clinoril
	Oxyphenylbutazone	Tandearil
	Mefenamic acid	Ponstel
	Meclofenamate	Meclomen
	Piroxicam	Feldene
Gold salts	Aurothioglucose	Solganol
	Aurothiomalate	Myochrysine
Penicillamine	Cuprimine	
Chloroquine	Chloroquine phosphate	Aralen
	Hydroxychloroquine sulfate	Plaquenil
Corticosteroids	Prednisone	
	Prednisolone	
Cytotoxic drugs	Azathioprine	Imuran
	Cyclophosphamide	Cytoxan)

upset and bleeding, skin rash, weight gain because of sodium retention, dizziness, as well as persistent headaches. These side-effects can be another reason for switching a patient from one drug to another. The newer anti-inflammatory medications may be better suited for the elderly patient than high doses of aspirin. Lower doses and less frequent dosage regimens can mean better compliance and fewer side-effects for the patient.[11] There is another problem associated with NSAID therapy, however, that relates to the drugs' therapeutic effects and not to their side-effects. Arthritic patients who are being treated with analgesics and anti-inflammatory medications always present the concern of "overuse" of their joints because pain and trauma is being masked by a drug's effects. Special care, therefore, must be provided in dealing with the arthritic patient who may be receiving drug therapy.

Thus far, the discussion of antiarthritic medications has been limited to the drugs that are used in both osteoarthritis and rheumatoid arthritis. The remaining medications reviewed, however, are very potent and are used primarily in rheumatoid arthritis. When the progression of rheumatoid arthritis in a patient is resistant to aspirin or NSAID therapy, more aggressive measures may be required to modify the course of the disease. Gold therapy with aurothiglucose or aurothiomalate may be beneficial, even in the elderly. The most common toxic reactions are rashes and mouth ulcers, of which less than 5% are serious.[6] Penicillamine, which is effective, can also cause rashes and mouth ulcers, in addition to a transient loss of taste. Most of its toxic effects disappear when the drug is stopped. Chloroquine and hydroxychloroquine, two antimalarial agents, have also been helpful in some patients. All of these medications, although necessary for some people, pose concern for the sensitive system of the elderly patient. They should be used only if absolutely necessary.

Steroids, such as prednisone or prednisolone, produce an immediate effect on inflammation. Their use in the elderly, however, is normally restricted to short-term therapy. Side-effects and toxicities are numerous and troublesome to the elderly, especially for those who already have a high prevalence of osteoporosis, fluid retention, hypertension, peptic ulcer disease, and thin, friable skin.[6]

Occasionally, cytoxic agents will be used in severe, progressive rheumatoid arthritis. Azothioprine and cyclophosphamide are the drugs frequently used. Because they have considerably toxic effects, they are used only for the more severe, life-threatening or crippling stages of the disease.

Gout, which is marked by hyperurecemia, is another arthritic disease that is common in the elderly. Drug therapy for the elderly is essentially the same as that for the younger patient. Side-effects, of course, may be more frequent in the older patient and, therefore, drug use must again be monitored. Indomethacin, ibuprofen, and colchicine, all induce a favorable response in acute attacks. Allupurinol and probenecid may help in long-term treatment. Aspirin should not be used for this condition.

CANCER

Pain management in the *cancer patient* is different from other types of chronic pain management. First of all, the concern of tolerance and addiction is not a consideration. Second, the pain is prevented from occurring by more frequent and varied dosages (as opposed to treatment as the pain occurs). There is no maximum effective dose, as a rule. Finally, the narcotic agents are usually prescribed, rather than the less-potent analgesics, which do not provide enough relief. Narcotic analgesics often include hydromorphone, codeine, oxycodone, methadone, meperidine, and pentazocine. Brompton's mixture is a liquid preparation that may include one of these drugs alone or in combination with other ingredients. The most worrisome side-effect of the narcotic analgesics is respiratory depression. Loss of diminished mental faculties can also be a problem for the patient who is older. The use of these drugs should not be eliminated because of these effects. Instead, extra care is needed in watching for the exaggeration of these effects. It is important that chronic pain of any origin be treated appropriately, not only for the comfort of the patient but also for the protection of the patient. Self-imposed immobility can easily cause further complications (joint contractures leading to disability, falls in avoiding use of the joint). Therapy, despite its concerns, therefore, is beneficial.

NEURALGIA

Trigeminal neuralgia can create an excruciatingly painful episode for the elderly patient who has this condition. Carbamazepine, the mainstay of treatment, is effective in 70% of patients.[28] Dizziness and drowsiness have been associated with its use. Phenytoin, an agent used primarily for seizures and other disorders, has also been used effectively.

Summary

As one reviews the drug therapy of common medical problems just discussed, it is easy to see that there are many drugs that can be prescribed for the older patient. This therapeutic intervention has added tremendously to the improved medical care provided over the years to increase the life expectancy of individuals. In 1900, an American could expect to die at an average age of 47 years. In 1981, that age had been increased to 73 years old.[29] The aim of continuing this trend for the future has to rest on educating the young and old alike, educating them not only about the diseases themselves and the proper use of the medications needed to treat those diseases but also teaching preventative measures.

The elderly, quite naturally, are the beneficiaries of good therapeutic intervention. The proper management of chronic illnesses (utilizing physician, pharmacist, physical therapist, occupational therapist, and nurses) can help greatly in improving the quality of life of our older people. In providing this good health care, all medical professionals must realize the uniqueness of the elderly patient. Furthermore, one must realize that despite the benefits of drug therapy, there are also some concerns.

The aged are more sensitive to drugs than younger individuals. This sensitivity lies with a combination of factors, which have already been discussed in detail. Briefly, though, the elderly are more likely to have multiple diseases that can alter the way the body handles the drug.[24,30,37] They are also more likely to take a large number of different drugs. This not only increases the risk of adverse drug reactions, but it also increases the risk of drug interactions. Add to this the aging processes with its physiologic changes that alter pharmacokinetics, and there is indeed a unique individual, one that may have difficulty in handling the drugs administered. Understanding this sensitivity to medications and combining it with the knowledge of how drugs actually do act in the body, can add to the medical care provided to the older patient. All health care professionals can take their part in providing quality care to the aged by being aware of these changes, being aware of how drugs affect the elderly differently, and being aware of all the factors that interplay to make the older patient different.

ADVERSE REACTIONS

Before we conclude this discussion of common concerns with drug therapy in the geriatric population, it is important that we discuss two additional problems. The first is adverse reactions from drug therapy. The second, to be discussed in the next section, is drug interactions. The elderly are highly susceptible to adverse drug reactions (side-effects and toxicities) and drug interactions. It is these responses that result in the unpredictability for the overall actions of the drugs.[24]

Side-effects are real. Besides the desired therapeutic effect of a drug (purpose for which the drug is given), there are, or can be, undesirable effects. These are untoward or adverse reactions of drug therapy. When prescribing a medication for a patient, the physician must decide whether or not the benefits of the drug's action outweigh the risk of the potential side-effects. This consideration is especially important for the elderly patient, as mentioned over and over again, who is sensitive to these effects.

The prevalence of adverse reactions does indeed increase with advancing age and, in addition, these effects seem to be more severe in the older patient than in their younger counterparts.[23] The reasons for the high prevalence of adverse drug reactions in old age again include all of the factors that have been discussed throughout this chapter. It has also been indicated that as the number of drugs used increases, so does the risk of the side-effects.[7,28] To combat this problem, the physician attempts to prescribe the smallest number of medications with the least number of side-effects.

Despite these attempts to improve the situation, some side-effects are going to occur. Side-effects are either allergic responses, exaggerated responses or the desired therapeutic effects (toxicities), or undesirable effects of the drug's activity. Sedation from antihistamines or anticholinergic actions of tricyclic antidepressants, for example, are responses to the drug's activity on other tissues or organ systems other than the intended site of action. Hypoglycemia from antidiabetic medications, on the other hand, may result from too much of the drug's intended effect. In all situations, side-effects can be anticipated and appropriately handled in the older patient if adjustments to therapy are made by taking into consideration the patient's altered drug responses and increased sensitivity to drugs.

There are several selected side-effects that are of special concern to therapists. These include postural hypotension, fatigue and weakness, depression, confusion, dementia, involuntary movements, dizziness and vertigo, ataxia, and bladder and bowel incontinence.[7,11] Almost any drug can cause one or more of these effects, but the drugs most commonly associated with adverse reactions in the elderly are analgesics, antibiotics, anticoagulants, antidepressants, antihypertensives, antiparkinsonian drugs, antipsychotics, bronchodilators, digoxin, diuretics, NSAIDs, oral hypoglycemia agents, and sedative–hypnotic drugs.[38] Unfortunately for the elderly, these are the same drugs used to treat the common medical problems found in their population. From the list of side-effects mentioned and the knowledge of the disease states themselves, it is sometimes hard to discern between drug effects and disease effects. If, however, the precipitating factor is due to a drug effect and the appropriate measures are taken, the patient can benefit greatly from behavioral changes and by having locomotor impairments or declines in mental and functional abilities reversed or returned to normal.

HYPOTENSION

Postural hypotension is probably more common in the elderly than in any other age group.[7] The term itself means that the systemic blood pressure falls upon assumption of an erect posture.[10] This is a serious disorder that can cause potential falls, fractures, immobility, and increased dependency, as well as cerebral and cardiac infarctions. Because the sensitivity of baroreceptors is decreased in the elderly such that there is already poor compensation for sudden postural changes or alterations in homeostatic mechanisms,[10,30] any additional impairment of this mechanism will further place the patient at risk for complications. There are many known causes of orthostatic hypotension, and this makes management of the condition difficult. Drugs should never be ruled out. Table 7-2 lists a number of drugs that can cause postural hypotension.

FATIGUE AND WEAKNESS

Other concerns for the therapist are the general complaints of *fatigue and weakness*. These are common complaints with the elderly and may have either physiologic or emotional causes.[7] Underlying disease can be a contributing factor. Among the diseases that are common to the older patient, cardiovascular disease, diabetes, depression, and arthritis might be seen to cause these complaints. Unfortunately, the role of drugs as an additional factor is often overlooked.

β-Blockers, because of their ability to slow down the heart and reduce blood flow to muscle, are a common source of fatigue. This effect may, or may not, disappear after time. Diuretics, too, are implicated in weakness and fatigue. They can cause dehydration, decrease blood volume, decrease cardiac output, or cause hypokalemia or hyponatremia, all of which produce the debilitating effects. Many drugs that have overall sedative effects can also add to these feelings. For the therapist, it is paramount to determine whether the effects can be alleviated through altered drug therapy or whether they are a cause of disease. Any attempt to treat the patient for drug-induced fatigue and weakness, if the drug is going to be continued in that patient, is hopeless. Vasodilators, digoxin, antihypertensives, and oral hypoglycemic agents may also interfere through various mechanisms and cause general weakness and a feeling of fatigue. In general, the drugs that are indicated in postural hypotension, can also cause these complaints.

DEPRESSION

Depressive illness is another concern with the elderly. Without going into the many factors involved in its presence, suffice it to say that drugs can cause *depressive reactions*. Because depressed individuals lack motivation, show disinterest, or even refuse to cooperate in therapy, recognition of drug-induced depression is important. Guanethidine, clonidine, hydralazine, methyldopa, and propranolol, all have been known to cause depression. Additionally, reserpine, levodopa, amantadine, diazepam, and glutethimide can also create a problem. Any drug that has adverse effects on brain function can contribute to depression. This includes drugs that have obvious direct effects, as well as those with effects that indirectly alter a patient's response.

CONFUSION

Sudden changes in cognitive function or behavior may result from adverse reactions to a number of drugs. Most drug-induced disorientation seen in geriatric practice is caused by cardiac glycosides, antiparkinsonian and antidepressant drugs, anticholinergic drugs, hypoglycemic agents, anti-inflammatory drugs, or analgesics.[38] Digitalis toxicity results in confusion, depression, and hallucinations. Barbiturates, diazepam, and oxazepam, by virtue of their central nervous system effects, can often cause drug-induced confusion; so can benztropine and trihexphenidyl, drugs used to manage parkinsonism, as well as amantadine, levodopa, and bromocriptine. Antidepressants, phenothiazines, and antispasmodic drugs, because of their anticholinergic activity, may also lead to delirium. Patients receiving cimetidine or

TABLE 7-2
Drugs That Can Cause Postural Hypotension

Drug Class	Examples
Tricyclic antidepressants (depression)	Amitriptyline
	Nortriptyline
	Desipramine
	Doxepin
	Imipramine
	Amoxapine
	Trimipramine
Tranquilizers (psychotic behavior)	Chlorpromazine
	Thioridazine
	Mesoridazine
Antihypertensive drugs	Prazosin
	Guanethidine
	Methyldopa
Diuretics (hypertension, CHF)	Hydrochlorothiazide
	Chlorthalidone
	Furosemide
Nitrates (angina)	Isosorbide dinitrate
	Nitroglycerin
	Pentaerythritol tetranitrate
Narcotic analgesics	Codeine
	Hydromorphone
	Meperidine
	Methadone
	Oxycodone
	Pentazocine
Vasodilators (peripheral vascular disease, hypertension)	Isoxsuprine
	Nicotinic acid
	Dipyridamole
	Hydralazine
	Nylidrin
	Cyclandelate
	Papaverine
β-Blockers (hypertension, cardiovascular disease)	Atenolol
	Metaprolol
	Nadolol
	Propranolol
	Timolol
Channel blockers (cardiovascular disease)	Verapamil
	Nifedipine
	Diltiazem
Levodopa (Parkinson's disease)	
Sedative–hypnotics (insomnia, anxiety, behavioral disturbances)	Diazepam
	Clorazepate
	Glutethimide
	Flurazepam
Antiarrhythmic drugs (cardiovascular disease)	Propranolol
	Disopyramide
	Procainamide
	Lidocaine

indomethacin have also manifested signs of confusion. It is interesting how large the list is of those drugs associated with confusional reactions in the elderly.

DEMENTIA

Dementia is a syndrome characterized by loss of intellectual abilities of sufficient severity to interfere with social and occupational functioning.[38] Both drug-induced confusion and drug-induced dementia are important to therapists. If an individual manifests any form of dementia, drug-induced changes that could result in that dementia cannot be ignored. Any drug that causes confusion can, with exaggerated drug levels, ultimately cause signs of dementia. This does not imply that it is not reversible. Sedative agents, hypnotics, and tranquilizers can cause concerns for the elderly, especially if the drugs are allowed to accumulate in the body. Diazepam, as one example, is a drug that is widely prescribed for the elderly, despite the fact that it can impair mental function and behavioral responses, even at normal adult doses. When the drug activity is prolonged because of pharmacokinetic changes, the excessive sedation, as well as paradoxic reactions of restlessness or psychosis, can often render the patient dependent and institutionalized.

DISORIENTATION AND MOVEMENT DISORDERS

The side-effect of drug induced *involuntary movements* has already been discussed for a number of drugs including chlorpromazine, fluphenazine, haloperidol, loxapine, perphenazine, trifluoperazine, and thiothixene.[7] These are all antipsychotic medications. Additionally, other drugs act to either exaggerate or initiate such effects: lithium carbonate, levodopa, anticholinergics, tricyclic antidepressants, and adrenergic drugs like isoproteronol and theophylline. The most troublesome drug-induced involuntary movements are those caused by the antipsychotic agents. Drug-induced parkinsonism (extrapyramdial symptoms) is a commonly encountered clinical problem after the administration of antipsychotic medication, especially in the elderly. Choreiform movement disorders are five times more frequent in the elderly than in the young and are not always reversible when the medication is stopped.[53] Other movement disorders, including tardive dyskinesia, akathisia, and tremor are also due to these agents. There is a wide spectrum of diability associated with these effects, disabilities that must be directly dealt with by the therapist.

Dizziness and vertigo are "real" symptoms for the geriatric patient. Although vertigo is defined separately from the nonspecific complaint of dizziness, both seem to appear together as one general problem. They are a concern primarily because of their ability to cause falls, produce feelings of inadequacy and dependency, as well as their ability to frustrate and confuse the patient. Patients themselves may not describe these effects in terms of dizziness but, rather, may complain of giddiness, light-headedness, or even faintness. Recent studies in patients over the age of 60 have shown drugs to be a major cause of dizziness.[7] Drugs can produce these symptoms by either direct effects on the brain or indirect effects that alter motor coordination and response. The list of drugs that can cause dizziness and vertigo in the elderly is almost as endless as those that cause confusion. Antibiotics, NSAIDs, benzodiazepines, β-blockers, cimetidine, barbiturates, and hypoglycemic agents are only the beginning. These symptoms should be very troublesome to the professional who must work directly with a patient's coordination and ability. If a drug-induced response is not corrected, no amount of therapy will help.

Ataxia concerns the irregularities in muscular coordination. Again, drugs can be a contributing factor. Almost any drug that has a sedative effect on the central nervous system can be a problem. Therefore, hypnotics and sedatives would be likely candidates. Benzodiazepines are especially troublesome; diazepam exerts exaggerated responses in the elderly population. Ataxia is just one of those responses. Other drugs of concern include alcohol, carbamazepine, levodopa, lithium, and indomethacin.

INCONTINENCE

Finally, one more problem that can be associated with drug use is *incontinence*. Although it is an effect that may have to be tolerated with many drugs, the therapist can find ways of working around the problem if it is drug-induced. Diuretics, for an example, can cause incontinence, especially for the geriatric patient who cannot move quickly enough to avoid it. It may be advisable, therefore, to suggest that the patients take their medicine well in advance of the therapy session or after the therapy. Bowel incontinence can similarly be avoided if laxatives are being used by the patient.

These are side-effects of primary concern to the therapist. Although they may not be all-inclusive, they are a start in the recognition that drugs "can present themselves as obstacles to successful rehabilitation."[7] The input from the therapist is extremely beneficial to the patient.

DRUG INTERACTIONS

Drug interactions are as real as side-effects, especially for the elderly. Their potential in causing problems for the geriatric patient cannot be emphasized enough. Drug interactions occur when the effect of one drug is inhibited or potentiated by the prior or concurrent administration of another drug.[32] With this basic concept in mind, it is easy to see the cause for concern with the elderly. Not enough drug means that the illness is not being treated: too much drug produces toxicities in patients who already have compromised systems. It is beyond the scope of this chapter to deal with all of the possible drug-to-drug interactions that occur. Perhaps, instead, an understanding of the mechanisms involved can help to develop an appreciation for the concern and the magnitude of the problem.

These mechanisms are easily discussed in list form:

1. *Alterations in absorption of the drug.* Any factor that alters the rate or degree of absorption may affect the performance of the drug. Therefore, changes in *p*H, changes in gastrointestinal motility, and the presence of interfering compounds, all can alter a drug's absorption. Antacids, for example, can alter the absorption of several drugs. They decrease the absorption of tetracycline by chelating the antibiotic, thereby making it unabsorbable. They can also change the *p*H of the stomach and alter absorption that way. Anticholinergics decrease gastrointestinal motility and can reduce the absorption or increase absorption of drugs. Most drug interactions interfering with absorption can be avoided by proper timing of dosage regimens.
2. *Alterations in distribution.* Because both pharmacologic and toxic responses are dependent on the amount of free drug in the plasma, any factor that alters

distribution will also alter the drug response. Because there are only a limited number of protein-binding sites available to a drug in the plasma, a competition will exist between two drugs that tend to bind with the same proteins. This ultimately results in the displacement of one drug from those sites. The drug having a greater affinity for the binding site will displace the other, resulting in the latter's exaggerated therapeutic response. Remember that this was a concern with warfarin (anticoagulant).

3. *Alterations in drug metabolism.* Many drug interactions result from the ability of one drug to stimulate the metabolism of another. Phenobarbital increases the rate of metabolism of warfarin, decreasing the anticoagulant effect. Other drug metabolism interactions are due to one drug inhibiting the metabolism of another. Tolbutamide metabolism is inhibited by warfarin, resulting in exaggerated hypoglycemia.

4. *Alterations in urinary excretion.* Because most drugs and drug metabolites are excreted by renal mechanisms, any drug-induced alteration in renal function may alter drug activity. Probenecid blocks the tubular excretion of penicillin and maintains higher levels in the body longer than normal. (This interaction is used to an advantage in some instances.) Urinary *p*H also can alter drug excretion. Basic drugs are excreted more rapidly in an acidic urine and more slowly in a basic urine. The converse is also true.

5. *Opposing pharmacologic effect.* This is a pharmacodynamic interaction resulting when two drugs have opposing effects either at one receptor site or different sites. Combinations of a narcotic with a narcotic antagonist or a vasoconstrictor with a vasodilator will result in no net effect on the intended response.

6. *Similar pharmacologic effect.* This is also a pharmacodynamic response. The result, however, is exaggerated pharmacologic effects or toxic effects of the drug. Benzodiazepines with alcohol can produce a profound oversedation, especially in the elderly. Antihistamines, antidepressants, and antipsychotics given together can cause real problems because of additive anticholinergic effects.

7. *Alteration of electrolyte levels.* Diuretics can cause hypokalemia. This presents a special problem to patients who are also being treated with digoxin. If the hypokalemia goes untreated, the heart may become more sensitive to the effects of digitalis, and arrhythmia may result. Sodium depletion, in addition, has been known to enhance lithium toxicity. Measures can be taken in both instances to compensate for the interaction.

There may be still other mechanisms of drug interactions. Open communication among all care givers is necessary in eliminating the potential for such interactions. Although it is impossible to recognize all of the interactions, it is important to know that they can and do exist.

Rehabilitation is the ultimate restoration of a disabled person to his maximum capacity (physical, emotional, and vocational).[7] For the elderly however, this may need to be slightly redefined. Because there are other factors involved in improvement of the patient, rehabilitation goals with the elderly may be set at returning the patients to their premorbid state. In addition, vocational considerations may not be a concern. To accomplish the task of rehabilitation in the elderly, then, the therapist must be able to assess the patient's ability as well as the patient's disabilities. Within this assessment, a patient's medication profile must be considered carefully and the many factors of drug therapy recognized. Proper rehabilitation, therefore, cannot be started effectively until a *total* assessment of the patient's condition is evaluated. Multiple abnormalities and multiple-drug therapy will dictate differences in patient handling and patient response. Certain treatment regimens may be indicated for some patients but contraindicated for others. The pace of the rehabilitation process may change because the patient may not be able to move as quickly as anticipated or may not have the endurance needed for the set activity. Prognosis, too, may be altered because of chronic illness or drug therapy. Whatever the changes are, patience is the key to helping the older person. Professionals must take the time required to investigate the entire history of the patient. Remember that drug interactions or side effects do occur, and although medications have improved a patient's health picture, they can also adversely influence the ability of a successful rehabilitation program. Whatever the indication is for drug therapy, or regardless of the therapist's position, any health professional who has a substantial contribution to make in the care and well-being of the older patient must recognize that drugs do play a part. A flexible, well-planned program with positive objectives must include this thought.

CASE 1   Mrs. RJ has been referred to an outpatient physical therapy clinic for treatment of cervical arthritis with resultant muscle spasms, pain, and functional difficulty. Mrs. RJ is recently widowed and has left her home to move into a retirement highrise in the city. She has been to several doctors for treatment of her complaints of weakness, tiredness, abdominal, occupital, neck, and arm pains as well as insomnia. The first doctor she saw gave her a prescription for flurazepam (Dalmane) 15–30 mg h.s. She felt this did not help and went to a second doctor who prescribed physical therapy and diazepam (Valium) 5–10 mg t.i.d. She has taken the medication for several days.

Her initial evaluation revealed somewhat unusual behavior, slight slurring of speech, as well as a rather odd staggering gait.

Upon returning home the evening of her first visit to physical therapy, she collapsed when entering her apartment building. She was immediately taken to the hospital where she became noisy and agitated. The hospital gave her 10 mg i.m. diazepam and returned her home with a referral to a geriatrician as a "social problem."

The geriatrician readmitted Mrs. RJ to the hospital where all drugs were discontinued. During the 10-day stay, her speech, gait, and mental functions all improved. She was discharged home without medications and directed to restart her physical therapy program.

CASE 2   Mrs. RW, a 72-year-old woman, was referred to a therapist by her family physician for treatment of an arthritic disability. She was doing quite well with her rehabilitation, showing improvement in mobility and capability. At that time she was receiving no long-term drug therapy except piroxicam (Feldene) once daily for her arthritis.

While on vacation, she visited a physician for treatment of a cold. She was found to have an elevated blood pressure — 170/110 mm Hg. Hydrochlorothiazide 50 mg was prescribed once daily. The doctor did not see the need to treat the cold.

Several days later, Mrs. RW returned from her vacation and went for another therapy session. Upon the start of her exercises, she fell and injured her hip. She was taken to her family doctor. X-ray examination revealed, fortunately, no fractures in the bone.

After questioning Mrs. RW at great length, it was found that she had been feeling light-headed, weak, and had fallen several times over the past few days. Hydrochlorothiazide was reduced to 25 mg daily and within a few days her normal physical ability had returned. Her blood pressure was under control, and her complaint, now discovered to be postural hypotension, had stopped.

REFERENCES

1. Barbagallo-Sangiorgi G, DiSciancia A, Frada G Jr et al: Diuretic therapy in old patients. In Barbagallo-Sangiorgi G, Exton-Smith AN (eds): Aging and Drug Therapy. New York, Plenum Press, 1984
2. Bienfang D, Glaucoma. In Walshe TM (ed): Manual of Clinical Problems in Geriatric Medicine. Boston, Little, Brown & Co, 1985
3. Blazer D: Depression in the Late Life. Philadelphia, CV Mosby, 1982
4. Boyd JR: Therapeutic dilemmas in the elderly. In Covington TR, Walker JI (eds): Current Geriatric Therapy. Philadelphia, WB Saunders, 1984
5. Brocklehurst JC: Gastrointestinal systems. In Brocklehurst JC (ed): Geriatric Pharmacology and Therapeutics. Boston, Blackwell Scientific Publications, 1984
6. Castleden CM: Analgesics. In Brocklehurst JC (ed): Geriatric Pharmacology and Therapeutics. Boston, Blackwell Scientific Publications, 1984
7. Chapron DJ: Drugs: An obstacle to rehabilitation of the elderly. In Jackson O (ed): Physical Therapy of the Geriatric Patient. New York, Churchill-Livingston, 1983
8. Chopra S, Curtis RL: Gastritis and peptic ulcer. In Walshe TM (ed): Manual of Clinical Problems in Geriatric Medicine. Boston, Little, Brown & Co, 1985
9. Christopher LJ, Ballinger BR, Shepherd AMM et al: Survey of hospital prescribing for the elderly. In Crooks J, Stevenson IH (eds): Drugs and the Elderly. London, Macmillan, 1979
10. Davison W: Treatment of orthostatic hypotension. In Barbagallo-Sangiorgi G, Exton-Smith AN (eds): Aging and Drug Therapy. New York, Plenum Press, 1984
11. Ehrlich: Diagnostic and management of rheumatic diseases in older patients. J Am Geriatr Soc 30:545-551, 1982
12. Evans RP, Hawkins DW: Bone and joint disorders. In Covington TR, Walker JI (eds): Current Geriatric Therapy. Philadelphia, WB Saunders, 1984
13. Gerbino PO, Gans JA: Antacids and laxatives for symptomatic relief in the elderly. J Am Geriatr Soc 30:S81-S87, 1982
14. Hodkinson HM: Common Symptoms of Disease in the Elderly, 2nd ed. London, Blackwell Scientific Publications, 1980
15. Hoy RH, Ponte CD: Cardiovascular disorders. In Covington TR, Walker JI (eds): Current Geriatric Therapy, Philadelphia, WB Saunders, 1984
16. Hyams DE: Central nervous system—antiparkinsonian and antiepileptic drugs, use of drugs in stroke. In Brocklehurst JC (ed): Geriatric Pharmacology and Therapeutics. Boston, Blackwell Scientific Publications, 1984

17. Hyams DE: Central nervous system—anxiolytics and hypnotics. In Brocklehurst JC (ed): Geriatric Pharmacology and Therapeutics. Boston, Blackwell Scientific Publications, 1984
18. Hyams DE: Central nervous system—dementia. In Brocklehurst JC (ed): Geriatric Pharmacology and Therapeutics. Boston, Blackwell Scientific Publications, 1984
19. Jacknowitz AI: Gastrointestinal disorders. In Covington TR, Walker JI (eds): Current Geriatric Therapy. Philadelphia, WB Saunders, 1984
20. KodaKimble MA, Katcher BS, Young LY (eds): Applied Therapeutics, 2nd ed. San Francisco, Applied Therapeutics, Inc. 1978.
21. LaBresh KA, Pietro DA: Hypertension in the elderly. In Walshe TM (ed): Manual of Clinical Problems in Geriatric Medicine. Boston, Little, Brown & Co, 1985
22. Lamy PP. Comparative pharmacokinetic changes and drug therapy in an older population. J Am Geriatr Soc 30:S11–S19, 1982
23. Lamy PP: Modifying drug dosage in elderly patients. In: Covington TR, Walker JI (eds): Current Geriatric Therapy. Philadelphia, WB Saunders, 1984
24. Lamy PP: Therapeutics and an older population: A pharmacists's perspective. J Am Geriatr Soc 30:S3–S5, 1982
25. Lamy PP: Prescribing for The Elderly. Littleton, Mass, PSG Publishing 1980.
26. Lye MDW: Cardiovascular system—digitalis glycosides. In Brocklehurst JC (ed): Geriatric Pharmacology and Therapeutics. Boston, Blackwell Scientific Publications, 1984
27. Lye MDW: Cardiovascular system—diuretics. In Brocklehurst JC (ed): Geriatric Pharmacology and Therapeutics. Boston, Blackwell Scientific Publications, 1984
28. MacLennan WJ, Shepherd AN, Stevenson IH: The Elderly. Berlin, Heidelberg, Great Britain, Springer-Verlag 1984
29. McGlone FB: Therapeutics and an older population: A physician's perspective. J Am Geriatr Soc 30:S1–S2, 1982
30. Moser M: The management of cardiovascular disease in the elderly. J Am Geriatr Soc 30:S20–S29, 1982
31. Myers-Robfogel MW, Bosmann HB: Clinical pharmacology in the aged—aspects of pharmacokinetics and drug sensitivity. In Williams TF (ed): Rehabilitation in the Aging. New York, Raven Press, 1984.
32. O'Hara NM, White DM: Drugs and the elderly. In Lewis CB (ed): Aging: The Health Care Challenge. Philadelphia, FA Davis, 1985
33. Palmore E: The myth of aging quiz. Gerontologist 19, 1980
34. Pietro DA: Treatment of congestive heart failure. In Walshe TM (ed): Manual of Clinical Problems in Geriatric Medicine. Boston, Little, Brown & Co, 1985
35. Pohl JEF: Hormones. In Brocklehurst JC (ed): Boston, Blackwell Scientific Publications, 1984
36. Pietro DA: Coronary disease in the elderly. In Walshe TM (ed): Manual of Clinical Problems in Geriatric Medicine. Boston, Little, Brown & Co, 1985
37. Price SA, Wilson LM: Pathophysiology—Clinical Concepts of Disease Processes. New York, McGraw-Hill, 1978
38. Robertson D: Adverse drug reactions in the elderly. In Brocklehurst JC (ed): Geriatric Pharmacology and Therapeutics. Boston, Blackwell Scientific Publications, 1984
39. Robertson D: Drug handling in old age. In Brocklehurst JC (ed): Geriatric Pharmacology and Therapeutics. Boston, Blackwell Scientific Publications, 1984
40. Rogers ES: Human Ecology and Health. New York, Macmillan, 1960
41. Sherter CB, Depew CC, Matthey RA: Pulmonary diseases and disorders of respiration. In Covington TR, Walker JI (eds): Current Geriatric Therapy. Philadelphia, WB Saunders, 1984
42. Simonson W: Medications and the Elderly, A Guide for Promoting Proper Use. Rockville, MD, Aspen Systems, 1984
43. Slovik DM: Carbohydrate metabolism and the diagnosis of diabetes mellitus in the elderly. In Walshe TM (ed): Manual of Clinical Problems in Geriatric Medicine. Boston, Little, Brown & Co, 1985
44. Slovik DM: Hyperthyroidism. In Walshe TM (ed): Manual of Clinical Problems in Geriatric Medicine. Boston, Little, Brown & Co, 1985

45. Stevenson IH: Pharmacokinetics in advancing age. In Barbagallo-Sangiorgi G, Exton-Smith AN (eds): Aging and Drug Therapy. New York, Plenum Press, 1984
46. Stevenson IH, Salem SAM, Shepherd AMM: Studies on drug absorption in the elderly. In Crooks J, Stevenson IH (eds): Drugs and the Elderly. Baltimore, University Park Press, 1979
47. Ullrich IH: Endocrine disorders. In Brocklehurst JC (ed): Geriatric Pharmacology and Therapeutics. Boston, Blackwell Scientific Publications, 1984
48. Walshe TM: Approach to cerebrovascular disease. In Walshe TM (ed): Manual of Clinical Problems in Geriatric Medicine. Boston, Little, Brown & Co, 1985
49. Walshe TM: Parkinson's disease. In Walshe TM (ed): Manual of Clinical Problems in Geriatric Medicine. Boston, Little, Brown & Co, 1985
50. Weg R: The Aged: Who, Where, How Well. Ethel Percy Andrews Gerontology Center, 1979
51. Williams T: Rehabilitation in the Aging. New York, Raven Press, 1984
52. Williamson J: Adverse reaction to prescribed drugs in the elderly. In Crooks J, Stevenson IH (eds): Drugs and the Elderly. Baltimore, University Park Press, 1979
53. Woo E: Drug treatment of the elderly. In Walshe TM (ed): Manual of Clinical Problems in Geriatric Medicine. Boston, Little, Brown & Co, 1985
54. Lewis CB: Clinical implications of neurology change with age. In Aging: The Health Care Challenge, pp 117–140. Philadelphia, FA Davis, 1985

Appendix
Drugs Commonly Used for Treatment
of the Elderly

GENERIC NAME	TRADE NAME(S)
Acetaminophen	Tylenol, Datril
Acetazolamide	Diamox
Acetohexamide	Dymelor
Albuterol	Proventil, Ventolin
Allopurinol	Zyloprim
Amantadine	Symmetrel
Amiloride	Midamor, (in) Moduretic
Amitriptyline	Elavil
Amobarbital	Amtyl Sodium
Antipyrine	(in) Auralgan
Aspirin	Ascriptin, Bayer, Bufferin
Aurothioglucose	Solganal
Aurothiomalate	Myochrysine
Azathioprine	Imuran
Baclofen	Lioresal
Beclomethasone	Vanceril, Beclovent
Benztropine	Cogentin
Bretylium	Bretylol
Bromocriptine	Parlodel
Bumetanide	Bumex
Captopril	Capoten
Carbamazepine	Tegretol
Chloral hydrate	Noctec
Chlordiazepoxide	Librium
Chloroquine	Aralen
Chlorpromazine	Thorazine
Chlorthalidone	Hygroton
Cimetidine	Tagamet
Clofibrate	Atromid-S
Clonidine	Catapres
Clorazepate	Tranxene
Codeine	Various preparations
Colchicine	Various manufacturers
Cortisone	Various manufacturers
Cromolyn	Intal, Nasalcrom
Cyclandelate	Cyclospasmol
Cyclophosamide	Cytoxan
Cyproheptadine	Periactin
Dantrolene	Dantrium

GENERIC NAME	TRADE NAME(S)
Desipramine	Norpramin
Dexamethasone	Decadron
Diazepam	Valium
Dicyclomine	Bentyl
Diltiazem	Cardizem
Diphenhydramine	Benadryl
Dipyridamole	Persantine
Disopyramide	Norpace
Doxepin	Sinequan
Doxycycline	Vibramycin
Ergot alkaloids (ergoloid mesylates)	Hydergine
Estrogen	Premarin
Ethanol	Lavacol
Ethosuximide	Zarontin
Fenoprofen	Nalfon
Fluoride, sodium	Luride
Fluphenazine	Prolixin
Flurazepam	Dalmane
Furosemide	Lasix
Glipizide	Glucotrol
Glutethimide	Doriden
Guanabenz	Wytensin
Guanethidine	Ismelin
Haloperidol	Haldol
Hydralazine	Apresoline
Hydrochlorothiazide	HydoDIURIL, Esidrix
Hydromorphone	Dilaudid
Hydroxychloroquine	Plaquenil
Ibuprofen	Motrin, Rufen
Imipramine	Tofranil
Indomethacin	Indocin
Isoproterenol	Isuprel, Norisodrine
Isosorbide dinitrate	Isordil, Sorbitrate
Isoxsuprine	Vasodilan
Labetalol	Normodyne, Trandate
Levodopa–carbidopa combination	Sinemet
Lidocaine	Xylocaine
Lithium carbonate	Lithobid, Eskalith
Lorazepam	Ativan
Levo-thyroxine	Synthroid
Meclofenamate sodium	Meclomen
Mefenamic acid	Ponstel
Meperidine	Demerol, (in) Mepergan

GENERIC NAME	TRADE NAME(S)
Metaproterenol	Alupent
Methadone	Dolophine
Methyldopa	Aldomet
Methylprednisolone	Medrol
Metoclopramide	Reglan
Metoprolol	Lopressor
Minoxidil	Loniten
Nadolol	Corgard
Naproxen	Naproxyn, Anaprox
Nicotinic acid	Various manufacturers
Nifedipine	Procardia
Nitroglycerin	Nitrostat, Nitro-Bid
Nortriptyline	Pamelor, Aventyl
Nylidrin	Arlidin
Oxazepam	Serax
Oxycodone	(in) Percodan, Percocet, Tylox
Pencillamine	Cuprimine, Depen
Pentaerythritol tetanitrate	Peritrate
Pentazocine	Talwin
Perphenazine	Trilafon
Phenelzine	Nardil
Phenobarbital	Various manufacturers
Phenylbutazone	Butazolidin
Phenytoin	Dilantin
Pilocarpine	(in) Pilocar, Isopto Carpine
Pindolol	Visken
Piroxicam	Feldene
Prazepam	Centrax
Prazosin	Minipress
Prednisolone	Various manufacturers
Prednisone	Deltasone
Primidone	Mysoline
Probenecid	Benemid
Procainamide	Pronestyl, Procan SR
Prochlorperazine	Compazine
Propranolol	Inderal
Protriptyline	Vivactil
Quinidine	Quinidex, Quinaglute
Quinine	Quinamm
Ranitidine	Zantac
Reserpine	Serpasil
Spironolactone	Aldactone
Sucralfate	Carafate

GENERIC NAME	TRADE NAME(S)
Sulfinpyrazone	Anturane
Sulindac	Clinoril
Temazepam	Restoril
Terbutaline	Bricanyl, Brethine
Theophylline	Theo-Dur, Elixophyllin
Thioridazine	Mellaril
Thiothixene	Navane
Timolol	Timoptic
Tolazamide	Tolinase
Tolbutamide	Orinase
Tolmetin	Tolectin
Trazodone	Desyrel
Triamterene	Dyrenium, (in) Dyazide
Triazolam	Halcion
Trifluoperazine	Stelazine
Trimipramine	Surmontil
Valproic acid	Depakene
Warfarin	Coumadin

Pediatrics 8

Barbara H. Connolly

The use of drugs in pediatrics represents a specific treatment approach to a variety of disorders. In addition to the drug therapy, rehabilitative therapy is commonly used as a general treatment approach to those disorders that involve the neuromuscular, the musculoskeletal, and the cardiopulmonary systems. In this chapter on pharmacology in pediatrics, a selected number of disorders seen in the pediatric population are briefly described and the types of medications used for the specific disorders are presented. In addition, a section on implications for rehabilitation therapy is also included.

In children with congenital or developmental disorders, more than one disorder or dysfunction may be present. In many cases, several drugs may be prescribed for a variety of problems. The physical or occupational therapist must be aware of the beneficial effects and of the adverse or toxic effects for each of the drugs that the individual child may be receiving. Additionally, the therapist should be aware of the effects of the drugs when they are given in combination.

The therapist has the responsibility to communicate to the child's family and to the child's physician any adverse reactions or lack of beneficial effects from the drugs that are being administered to the child. Many times, the physician may rely heavily on the observations made by the therapist about the effectiveness of a drug that has been prescribed, for example, muscle relaxers or seizure medications.

This chapter primarily focuses on disorders of the neuromuscular and musculoskeletal system. Information on disorders of the cardiopulmonary system are included in the chapters on cardiopulmonary problems. Disorders that are often seen in children with neuromuscular or musculoskeletal problems, such as urologic and endocrinologic problems, are also included in this chapter. A section on immunizations is included because all children are required to undergo immunization against certain diseases as a part of routine health care.

IMMUNIZATIONS

Immunization against infectious diseases is an important part of routine child care. Even for the child with congenital or acquired developmental disorders, a schedule of immunization is important. The schedule for the administration of immunizations as recommended by the American Academy of Pediatrics is shown in Table 8-1.[1] For children with central nervous system disorders that are stable, however, an individual assessment of need must be made before immunizations are initiated. In the past, the use of the pertussis vaccine was contraindicated in those children with seizure disorders. The current recommendation is that a static neurologic disease in infants does not constitute a contraindication; however, an evolving neurologic disease does. Additionally, immunizations should be deferred in children with acute febrile respiratory infections or with any other major infection.

The immunization schedule for older children is different from that for younger children[1] (Table 8-2). The rationale for this different schedule is based on the following factors:

1. Older children have a greater risk of febrile reactions to the pertussis vaccine and a lower risk of severe pertussis.

TABLE 8-1
Recommended Schedule for Immunization of Infants and Children

Age of Child	Types of Immunization
2 mo	Diphtheria–tetanus–pertussis
	Trivalent oral poliovirus
4 mo	Diphtheria–tetanus–pertussis
	Trivalent oral poliovirus
6 mo	Diphtheria–tetanus–pertussis
	Trivalent oral poliovirus (optional)
1 yr	Tubercillin test
15 mo	Measles–rubella or
	Measles–rubella–mumps
18 mo	Diphtheria–tetanus–pertussis
	Trivalent oral poliovirus
4–6 yr	Diphtheria–tetanus–pertussis
	Trivalent oral poliovirus
14–16 yr	Tetanus–diphtheria (repeat every 10 yr)

(From the Report of the Committee on Infectious Diseases, 19th ed. American Academy of Pediatrics, 1982.)

TABLE 8-2
Recommended Schedule for Immunization for
Persons Not Immunized in Infancy
(After Age 6 Years)

Schedule	Type of Immunization
Initial visit	Tetanus–diptheria
	Trivalent oral poliovirus
1-mo later	Measles
	Mumps
	Rubella
2-mo later	Tetanus–diphtheria
	Trivalent oral poliovirus
6–12-mo later	Tetanus–diphtheria
	Trivalent oral poliovirus
14–16 yr	Tetanus–diphtheria (repeat every 10 yr)

(From the Report of the Committee on Infectious Diseases, 19th ed. American Academy of Pediatrics, 1982.)

2.   Older children are able to obtain an effective immunization against diphtheria with a reduced dose of highly purified diphtheria toxoid that ensures a lower rate of hypersensitivity reaction.
3.   Live polio vaccine strains carry a slightly higher risk of disease if administered to adults not previously immunized.

ADVERSE REACTIONS

If a mild febrile reaction occurs, aspirin may be administered to the child. However, if a severe reaction occurs as a result of the diphtheria–pertussis–tetanus (DPT) injection, careful evaluation must be made before further immunization is considered. Further immunizations may have to be deferred or given in smaller doses. Severe reactions to the immunizations include high fever, seizures, and CNS involvement.

IMPLICATIONS FOR THERAPY

Therapists working with the pediatric population should alert parents to the importance of their children receiving immunizations, even if the child has a neurologic disorder. After the child receives an immunization, the therapist should be aware of the potentially severe adverse affects from the injection and advise the parents to contact their physician about further inoculations if such effects are noted.

ENDOCRINE DISORDERS

Hypothyroidism

Hypothyroidism is one of the most common endocrine abnormalities in childhood. The disorder may either be congenital or acquired. In most states, a newborn-screening program has been developed for the detection of congenital hypothyroidism because the incidence is approximately 1:4000 newborn infants.[5]

The functional signs and symptoms noted in hypothyroidism include physical and mental sluggishness; cool, gray, pale skin; decreased intestinal activity; large tongues; poor muscle tone with protuberant abdomens, umbilical hernias, lumbar lordosis; hypothermia; bradycardia; decreased sweating; carotenemia; decreased pulse pressure; hoarse voice or cry; and transient deafness. Retardation of growth and development also occurs with the following signs and symptoms noted: shortness of stature, infantile skeletal proportions, infantile nasoorbital configuration; retarded bone age and epiphyseal dysgenesis; retarded dental development; and slowing of mental responsiveness. Other signs and symptoms include sexual precocity; myxedema of tissue; dry, scaly, coarse skin; and dry, coarse, brittle hair.

Juvenile myxedema (acquired hypothyroidism) usually presents with the classic signs of hypothyroidism plus myopathy, ataxia, and peripheral neuropathy.

SPECIFIC TREATMENT

Desiccated thyroid (USP) or synthetic sodium salt of L-thyroxine (L-T_4) are used as a thyroid replacement. One grain of desiccated thyroid is equal in strength to 100 μg of L-T_4.

In neonates and infants, 1/8 to 1/4 grain of desiccated thyroid or the equivalent in L-T_4 are initially given for 4 to 7 days. An increase of 1/8 to 1/2 grain (or the equivalent L-T_4) is given at weekly intervals until a daily dosage of 3/4 to 1 grain is given to children up to 1 year of age. In older children, the following dosages of desiccated thyroid are suggested:[5] 1 to 6 years of age, 1 to 2 grains daily; 6 to 12 years of age, 1-1/2 to 2-1/2 grains daily; and over 12 years of age, 2 to 3 grains daily.

The therapeutic range is evaluated by the child's clinical response (appearance, growth, and development), sleeping pulses, and thyroid function tests. The prognosis for mental development is guarded if treatment is delayed beyond 3 years of age.

ADVERSE EFFECTS

Overdoses of desiccated thyroid or L-T_4 may produce signs of hyperthyroidism. These include nervousness, emotional instability, irritability, hyperactivity, tremor, insomnia, muscle weakness, loss of weight, vomiting, diarrhea, and increased frequency of stools. Overtreatment may also produce accelerated skeletal maturation and craniosynostosis.

IMPLICATIONS FOR THERAPY

Therapists should be aware of the adverse effects of overmedication, particularly in the areas of hyperactivity, tremor, and muscle weakness because these effects should be easily observable during therapy sessions. Inadequate doses in infants is manifested by bradycardia, circulatory mottling, hoarse cry, constipation, and a delay in the relaxation phase of the deep tendon reflexes. These effects are also easily observable and should be noted by the therapist and reported to the child's family and physician.

Parents of children with juvenile-onset hypothroidism should be alerted to a rapid response to the medication in the child. The effects noted after the initiation of treatment include excessive shedding of hair, increased alertness in the child, initial rapid weight loss, and rapid catch-up growth.[4]

DIGESTIVE DISORDERS

Gastroesophageal Reflux

Gastroesophageal reflux occurs occasionally in most people. In certain groups of children (especially those with neuromotor dysfunction), however, the reflux of gastric material may occur after every meal. This pathologic gastroesophageal reflux occurs when abnormalities in the lower esophageal sphincter function are present or when increases in intragastric pressure occur.

SPECIFIC TREATMENT

Conservative treatment is tried initially, with the child being given small meals and being placed in a upright position of approximately 60° after each meal. The avoidance of fats, chocolates, peppermint, spearment, theophylline, isoproterenol, sedatives, irritants, and acid foods is suggested because these substances have a detrimental effect on lower esophageal sphincter pressure. Antacids and proteins may be suggested because of their beneficial effects on lower esophageal sphincter pressure.

Medical treatment includes the use of antacids or cimetidine; alaginic acid; and bethanechol or metoclopramide hydrochloride for lower esophageal sphincter pressure.

Cimetidine in pediatrics is given in dosages of 20 mg/kg to 40 mg/kg per day in divided doses at 6-hr intervals. Bethanechol is given in dosages that are highly individualized but vary from 0.15 mg/kg to 0.2 mg/kg three times daily. Metoclopramide is administered at a dosage of 0.1 mg/kg intravenously for children under 6 years of age and 2.5 mg/kg to 5 mg/kg intravenously in children from 6 to 12 years of age.

ADVERSE EFFECTS

Cimetidine

The most frequently reported side-effects of cimetidine include headache, tiredness, diarrhea, constipation, dizziness, rash, muscle pain, and mild gynecomastia.

Bethanechol

The most commonly seen side-effects are hypotension with dizziness, faintness, nausea, vomiting, abdominal cramps, flushing of the skin, increased sweating, salivation and lacrimation, malaise, and headache.

Metoclopramide

Side-effects noted with metoclopramide include mild sedation, fatigue, restlessness, agitation, headache, nausea, constipation, diarrhea, and dry mouth. A urticarial or maculopapular rash may also be seen.

IMPLICATIONS FOR THERAPY

If the child is receiving cimetidine, the therapist should instruct the parent to administer the drug with a meal to reduce the chance of vomiting and nausea. Therapy should not be scheduled for the child immediately after meals because of the importance of upright positioning of the child as well as the use of the medications.

If the child is receiving bethanechol, the therapist should remind the parent to administer the drug at least 1 to 2 hr before a meal to decrease the possibility of nausea and diarrhea. Orthostatic hypotension is a side-effect noted with the drug. Therapists should be careful not to make rapid position changes with the child, particularly in taking the child from a supine to an upright position. Early signs of overdose, such as salivation, sweating, flushing, and abdominal cramping, should be reported to the child's physician.

The major consideration to be made with the administration of metoclopramide is that the medication should be given 30 min before meals.

INBORN ERRORS OF METABOLISM

Phenylketonuria

Phenylketonuria (PKU) is the most common disorder of the hyperphenylalanine-mias occurring in the United States, with an incidence of approximately 1:11,000 births. The disorder is autosomal recessively inherited. Diagnosis of the disorder is made after assessment of plasma phenylalanine values and of urinary phenylke-tones when the child is receiving a regular protein diet. Treatment is initiated im-mediately after a presumptive diagnosis of PKU is made.

For untreated patients, symptoms or sequelae include developmental delays; neurologic problems such as hyperactivity, microcephaly, and seizures; "musty" odor; and pigment dilution such as fair skin and light hair. The pathophysiologic basis of the neurologic dysfunction assumed to be the toxic effects of phenylalanine and phenylketones on myelin formation.

SPECIFIC TREATMENT

For the child with classic PKU, a diet low in phenylalanine is implemented. Lofe-nalac, plus supplemental protein, is given to the child to maintain a plasma pheny-lalanine level between 4 mg/dl and 10 mg/dl.[7] Phenylalanine levels should be mon-itored weekly during the first few months and every few months therafter. The special diet may have to be followed for as long as 10 years in some patients.

ADVERSE EFFECTS

Adverse effects are not reported for the use of Lofenalac.[7] However, Lofenalac should not be used with normal infants and children. This supplement is not nutritionally complete for these children.

IMPLICATIONS FOR THERAPY

Therapists typically see only those children with untreated or late-treated PKU. The emergence of more neurologic signs during the time that the therapist works with the child with PKU may signal problems with the child's diet. Referral of the child for dietary assessment by a metabolic nutritionist may be indicated. Additionally, the parent or care giver should be informed if the child vomits during therapy because the calculation of intake and output is important in the dietary management of the child.

Maple Syrup Urine Disease

Maple syrup urine disease (MSUD) is an inherited deficiency of branched-chain ketoacid decarboxylase, an enzyme in the catabolism of the branched-chain amino acids: leucine, isoleucine, and valine. The disorder is autosomal recessively inherited.

Symptoms of the disorder occur classically within the first week of life and include lethargy, anorexia, vomiting, seizures, coma, and death. A sweet odor similar to that of maple syrup is present in body sweat and urine. Clinically, an elevation of the amino acids and their ketoacids (isocaproic, 2-methylvaleric, and isovaleric) occurs, as well as hypoglycemia and profound metabolic ketoacidosis. Neurologic symptoms appear to be caused by the elevation of leucine and its organic acid.

SPECIFIC TREATMENT

Immediate treatment consists of vigorous fluid and alkali therapy along with the introduction of a high caloric, nonprotein formula. If the child survives, the dietary treatment continues to consist of restricting the branched-chain amino acids to an amount that maintains growth with the least ketoacidosis. The most commonly utilized dietary formula is the Mead Johnson MSUD diet powder.[7] Patients with MSUD must continue on the diet therapy for their entire lives.

ADVERSE EFFECTS

Adverse effects are not reported for the use of the MSUD dietary powder. However, this powder should not be used with normal infants and children. The MSUD dietary powder is not nutritionally complete for these children.

IMPLICATIONS FOR THERAPY

Infants who survive the newborn period manifest neurologic deficits in varying degrees dependent upon their dietary management and the resulting levels of leucine. Neurologic problems seen in the infants include increased muscle tone, seizures, and absence of automatic postural reactions. Therapists should be mindful that the neurologic signs and biochemical alterations seen in children with MSUD may be regulated by dietary management. If the child's neurologic signs worsen over a short period, the therapist should contact the child's physician or metabolic nutritionist for reassessment of the child's diet.

Homocystinuria

Homocystinuria, an autosomal recessively inherited disorder, is one of the more common defects in transsulfuration, cystathionine β-synthase deficiency. In patients with homocystinuria, symptoms occur in the ocular, skeletal, central nervous, vascular, and other systems. These children have fair, sparse hair, blue eyes, malar flush, and livido reticularis. Mental retardation is present as is seizure disorders. Skeletal findings of osteoporosis and vertebral abnormalities are also prominent. Increased platelet adhesiveness is a factor in the development of occlusive vascular disease, which is associated with seizures, hemiplegia, renal hypertension, and death.

SPECIFIC TREATMENT

Specific drug treatment has consisted of a diet low in methionine or cysteine. Various chemical studies have indicated minimal responsiveness to the use of pyridoxine or vitamin B_{12} with certain children.[6]

ADVERSE EFFECTS

Side-effects are rarely seen with the administration of pyridoxine. Adverse reactions that have been reported include paresthesias, somnolence, slight flushing or feelings of warmth, low folic acid levels, and temporary burning or stinging pain at the injection site.[4]

IMPLICATIONS FOR THERAPY

Therapists who treat children with homocystinuria should be told if the individual child is receiving pyridoxine. If so, the therapist should be aware that paresthesias are seen as rare adverse reactions to the medication. If a paresthesia is suspected, the therapist should contact the child's physician.

Mucopolysaccharidoses

The lysosomal storage diseases that compose the mucopolysaccharidoses category are all clinically characterized by disturbances in the connective tissue caused by accumulation of mucopolysaccharides. The exact expression of the disorder is dependent upon the particular mucopolysaccharide stored and the tissue in which it normally occurs. Tissues most often involved are the eyes, brain, liver, skin, and musculoskeletal. Varying degrees of dysostosis multiplex are seen radiographically in the disorders: the major problems being an elongated sella turcica, anterior spatulate ribs, anterior vertebral wedging, diaphyseal flaring of the long bones, and proximal narrowing of the diaphyses of the shortened metacarpal bones.

SPECIFIC TREATMENT

No known medical treatment is effective in preventing the progression of the diseases. Most children have a progressive course with an early death.

IMPLICATIONS FOR THERAPY

Children with mucopolysaccharide disorders are frequently seen by therapists because of their musculoskeletal involvement. Although no medications may be given for the primary disorder (i.e., lysosomal storage disease), some of the children may be taking cardiac medications if they have either Hurler's syndrome or Scheie's syndrome which usually has a cardiac involvement.

INFECTIONS

Bacterial Meningitis

Bacterial meningitis in children is most commonly caused by *Haemophilus influenzae*. Bacterial meningitis usually occurs in children under 2 years of age and is rarely seen in children older than 10 years of age. The mortality from bacterial meningitis is approximately 11%.[2] In neonates, a higher mortality may be seen because of the additional involvement of staphylococci, enterobacteria, and pseudomonas.[3]

Signs and symptoms associated with meningitis include

1. Meningeal signs: stiffness of the neck, stiffness of the back, positive Kernig sign, positive Brudzinski sign
2. Increased intracranial pressure: bulging fontanelles (infants), headache, irritability, projectile vomiting, diplopia
3. Changes in sensorium: decreased consciousness
4. Seizures: occur in approximately 25% to 40% of patients
5. Fever
6. Shock

Later complications from the central nervous system infection may include hydrocephalus, deafness, paralysis, mental retardation, and focal seizures. Arthritis may be a late complication of meningococcal meningitis.

SPECIFIC TREATMENT

If the menigitis is of *H. influenzae* origin, the treatment of choice for infants over 1 month of age is chloramphenicol and ampicillin. Ampicillin is initially given intravenously 100 mg/kg followed by 300 mg/kg daily intravenously in six divided doses. Chloramphenicol is administered at a dosage of 100 mg/kg daily in divided doses every 12 hr. In neonates, care must be used if the chloramphenicol is given in the presence of hemolytic anemia, granulocytopenia, or in the presence of liver disease.[3] Ampicillin and chloramphenicol are both continued for 10 days after initiation.

In meningococcal meningitis, the aforementioned drugs may be used in combination with pencillin G. If the meningitis is of pneumococcal, streptococcal, or staphylococcal origin, pencillin G in large doses is given. Dosage of 300,000 units/kg per day are given intravenously in divided doses for 10 days. If staphylococcal infection is present, methicillin, oxacillin, or nofcillin may also be used.

In gram-negative bacterial infections seen in neonatal meningitis and infections secondary to congenital defects, gentamicin may be used. For neonates, intramuscular injections of 3 mg/kg to 6 mg/kg daily are given along with 1 mg/day intrathecally.

ADVERSE EFFECTS

Chloramphenicol

Toxic reactions include stomatitis, encephalopathy, optic neuropathy, and marrow aplasia. In the infant, the "gray" syndrome, which comprise vomiting, abdominal distention, sweating, and pallor, may be noted.

Gentamicin

Adverse reactions to gentamicin include ototoxicity, which usually involves the vestibular system but sometimes the auditory system as well; renal or hepatic damage; convulsions; and hypersensitivity.

Ampicillin

Adverse reactions to ampicillin are rare. However, in some cases, diarrhea, skin rash, or fever may be seen. Hypersensitivity may develop in a few patients.

Pencillin G

Hypersensitivity may occur in children who receive pencillin G. Anaphylaxis, urticaria, rash, and drug fever may be seen if the hypersensitivity occurs.[4] Changes in bowel flora, candidiasis, diarrhea, and hemolytic anemia may also be adverse reactions to pencillin G.

IMPLICATIONS FOR THERAPY

With children receiving ampicillin, the therapist should be aware of the rash that can occur. The ampicillin rash is characteristically dull red, macular or maculopapular, and mildly pruritic. It usually begins in pressure areas, such as the knees, elbows, palms, and soles, and then spreads over most of the body. It may develop immediately after administration of the drug but often does not appear until after 5 to 14 days of treatment. If a rash is seen, the physician should be notified. Parents should be instructed that ampicillin should be given to the child at least 1 hr before or 2 hr after meals.

Therapists should be aware of the early signs of the "gray" syndrome in neonates and infants receiving chloramphenicol. These early signs include abdominal distention, failure to feed, pallor, and changes in vital signs. If the therapist suspects the gray syndrome, contact should be made with the child's physician. The therapist should also be on the alert for abnormal bleeding problems in children taking this drug. Problems such as fever, petechiae, nose bleeds, bleeding gums, or any other unusual bleeding or bruising should be reported immediately.

Because the major side-effects of gentamicin involve the vestibular and auditory systems, the therapist should be alert to any newly occurring problems with either of these systems after the initiation of gentamicin therapy.

The therapist should immediately report to the child's physician any reaction to pencillin G that is noted in the child. These early reactions include onset of rash, pruritus, fever, chills, and breathing difficulties.

Viral Meningoencephalitis

Viral infections of the central nervous system have signs and symptoms similar to those occurring with bacterial meningitis. The infection may involve either the meninges or the brain, but usually both are affected.

Specific symptoms include headache, confusion, fever, neck stiffness, seizures, ataxia, photophobia, and weakness. Focal deficits, such as hemiparesis or dysphasia, may also be present. Usually the symptoms evolve slowly over a period of 7 to 10 days and then subside.

Residual dysfunctions resulting from the viral infections include psychomotor retardation, behavioral disorders, seizures and, occasionally, blindness, hemiparesis, or speech impairment.

SPECIFIC TREATMENT

Vidarabine is an antiviral agent that has proved effective against herpes simplex viral encephalitis.[5] Otherwise, specific treatment is composed of supportive care and minimization of serious complications. Vidarabine is given intravenously at a dosage of 15 mg/kg daily, infused over a 12-hr period.[4]

ADVERSE EFFECTS

Thrombophlebitis is a common side-effect of vidarabine. Other adverse reactions include gastrointestinal disturbances, tremor, and weakness.

IMPLICATIONS FOR THERAPY

The therapist should report any sudden onset of tremors and weakness in the patient who is receiving vidarabine as a medication for viral meningitis. Therapists working with the patient during the acute phase of the viral infection would more likely be working with the patients who are receiving vidarabine.

Acute Otitis Media

Acute otitis media is common during infancy and childhood. Otitis media is a common complication of an upper respiratory tract infection because of three factors: the eustachian tubes are relatively short; the immunity against particular organisms has not yet been established through previous exposure; and tubal blockage is frequently fostered by allergic rhinitis, adenoid enlargement, and infection.

The most common bacterial pathogens causing otitis media are *H. influenzae* (especially in children under 6 years of age), β-hemolytic streptococci, and the pneumococcus. In approximately one-third of the cases, no pathogen is found, and a viral cause is likely. Acute otitis media in infants may also be related to being fed with a bottle while lying in a horizontal position.

The clinical signs and symptoms in infants include irritability, restless sleep, and rubbing or pulling of the ears. Fever may be high in infants, and even febrile seizures may be seen in some children. In older children, pain, dizziness, and headaches may be reported. Upper respiratory tract infection signs may be present in children of all ages.

SPECIFIC TREATMENT

Aspirin or analgesics may be used as a general measure to decrease discomfort and fever. Both ampicillin and amoxicillin have been found to be effective against *H. influenzae*, β-hemolytic streptococci, and the pneumococcus. Ampicillin is given in oral dosages of 50 mg/kg to 110 mg/kg a day in four divided doses for 7 days, if the treatment is initiated early; 10 to 14 days, if the treatment is initiated later.

If amoxicillin is the drug of choice, it is given orally in dosages of 20 mg/kg a day in three divided doses for the same duration as outlined for ampicillin. Amoxicillin is used instead of ampicillin if better middle-ear penetration is desired. Amoxicillin may also be used instead of ampicillin because it permits smaller doses and decreases the frequency of diarrhea and secondary candidal rashes.

ADVERSE EFFECTS

Ampicillin

The adverse effects of ampicillin are discussed in the section on bacterial meningitis.

Amoxicillin

Amoxicillin has fewer side effects than ampicillin. Amoxicillin is better absorbed than ampicillin and, therefore, few gastrointestinal effects are seen.

IMPLICATIONS FOR THERAPY

The therapist should note any hypersensitivity reactions in the child such as itching, skin rash or hives, wheezing, diarrhea, or fever. The parents should be urged to contact the physician if any of these signs occur.

Urinary Tract Infections

Urinary tract infections may be caused by a variety of organisms, with the most frequent causative organism being *Escherichia coli.* Any lesion or disorder that hinders periodic bladder emptying leads to stasis and residual urine, causing an increased susceptibility to infection. In pediatrics, those children who have either an atonic or neurogenic bladder may have repeated incidents of urinary tract infections. Neurogenic bladders are caused by congenital anomalies of the spinal cord. The most common causes of these congenital anomalies in children are myelomeningocele, spinal dysraphism, and sacral agensis. Children with myelomeningocele constitute the majority of children with neurogenic bladders. Early assessment of the urinary tract is mandatory because these children are at risk for urinary tract infections. Frequent urinalyses with bacterial cultures are important to the overall management. Seventy-five percent of these children will have a urinary tract infection by 4 years of age.[5]

In infants and young children, the signs and symptoms may be nonspecific and may include failure to thrive, gastrointestinal disturbances, weight loss, and malodorous urine. Dull or sharp pains and tenderness in the kidney area or abdomen may also be present. Fever may be present if pyelonephritis, not only cystitis, is the culprit. In older children, who can communicate, frequency, urgency, and painful urination may be the chief complaints.

Upon urinalysis, pyuria is characteristically present. However, the exact causative organism can be identified by a urine culture.

SPECIFIC TREATMENT

The specific drug treatment is based upon the outcome of the urine culture and the bacterial sensitivity to the antibiotic. Chemotherapeutics or antibiotics have

classically been prescribed for 10 days. Initial therapy in the nonfebrile child is
initiated with oral sulfonamides or nitrofurantoin. If the child is febrile, one of the
penicillin derivatives, such as cephalosporin, may be indicated. If the child is febrile,
clinically septic, and unable to take oral medications, hospitalization and parenteral
antibiotics, such as an aminoglycoside along with carbenicillin or ampicillin, are
necessary.

ADVERSE EFFECTS

Sulfonamides

Adverse reactions to the sulfonamides include crystalluria (mechanical obstruction
to the bladder), hypersensitivity (fever, rash, hepatitis, lupuslike state, and vasculitis),
neutropenia, agranulocytosis, aplastic anemia, and thrombocytopenia.

Nitrofurantoin

Adverse reactions to nitrofurantoin include primaquine-sensitive hemolytic anemia,
peripheral neuropathy, rash, and chills.

Carbenicillin

Adverse reactions to carbenicillin include allergic reactions, thrombophlebitis, and
thrombasthenia.

Cephalosporin

Common adverse reactions to the cephalosporin family of drugs include gastrointestinal problems, such as diarrhea, vomiting, nausea, anorexia, and abdominal pain;
hematologic problems, such as transient leukopenia, granulocytopenia, thrombocytopenia, and neutropenia; hypersensitivity problems, such as rash, pruritus, and
fever; and other problems including phlebitis, thrombophlebitis, pain, induration,
and tenderness at the injection site.

Ampicillin

The adverse reactions to ampicillin were discussed in the section on bacterial
meningitis.

IMPLICATIONS FOR THERAPY

Urinary tract infections are common occurrences in children seen in therapy,
especially in children who have myelodysplasias and who have neurogenic bladders.
Urinary tract infections are also common in children with severe spasticity, a result
of the spastic nature of the bladder in these children. Therapists should be aware
of the type of medication that the child is taking for any urinary tract infection
and of the signs of hypersensitivity in the children to the medications. With the
sulfonamides, fever with a sore throat, malaise, unusual fatigue, joint pains, pallor,
bleeding tendencies, rash, and jaundice are early signs of blood dyscrasias or
hypersensitivity. Parents should be urged to administer nitrofurantoin with meals
or with milk to decrease gastric irritation. Additionally, the therapist might suggest
that the medication be given a few hours before the therapy treatment time to
decrease the chance of nausea and vomiting interfering with the treatment session.

Hypersensitivity reactions to the cephalosporin group of drugs should be reported to the physician immediately by either the therapist or by the parent. The therapist should be aware that diarrhea, vomiting, and nausea are commonly occurring side-effects of the medication and that these disturbances may be seen in children receiving cephalosporins.

Pyogenic Arthritis

Pyogenic arthritis is a fairly common occurrence in children, particularly in those who have chronic illnesses or immunodeficiency states. The arthritis that occurs is due to the infection of one or more joints by hematogenous spread or by direct extension of a pathogenic bacteria. A history of preceding trauma is obtained in approximately one-third of the cases.[10] The most common organisms that cause the infection include *Staphylococcus aureus*, gonococci, meningococci, pneumococci, and *H.* influenzae. Usually, the child has monoarticular involvement, most frequently the knee, then the ankle, and the elbow in that order of frequency.

The onset is usually acute with chills, high fever, and pain in the affected joints. The overlaying tissue at the joint may be swollen, tender, and warm. The joint may also be "splinted" because of muscle spasms.

SPECIFIC TREATMENT

The joint sepsis must be identified and promptly treated. Broad-spectrum antibiotics are used until the organism is identified. Additionally, joint aspiration is done daily to minimize any articular damage resulting from the proteolytic enzymes present in the exudate. Severe cases of gonococcal arthritis respond particularly well to intravenous penicillin or to intramuscular penicillin in milder cases.

ADVERSE EFFECTS

Adverse reactions to the penicillin group of drugs include hypersensitivity reactions, such as pruritus, urticaria, and other skin eruptions; chills; fever; wheezing; anaphylaxis; eosinophilia, hemolytic anemia, and other blood abnormalities; neuropathy; and nephrotoxicity. Local pain and tenderness, as well as fever, may be associated with intramuscular injections.

IMPLICATIONS FOR THERAPY

The therapeutic implications are the same as those dicussed under the section on bacterial meningitis.

Osteomyelitis

Osteomyelitis is an infectious process that may include all parts of the bone, but that usually involves only the metaphysis of the bone. In the United States, approximately 80% of the cases are caused by staphylococci.[5] Other cases may be caused by streptococci or salmonellae. The infection is usually the result of an hematogenous spread, but it may be a local extension of an infected focus. Considerable areas of the cortex of the bone may necrose and the sequestra may not be absorbed. Should this happen, surgical intervention is necessary.

Early signs and symptoms include localized tenderness over the metaphyseal area and pain on weight-bearing. Later signs and symptoms include localized erythema, warmth, tenderness, swelling, fever, elevated pulse, pain over the end of the shaft, and joint motion limitations.

SPECIFIC TREATMENT

A synthetic penicillinase-resistant penicillin, such as nafcillin, is given intravenously until the results of the sensitivity tests are available. Intravenous antibiotics, specific to the organism responsible for the infection are given for 10 to 21 days, with subsequent oral antibiotics. Nafcillin, 50 mg/kg to 250 mg/kg a day, may be given intravenously in divided doses every 4 hr. For adolescents, the dosage may be up to 18 g/day.

ADVERSE EFFECTS

Adverse reactions to nafcillin include hypersensitivity reactions such as fever, rash and vomiting; kidney damage; and hematuria.

IMPLICATIONS FOR THERAPY

Therapists should advise the patient or family that the medication, nafcillin, should be taken on an empty stomach at least 1 hr before, or 2 hr after, meals for it to be absorbed. Therapists should be aware that nausea and vomiting are commonly seen as a side-effect of the drug and that patients may experience these effects during therapy. Rash is also a common occurrence. Therapists should particularly note any signs of neutropenia, such as malaise, fever, sore mouth or throat, and have the patient contact the physician immediately if these symptoms occur.

COLLAGEN DISEASES

Rheumatoid Arthritis

Juvenile rheumatoid arthritis (JRA), a chronic illness in childhood, the etiology of which is unknown, is one of the leading causes of childhood disability. Approximately 75% of children who have a major generalized rheumatoid disease have JRA.[5]

In general, rheumatoid arthritis has its onset between 2 and 5 years of age, with a peak incidence between 2 and 3 years.[5,10] An onset of the disease before 6 months of age is very rare. Overall, girls are affected twice as often as boys.

Three types of JRA have been described: systemic, oligoarticular, and polyarticular. The oligoarticular (also known as pauciarticular) type is the most common and most benign. The large joints of the body are usually involved, with the knees being most commonly affected. Approximately one-half of the children affected have a monoarthritis at onset, but signs may appear later in other joints. Children affected usually have considerable swelling in the joint, but approximately 50% of the children have little or no pain. The onset may be insidious or abrupt. The joints are usually warm, tender, and painful on movement. A large effusion may be present. The natural history of the oligoarticular type is one of continuing synovitis over several years, with periods of remissions and exacerbations. Complications include the development of flexor contractures, knee instability with valgus deviation or subluxation of the knee, and leg length discrepancy caused by the overgrowth of the affected limb.

Children with the polyarticular type may also have either acute or insidious onset. The patient may experience malaise, low-grade fever, fatigue, anorexia, weight loss, and morning stiffness. Tenderness and soft-tissue swelling is present in both large and small joints. Joint involvement is usually symmetric. Temporomandibular joint involvement is common. Over a period of years, joint contractures may occur.

The systemic type of JRA is also known as Still's disease. Systemic manifestations include fever, rash, and joint swelling for 6 weeks or longer. The characteristic rash involves pink, macular skin lesions on the trunk and proximal extremities. The temperature is usually seen in a remitting pattern with daily or twice daily elevations of 102° to 104°F.

Laboratory findings on all types of JRA include polymorphonuclear leukocytosis and accelerated sedimentation rates. Synovial fluid may show an inflammatory reaction.

SPECIFIC TREATMENT

The aims of treatment are to presserve function, prevent deformity, and to ameliorate discomfort. In most cases of JRA, conservative treatment is initially undertaken, and hazardous drugs are not used. Specific measures of treatment include:

Nonsteroidal Anti-inflammatory Drugs

Aspirin is used most commonly. The average dosage of aspirin is 90 mg/kg to 120 mg/kg a day, every 4 to 6 hr.[10] Symptomatic improvement, blood levels, and signs of toxicity are used as a means of regulating the dosages. In children who do not tolerate aspirin or who show no benefit, other nonsteroidal anti-inflammatory drugs are available.

Tolmetin, given at a dosage of 20 mg/kg to 30 mg/kg a day, or naproxen given at a dosage of 10 mg/kg a day in two divided doses, are both FDA approved and have the most extensive therapeutic background. Flurbiprofen, administered at 4 mg/kg a day, a medication used in England and shortly to be approved in the United States, will be the first liquid medication available for very young children.[10]

Corticosteroids

Corticosteroids do not alter the course of prognosis of JRA and are seldom indicated in the treatment. However, corticosteroids may be used (especially prednisone at 2 mg/kg to 3 mg/kg a day) for children with systemic JRA who fail to respond to salicylates. Large doses may be needed to suppress fever and other systemic manifestations such as myocarditis or iritis. Intraarticular steroid injections may be used sparingly with symptomatic joints. However, repeated injections may accelerate the destructive process because steroids suppress synthesis of the articular cartilage matrix.

Gold Salts and Penicillamine

Gold salts and penicillamine are being used more frequently with patients who do not respond to salicylates.

ADVERSE EFFECTS

Aspirin

Signs of toxicity include tinnitus, nausea, vomiting, and hyperpnea. Gastrointestinal symptoms that may accompany aspirin use are avoided by giving the aspirin with milk or meals, by using buffered or enteric coated preparations, or by using nonacetylated salicylates such as salsalate or choline magnesium trisalicylate. Mild hepatoxicity caused by salcylates (aspirin) is noted frequently in children with JRA

Tolmetin

Adverse effects include headache, dizziness, vertigo, light-headedness, mood elevation or depression, nervousness, weakness, drowsiness, insomnia, tinnitus, epigastric or abdominal pain, nausea, vomiting, constipation, transient and small decreases in hemoglobin and hematocrit, and fever.[4]

Naproxen

Side-effects noted with the use of naproxen include headache, drowsiness, dizziness, depression, dyspnea, blurred vision, tinnitus, anorexia, heartburn, nausea, vomiting, agranulocytosis, and rash.

Corticosteroids

The side-effects of corticosteroids are inevitable with the use of the drug. However, a trial period of alternate-day therapy may be used in an attempt to decrease the side-effects. Side-effects include fluid accumulation, increased occurrence of oral candidal infection, anorexia, paresthesias, drowsiness, muscle weakness, nausea, polyuria, postural hypotension, and mental depression.

IMPLICATIONS FOR THERAPY

Therapists working with children with JRA must be aware that most of the medications used with these children may have gastrointestinal side-effects. The resulting nausea and vomiting from the medications may limit the amount of therapy that can be accomplished with the children during times of acute flares in the disease. Additionally, drowsiness and dizziness may be side-effects seen with the ingestation of tolmetin, naproxen, and corticosteroids. Patients should be cautioned about participating in activities that could be potentially hazardous because they require normal balance and equilibrium.

With the medications, the therapist should begin to see progressive improvement in the patient, generally within 1 week.[4] Reduced joint pain, decreased joint swelling, and improved functional abilities are therapeutic responses that should be noted with the medications.

NEUROMUSCULAR DISORDERS

Dermatomyositis

Dermatomyositis is an inflammatory disease affecting the muscular system in children, with girls being more frequently affected than boys. The disease occurs with a sudden onset, although many of the patients have a history of an upper respiratory or gastrointestinal infection.

Signs and symptoms of dermatomyositis include skin lesions (violaceous color of the eyelids, red and violaceous patches around the fingernails and interphalangeal joints of the hands); tenderness and soreness of muscles; nasal speech; difficulty in swallowing; and muscle atrophy in the later stages.

SPECIFIC TREATMENT

Steroid therapy and ACTH have been effective in controlling the effects of dermatomyositis. With the drug therapy, the child may have a disease course that is characterized by remissions and exacerbations.

ADVERSE EFFECTS
Corticosteroids

The adverse effects of corticosteroids are discussed in the section on rheumatoid arthritis.

ACTH

The side-effects seen with ACTH are usually reversible upon discontinuation of the medication. Adverse effects noted with the use of ACTH include hypersensitivity, sodium and water retention, increased potassium excretion, calcium loss, and impaired wound healing.

IMPLICATIONS FOR THERAPY

The use of corticosteroids and ACTH in children with dermatomyositis does not cure the disorder, but a dramatic improvement in the symptoms should be seen with the administration of the drugs.[6] Therapists should be aware that prolonged use of ACTH increases the risk of hypersensitivity in the child and should be alert to the early signs of this hypersensitivity — skin reactions, dizziness, nausea, vomiting, mild fever, anaphylactic shock, wheezing, and circulatory failure. The child's physician should be contacted immediately if any of the signs of hypersensitivity are noted. Growth and development of the child receiving ACTH must also be carefully monitored because of the effects of hormone therapy on the child.

Dystonia Musculorum Deformans

Dystonia musculorum deformans begins gradually with the child initially experiencing mild gait difficulty that progresses to dystonia in the trunk, extremities, and head. Facial grimacing and gross motor incoordination may also be present. By 5 to 6 years of age, the child may be totally dependent.

SPECIFIC TREATMENT

Medical treatment of the disorder with L-dopa has provided relief to some patients.[6] The dosage is highly individualized for each child.

ADVERSE EFFECTS

Frequent side-effects seen with L-dopa include orthostatic hypotension, anorexia, nausea, vomiting, abdominal distress, dry mouth, dysphagia, choreiform and involuntary movements, increased hand tremor, ataxia, muscle twitching, weakness, fatigue, headache, confusion, agitation, and blurred vision.

IMPLICATIONS FOR THERAPY

The therapeutic effects may show substantial improvement in some patients during the second or third week of therapy, but in others, the improvement may not be seen for up to 6 months. A large percentage of patients taking L-dopa for longer than 1 year begin to show abnormal involuntary movements. For the child with dystonia musculorum deformans, it may be difficult to determine if the disease is causing the abnormal movements or if the L-dopa is having adverse effects. A reduction of the dosage seems to decrease the abnormal movements caused by the medication.

Spasticity

Management of the child with spasticity usually begins with a vigorous program of physical and occupational therapy. However, many children may additionally benefit from medications to reduce spasticity. No drug is capable of achieving sustained reductions in spasticity without some sedative effects. However, some drugs are available that provide benefits to the child with severe spasticity.

The three most commonly used drugs to reduce spasticity are diazepam, dantrolene and baclofen. Diazepam (Valium) has traditionally been used as a tranquilizer with adults. With children, however, small doses have little tranquilizing effects. In children, diazepam acts primarily as a muscle relaxant by blocking the nerve impulses at the spinal cord. The improvements seen in performance in patients with spasticity is thought to be related to the reduction in abnormal excitation to the muscle.[9] The neurophysiologic effects of diazepam include: (1) inhibition of the brain stem-activating system, (2) increase of presynaptic inhibition, (3) inhibition of polysynaptic spinal reflexes, and (4) inhibition of fusimotor activity.[2] Diazepam tends to interact with seizure medications, which increases the likelihood of drowsiness. Drowsiness may occur at low levels in some children, but others may take up to 45 mg/day without drowsiness. The recommended dosage are 1 mg t.i.d. for children under 6 months of age, 2 mg t.i.d. for children over than 6 months of age, and 2 mg to 5 mg t.i.d. for children older than 1 year.

Dantrolene (Dantrium) is a hydantoin derivative that provides peripheral muscle relaxant action. It acts directly on the spastic muscle by interfering with the calcium ion release from the sarcoplasmic reticulum. The clinical dose produces a reduction in the contractability of skeletal muscle but has no effect on smooth or cardiac muscle. If dantrolene is used in combination with other medications, however, it tends to bring out the "drowsiness" effects of these medications. The recommended dosages for dantrolene for relief of spasticity are 25 mg b.i.d. for children under 1 year of age and 25 mg to 50 mg q.i.d. for children over 1 year of age.

Baclofen (Liorisal) is a centrally acting skeletal muscle relaxant. The drug depresses polysynaptic afferent reflex activity at the spinal cord level and, thus, reduces spasticity caused by upper motor neuron lesions. Although baclofen works with children with brain damage, it has been shown to be more effective in patients with spinal cord lesions and multiple sclerosis. The drug is given initially as 5 mg t.i.d. and increased by 5 mg per dose every 3 days until an adequate response, or adverse reactions, develops. In children, the dosage should be no higher than 10 mg t.i.d. or q.i.d.

ADVERSE EFFECTS

Diazepam

The common side-effects noted with diazepam use include drowsiness, fatigue, ataxia, confusion, paradoxic rage, dizziness, vertigo, headache, hypotension, xerostomia, nausea, incontinence, blurred vision, diplopia, and nystagmus.

Dantrolene

Adverse effects noted with dantrolene include drowsiness, muscle weakness, dizziness, tachycardia, diarrhea, constipation, bloody or dark urine, blurred vision, diplopia, and hypersensitivity. In 2% to 3% of the children who take dantrolene, the drug produces jaundice; the tubules in the liver are apparently blocked by the drug. However, the dysfunction is reversible with discontinuance of the drug.

Baclofen

The most commong side effects noted with baclofen include transient drowsiness, vertigo, dizziness, weakness, fatigue, ataxia, headache, confusion, and insomnia. Gastrointestinal effects may include nausea, vomiting, constipation, and diarrhea. A reduction in blood pressure may also occur with the use of baclofen.

IMPLICATIONS FOR THERAPY

Therapists dealing with children with spasticity must be aware of the effects of muscle relaxants on these children. In many cases, the child's physician depends upon the therapist to aid in regulating the amount of muscle relaxant that the child can tolerate without becoming too drowsy or too relaxed. The therapist is able to relay information to the physician about the ability of the child to participate in therapy as the drug (or drugs) is being regulated and about the benefits that the child is achieving from use of the drug. In addition to the effects of relaxation and drowsiness, the therapist should also be aware that these drugs may cause dizziness, vertigo, and ataxia in certain children. These adverse effects of the medication may interfere with the child's participation in therapy and need to be reported to the child's family and physician.

SEIZURES

A convulsion or seizure disorder represents an excessive neuronal discharge that is a sign of disordered brain function. An estimated 3% of all children experience at least one seizure episode during their early life.[5]

Seizure classifications from the International Classification of Epileptic Seizures now lists the major types of seizures as partial seizures, generalized seizures, unilateral seizures, and unclassified seizures. Treatment for a seizure disorder is initiated as soon as the type of seizure is determined. Usually, a single drug is begun, and other drugs are then added if the seizures are not controlled after the first drug has been increased to a maximum tolerated dosage. A variety of drugs and combinations of medications may be required for adequate seizure control. Changes in dosages and drugs are often necessary because children often "outgrow" the drugs during the first 2 years of life, pubescence, and adolescence. When a drug is discontinued, the dosage is gradually reduced over a period of 1 to 2 weeks. The new drug is then given in full dosage as the old drug is being discontinued.

SPECIFIC MEASURES

The medications for seizure disorders vary depending upon the type of seizure. Table 8-3 lists the types of medications administered for the different types of seizure disorders. The recommended dosage for each type of medication is also shown in the table.

ADVERSE EFFECTS

The most frequently occurring side-effects for each of the medications that may be prescribed for seizure disorders are listed in Table 8-3. Although the side-effects are listed for each individual medication, many children receive more than one medication for the control of their seizure disorder and, thus, may experience numerous side-effects.

IMPLICATIONS FOR THERAPY

Seizure medications in children present a variety of problems for the therapist. Often, the child must receive very high doses of the medications to regulate the seizure activity. When this occurs, the child may be so drowsy that the therapist may be unable to get the child to participate in the therapy program. Occasionally, the high dosages of medication may cause the child to be so hyperactive that the therapist cannot get the child to attend to the therapy activities; or the child may become ataxic in addition to other neuromotor problems because of the side-effects of certain medications such as phenobarbital or primidone (Mysoline). Because the child must receive some type of medication for control of his seizures, the therapist must work with the child's physician to accomplish the goals of both disciplines, i.e., controlling the seizures and working on developmental activities.

CASE STUDIES

The following two case studies demonstrate the importance of the therapist knowing what types of medications the child is receiving and what adverse effects might

TABLE 8-3
Seizure Medications

Drug	Indication	Side-Effects	Dosage
Phenobarbital	Tonic–clonic seizures; partial seizures; status epilepticus; febrile seizures	Drowsy, hyperactivity, rash, ataxia	4–6 mg/kg/day
Phenytoin (Dilantin)	Grand mal seizures; psychomotor seizures	Gum hyperplasia, nystagmus, rash, ataxia, lethargy, thrombocytopenia	4–8 mg/kg/day
Diazepam (Valium)	Generalized seizures; myoclonic seizures; status epilepticus	Drowsiness, fatigue, ataxia, hypotension, blurred vision, xerostomia	0.5–1.0 mg/kg/day
Valproic acid (Depakene)	Absence seizures; mixed seizures; status epilepticus; febrile seizures	Breakthrough seizures, drowsiness, nausea, depression, dizziness, ataxia	15–? /day Not to exceed 60 mg/day
Carbamazepine (Tegretol)	Grand mal seizures; psychomotor seizures; mixed seizures	Dizziness, vertigo, drowsiness, disturbances of coordination, rash, ataxia	200–? /day Not to exceed 1000 mg/day
Clonazepam (Clonopin)	Absence seizures; akinetic seizures; myoclonic seizures	Drowsiness, ataxia, hirsutism, xerostomia, confusion, leukopenia,	0.02–0.2 mg/kg/day
Primidone (Mysoline)	Complex partial seizures; tonic–clonic seizures	Ataxia, drowsiness, leukopenia, rash	15–25 mg/kg/day
Ethosuximide (Zarontin)	Absence seizures; akinetic seizures; atonic seizures	Ataxia, nausea, drowsiness, leukopenia, eosinophilia, blurred vision	20–25 mg/kg/day
Clorazepate (Tranxene)	Partial seizures	Drowsiness, GI disturbances, diplopia, ataxia, dizziness, headache	9–60 mg/day
Mephobarbital (Mebaral)	Generalized seizures; focal seizures	Drowsy, ataxia, irritability, nausea, hypersensitivity	8–10 mg/kg/day
ACTH	Infantile spasms	Cushingoid state, growth suppression, peptic ulcer, fluid retention	5–50 units/day

be anticipated. These two case studies also illustrate the importance of the therapist working in conjunction with the primary physician in the overall management of the child's medical and developmental problems.

CASE 1   Kimberly is a 7-year-old child with a diagnosis of severe spastic quadriparesis. She is currently enrolled in a school program on a daily basis and is receiving both physical therapy and occupational therapy. During the therapy sessions, the therapists noted that Kimberly was extremely difficult to handle as a result of her overall increased tone. Even with relaxation techniques, Kimberly's tone was lowered for only a few minutes. In addition to the neuromotor disorder, Kimberly also has a seizure disorder consisting of generalized and myoclonic seizures. She is currently receiving both phenytoin (Dilantin) and phenobarbital for her seizures and has good control with these drugs.

Both the physical therapist and the occupational therapist working with Kimberly felt that she might benefit from receiving a muscle relaxant. In addition to the benefits that would be gained in physical therapy, the therapists felt that the mother would be better able to handle Kimberly at home if she were more relaxed.

On evaluation, the pediatric neurologist concurred with the therapists that a muscle relaxant might be beneficial for Kimberly. Diazepam (Valium) was prescribed as the drug of choice because it appeared to have the least sedative effects.

After implementation of Valium therapy, Kimberly was seen in physical therapy within 1 week. She was more relaxed and was able to participate in more developmental activities. However, by the second physical therapy visit, Kimberly was beginning to react adversely to the medication. The mother reported that Kimberly was becoming difficult to arouse during the day and that she seemed to have lost many of her developmental skills. She was having a difficult time lifting her head from a prone position and was not alert to the environment, even after she had lifted her head from this position. The mother additionally stated that Kimberly seemed "tired" all of the time and that she had difficulty getting her to eat.

Both the occupational and physical therapists felt that Kimberly was receiving too much of the muscle relaxant and that the pediatric neurologist should be contacted. During the next 2 months, multiple contacts were made with the neurologist to obtain the appropriate amount of relaxation from the Valium while decreasing the adverse effects of drowsiness, fatigue, and decreased alertness that were being noted in Kimberly.

With the cooperation of parents, the therapists, and the neurologist, eventually Kimberly was able to participate more fully in the therapy programs without experiencing adverse reactions from the medications. However, as Kimberly grows, the therapists are anticipating that the "trial-and-error" period of adjusting the relaxation medication will again occur.

CASE 2   Jeremy is a 4-year-old child with a diagnosis of porencephalia and spastic quadriparesis. Additionally, he has a seizure disorder resulting from the porencephalia. Jeremy has been followed in physical therapy since he was 6 months old and has been followed since birth by pediatric neurology.

With weekly physical therapy, Jeremy had been making slow but steady progress with head control and with upper body movement. His mother was very active in the program and worked with Jeremy on a daily basis. During this period, Jeremy was taking clonazepam (Clonopin) and valproic acid (Depakene) for control of his myoclonic seizures.

During a 4-week period, a steady decline was noted in Jeremy's overall abilities. The mother reported that he was fussy all of the time and that he acted as if his head "hurt." She felt that perhaps he had an ear infection but when examined by the family physician, no evidence of otitis media was noted. In addition to his mother's evaluation, the therapist noted that Jeremy was no longer interested in lifting his head or participating in any of the gross motor activities. He appeared to be disoriented and disinterested. Eventually, the mother noted that Jeremy seemed to be sleeping almost constantly. He was difficult to arouse at mealtime and was eating very little. The mother reported that his seizure activity had increased but only from approximately three myoclonic seizures a day to ten seizures a day.

At the end of the 4-week period and after a second visit to the family physician, the mother returned to the pediatric neurologist, fearing that Jeremy was developing hydrocephalus because this had been explained to her in the past as a possibility. On examination, the pediatric neurologist determined that Jeremy was reacting adversely to the Clonopin and immediately discontinued this medication and started treatment with clorazepate (Tranxene) and Depakene instead. Within 24 hr, Jeremy was again alert and reactive to the environment. He was eating well and again participating without difficulty with the physical therapy program. Had Jeremy been referred to the pediatric neurologist sooner, his problems during the 4-week period could have been reduced and his participation in physical therapy would not have been hindered.

REFERENCES

1. American Academy of Pediatrics: Report of the Committee of Infectious Diseases, 19th ed. 1982
2. Calne DB: Therapeutics in Neurology. Oxford, Blackwell Scientific Publications, 1975
3. Cloherty JP, Stark AR (eds): Manual of Neonatal Care. Boston, Little, Brown & Co, 1980
4. Govoni LE, Hayes JE: Drugs and Nursing Implications, 5th ed. Norwalk, Appleton-Century-Crofts, 1985
5. Hughes JG, Griffith JF (eds): Synopsis of Pediatrics. 6th ed. St Louis, CV Mosby, 1984
6. Jabbour JT, Duenas DA, Gilmartin RC et al: Pediatric Neurology Handbook. Flushing, NY, Medical Examinations Publishing, 1973

7. Physicians Desk Reference for Nonprescription Drugs, 6th ed. Oradell, NJ, Medical Economics, 1985

8. Physicians Desk Reference, 37th ed. Oradell, NJ, Medical Economics, 1983

9. Pinelli P: In Garattini S, Mussini E, and Randall LO (eds). The Benzodiazepines. New York, Raven Press, 1973

10. Silver HK, Kempe CH, Bruyn HB: Handbook of Pediatrics. 14th ed. Los Altos, Calif, Lange Medical Publications, 1983

Psychiatry

Claudia K. Allen

9

The discovery of psychotropic drugs has changed the care of the mentally ill. In many instances, the drugs have reduced the length of hospitalization and returned people to productive roles in society. The drugs are associated with four major neurotransmitters: acetylcholine, norepinephrine, dopamine, and serotonin. Knowledge about how the neurotransmitters work has been emerging at an incredible rate during the last 3 decades, and the field seems to be ready for even greater achievements.[29] The process of recognizing and adapting to these changes is a challenge for all health care professionals.

The scope and the rate of knowledge development have had a revolutionary effect on the practice of psychiatry. This chapter will begin with an overview of the dramatic changes in psychiatry, including a discussion of potential implications for rehabilitation professionals. Three prevalent mental disorders will be described: affective disorders (mania and depression), schizophrenic disorders, and personality disorders. Drug effectiveness will probably have a revolutionary effect on rehabilitation objectives as well, and the relationships between rehabilitation and psychiatry will be discussed. Case examples will be included.

PSYCHIATRIC REVOLUTION

Stigma is a problem for all people who have a disability, and the stigma linked with mental illness is usually greater than that linked with physical disabilities. Stigma generalizes to professionals who work with the disabled, and psychiatrists ("shrinks") have acquired a reputation as oddballs. The problem was not helped by the fact that American psychiatrists adopted Freud's view of mental illness, using terms such as *oral* and *anal* while drawing analogies to Alice in Wonderland. Many people assume that this is still the state of the art in psychiatry; it is not.

A relatively rapid way of seeing, first hand, the revolution that has occurred in psychiatry can be suggested: Go to the library and compare a journal published in the 1950s with one published in the 1980s; note the title, tables, graphics, descriptions of behavior, use of the scientific method, and reference to the basic neurosciences. Journals that you might want to consider include *American Journal of Psychiatry*, published by the American Psychiatric Association; *Archives of General Psychiatry*, published by the American Medical Association; *Journal of Clinical Psychiatry*, boasting the largest readership; and the *British Journal of Psychiatry*, containing a prestigious, other-than-American view of mental illness. The differences are astonishing. The titles in the 1980s contain words such as *neurotransmitter* that did not exist 30 years ago. Graphic, theoretical descriptions have been replaced by statistical tables. The number of credible research instruments that have been developed to measure aspects of mental illness objectively is remarkable. I also suggest that you compare the letters to the editor. The 1980s list of concerns includes new drug uses, cautions about drug side-effects, disquiet about loss of humanistic approach to patient care, and debate about what the tests are actually measuring. The topics of concern in present-day psychiatry are more closely connected to the biologic topics of other medical specialties. As a medical specialty, the psychiatric literature formerly contained numerous anomalies; those anomalies have been markedly reduced.

The understanding of the revolution in psychiatry helps in establishing a working relationship with a psychiatrist. A physician who was trained in the 1980s will probably be thinking about the connections between psychotropic drugs and changes in functional behavior. A physician trained in the 1950s is more likely to use psychodynamic terminology to explain behavior. Individuals vary but, over all, there often seems to be a generation gap in current practice.

Psychotherapy or Drugs

Another major change has occurred in the use of psychotherapy. Psychotherapy was formerly the form of treatment for all psychiatric patients. Research studies have shown that psychotherapy is not effective, and may even be harmful, in severe or acute cases of depression, mania, and schizophrenia. Basically, the studies have shown that it does no good to talk to someone who is too sick and confused to form an intelligible sentence. Psychotherapy has been shown to be as effective as an antidepressant medication when treating outpatients with mild depression. Credible studies that show psychotherapy to be more effective than drugs have not been conducted (attempts are underway). Thousands of studies that demonstrate the effectiveness, as well as the side-effects, of psychotropic drugs exist.[7]

The use of psychotherapy or drugs is at the heart of a long conflict between psychiatrists and other mental health professionals. Psychiatrists have made considerable progress in verifying the efficacy of psychotropic drugs. Psychotherapists are just beginning to translate treatment theories into standardized procedures, control groups, and objective outcome measures.

The uses for psychotherapy and drugs are based on different assumptions about the cause of mental illness. Psychotherapy assumes that the cause is learned during the patient's interactions with the social environment. The use of drugs assumes that the problem is a biologic abnormality. There are a mounting number of studies to support the biologic assumption; these studies are enhanced by recent technologic advances. Researchers are using CAT, PET, and MRI. Computerized axial tomography (CAT) provides an anatomic picture of the brain. A number of studies, conducted in a variety of settings in the United States and Britain, have found morphologic abnormalities in schizophrenia and mania.[4,5,13,16,17,23,27,28,35,36] Positron emission tomography (PET) provides a colorful picture of brain metabolism. One of the neurotransmitters, dopamine, has been traced in normal subjects, and in subjects with schizophrenic and affective disorders. These scans have also demonstrated abnormalities in schizophrenia and affective disorders.[8,9] Magnetic resonance imaging (MRI) uses electromagnetic force and radio frequencies to form anatomic images; the chief advantage over CAT is that MRI does not involve radioactive materials. As of this writing, PET and MRI are recent developments. Several years have been spent ironing out technical difficulties and, at last, the technology is ready to address human disorders. The initial studies suggest that biologic abnormalities may be definable.

The CAT, PET, and MRI scans seem to be describing where and what is wrong but, not necessarily, why it went wrong. A few years ago an alert researcher was looking at some data concerning adopted children who developed schizophrenia. He noticed that many of them were born during the same season, raising questions about viruses and other infectious diseases. Watson and coworkers[33] found that schizophrenic birth seasonality does seem to be related to the incidence of infectious disease (diphtheria, pneumonia, and influenza are suggested). So far, researchers have been frustrated in their attempts to find a virus or autoimmunity associated with schizophrenia.[30,31] Some success seems to be evident in locating a virus associated with depression: Epstein-Barr, a herpes virus, is also associated with mononucleosis.[24] It is too soon to tell if viruses cause mental illness, but the possibility does exist. The viral implications for psychotherapy are substantial.

More and more of the so-called functional disorders are resembling regular diseases. In addition, the medical problems that can be corrected by psychotherapy are being reexamined. Psychotherapy is conducted by talking to the patient. Talking, in the sequence of probable success, may be as follows: getting the patient to stop eating salt, to lose weight, to stop smoking, to stop drinking, to stop feeling depression, to stop having schizophrenia, and to stop having Alzheimer's disease. One cannot talk someone out of having dementia or schizophrenia. It can also be very difficult to get some people to reduce their salt intake, even when medical indications are clearly evident.

The difficulties that the psychotherapists have encountered should be noted by all health professionals. We have adopted a tendency to tell people what they ought to do; noncompliance rates for prescribed medications run as high as 50%, and even higher for other recommendations. Getting people to change their behavior is difficult. Treatment objectives, as a general rule, need to be less sanguine and more tough-minded when the objective is to be achieved by talking to the patient. I do not mean to suggest that these objectives should be abandoned. Actually, the reverse is true. I suspect that rehabilitation professionals need to be more selective about stating these objectives, and when the objective is very important, more time needs to be allotted to the fulfillment of "talking" objectives.

Character Assassination

Freud's efforts to describe aberrant thought had an unfortunate side-effect, character assassination. The terms he developed can be used to unjustly label behavior as deviant. The problem is well known and great strides in correcting it were made with the most recent diagnostic criteria (*DSM–III–R*, 1987).[10] The problem, however, is far from rectified. In psychiatric circles, the diagnosis that is of gravest concern for abuse is *borderline personality disorder*. All of the personality disorders (especially antisocial, narcissistic, histrionic, passive–aggressive, dependent) can be used in a libelous fashion. Alcoholism and drug abuse can be labeled unjustly, too. It is my impression that these terms are much abused by nonpsychiatric health professionals. My advice is to avoid using the label unless one is using the *DSM–III–R*[10] and the patient's behavior fulfills the diagnostic criteria. The concern is that effective treatment methods for these disorders are largely unknown and the prognosis is usually poor. When abused, these diagnostic categories are used to blame the patient for the health professional's failure to attain or even pursue a treatment objective. Clearly, precautions need to be taken to avoid this possibility.

An additional lesson can be learned from these problems with diagnostic criteria and ambiguous treatment effectiveness. Medical professionals speak of *abuse* when ambiguities in diagnosis and treatment exist. Many ambiguities in rehabilitation objectives currently exist — controlled, replicated efficacy studies with reliability and validity are far too rare, much rarer than in psychiatry. The rehabilitation professional is forced to rely on a *belief* that an objective can be fulfilled. A belief is unsubstantiated dogma. The history of psychiatry is filled with examples of atrocities occurring when one is forced to rely on a belief system.

Adapting to all of these changes in psychiatry is not easy because the changes have been so rapid and so fundamental. This chapter outlines the major changes that have occurred. Basic references that condense psychiatric information into brief and lucid material can be suggested. I would recommend *Psychiatric Diagnosis* by Goodwin and Guze[14] as a comprehensive text. Hollister's *Clinical Pharmacology of Psychotherapeutic Drugs*[15] has a narrower focus but is still a good, basic text. The neurologist's point of view is presented by Klawans and Weiner in a *Textbook of Clinical Neuropharmacology*.[19] The divisions between neurology and psychiatry are diminishing, and this last text helps the reader to gain perspective on this change.

The rest of this chapter will be devoted to the treatment of three prevalent and severe mental disorders: unipolar affective disorders, bipolar affective disorders, and schizophrenic disorders.

AFFECTIVE DISORDERS

Mood disorders are characterized by two extremes, either depression or euphoria. When mania occurs, with or without depression, the diagnosis is *bipolar mood disorder*. Depression only is diagnosed as *unipolar mood disorder*. Mood disorders were first described by Hippocrates, but throughout recorded history it has been difficult to identify behavioral observations that distinguish between a pathologic condition and a normal condition, such as bereavement or loss. Mood is an ambiguous concept. The most recent diagnostic criteria have included vegetative signs that permit more objective evaluation: sleep disturbance, weight loss, loss of energy, hyperactivity, pressured speech, distractibility (*DSM–III–R*, 1987).[10] The additional criteria make it easier to identify a pathologic condition.

Bipolar Mood Disorders and Lithium

An elevated, expansive, or irritable mood characterizes a *manic* episode. Not all manic patients are euphoric, and irritability with, or without, euphoria is common. Irritability is likely to be elicited when someone attempts to direct the patient's behavior; noncompliance or angry outbursts may occur. Before seeking treatment, these patients' behavior is disruptive — they may be in perpetual motion day and night; talk incessantly; neglect sleeping and eating; have unrealistic ideas of what they do, although they accomplish virtually nothing; start ambitious projects and quit after creating a terrible mess; get involved in foolish spending sprees or financial investments; solicit and engage in sexual indiscretions; drive recklessly or attempt to direct traffic. They are frequently brought to a hospital by the police or family members when their behavior is so disruptive that it cannot be tolerated in the community. If so, they seldom think there is anything the matter with them. In more fortunate cases, the patient recognizes the disturbance and seeks help.

Since 1970, lithium salts have been used to normalize the acute manic episode. Lithium is absorbed into the body fluid within about 6 to 8 hr after an oral dose, but absorption into the brain is slow. No protein binding occurs. The lithium has an effect on mania within about 10 days, and about 3 weeks are required for total normalization to occur. The dosage is gradually increased until a therapeutic blood level is reached, ranging between 0.9 mEq/liter and 1.4 mEq/liter. A neuroleptic drug, chlorpromazine, is frequently administered with lithium during the first 10 days and discontinued as the lithium takes effect.

Lithium produces a number of side-effects while drug tolerance is being developed. Patients who think there is nothing the matter with them are likely to complain vehemently about these side-effects. Gastrointestinal effects may include diarrhea, nausea, vomiting, and abdominal pain. Renal symptoms may include polyuria, dry mouth, and thirst. These side-effects are transient and disappear as the lithium takes effect. The difficulties reside in convincing the patients of any or all of the following: (1) there is something disruptive about their behavior; (2) lithium does work; and (3) the side-effects will go away. In a study conducted by Taylor and Abrams[32] the only factor that was significant in predicting a poor response to lithium was a premature termination of treatment. My clinical experience suggests that talking about treatment termination intensifies when patients begin to experience side-effects. Sometimes the only way to get persons through this difficult period is to have them involuntarily committed to a psychiatric hospital.

COGNITIVE LEVELS

This brings us to a central problem in the treatment of brain disorders: When is a person competent to manage his or her affairs, and when does a care giver have to make the decisions? The legal definitions of competency are unclear; forensic psychiatry has just begun to address this problem. I suspect that competence can be determined by using the cognitive levels and task analyses found in Tables 9-1 and 9-2. The cognitive levels and task analyses are ordinal scales designed to measure

(*Text continues on p. 214*)

TABLE 9-1
Cognitive Levels

Attributes	Level 1: Automatic Actions	Level 2: Postural Actions	Level 3: Manual Actions	Level 4: Goal-Directed Actions	Level 5: Exploratory Actions	Level 6: Planned Actions
ATTENTION TO SENSORY CUES	Subliminal cues	Proprioceptive cues	Tactile cues	Visible cues	Related cues	Symbolic cues
MOTOR ACTIONS						
Spontaneous	Automatic	Postural	Manual	Goal-directed	Exploratory	Planned
Imitated	None	Approximations	Manipulations	Replications	Novelty	Unnecessary
CONSCIOUS AWARENESS						
Purpose	Arousal	Comfort	Interest	Compliance	Self-control	Reflection
Experience	Indistinct	Moving	Touching	Seeing	Inductive reasoning	Deductive reasoning
Process	Habitual or reflexive	Effect on body	Effect on environment	Several actions	Overt trial and error	Covert trial and error
Time	Seconds	Minutes	Half hours	Hours	Weeks	Past and future

Allen CK: Occupational Therapy for Psychiatric Diseases: Measurement and Management of Cognitive Disabilities, p 34. Boston, Little, Brown & Co, 1985

TABLE 9-2
Task Analysis

Attributes	Level 1: Automatic Actions	Level 2: Postural Actions	Level 3: Manual Actions	Level 4: Goal-Directed Actions	Level 5: Exploratory Actions	Level 6: Planned Actions
MATTER						
Sensory cue	Threshold of consciousness	Proprioceptive cues	Tactile cues	Visible cues	Related cues	Symbolic cues
Perceptibility	Penetrates subliminal state	Own body Furniture and clothing	Exterior surfaces	Color and shape	Space and depth	Intangible
Setting	Internal	Range of motion	Arms reach	Visual field	Task environment	Potential task environment
Sample	Alerting stimuli	Demonstrated action	Material object	Exact match	Tangible possibilities	Hypothetical ideas
BEHAVIOR						
Motor actions Number	Automatic One action	Postural One action	Manual One action	Goal-directed One step at a time	Exploratory Several steps at a time	Planned Infinite
Tool use	Stimulated use of body parts	Spontaneous use of body parts	Chance use of found objects	Hand tools used as a means to an end	Hand tools used to vary means and end	Tool making Power tools
Other people	Shouting Touching	Moving	Manipulating objects	Sharing goals	Sharing explorations	Sharing plans and recognizing autonomous plans
Direction Verbal	Verbs Introjections	Pronouns Names of body parts	Names of material objects	Adjectives Adverbs	Prepositions Explanations	Conjunctions Conjectures
Demonstrated	Physical contact	Gross motor and guided movements	Action on an object	Each step in a series	Each step and precautions for potential errors	Not required

Allen CK: Occupational Therapy for Psychiatric Diseases: Measurement and Management of Cognitive Disabilities, p 34. Boston, Little, Brown & Co, 1985 the functional abilities and social welfare needs of persons with mental disorders.[1-3] The congnitive levels measure sensorimotor performance abilities.

A brief profile of the cognitive levels, as they relate to the need for care giver assistance, is required. Level 1 is *responding*: automatic actions are associated with subliminal cues. At level 1 the patient is conscious and can perform voluntary motor actions like chewing, swallowing, and picking up food. All other activities required to sustain life must be done by a care giver. Level 2 is *performing*: postural actions are associated with proprioceptive cues. At level 2 the patient imitates postural actions and cooperates by moving hands, feet, head, as the care giver assists with grooming, dressing, and bathing activities. Food is prepared by the care giver. The patient may need to be escorted to the table and the bathroom. Aimless pacing and wandering may occur and protection from getting lost may be required. Level 3 is *repeating*: manual actions are associated with tactile cues. At level 3 the patient imitates a manual action that has an effect on an external object. Daily grooming tasks, like brushing teeth, washing hands, showering, and getting dressed, can be done independently. Gross errors in clothing selection and using fasteners, like zippers, may need to be corrected by the care giver. While pacing or wandering, the patient may get into things or get lost. Food is prepared by the care giver but some assistance from the patient may be obtained when repetitive manual actions, such as peeling potatoes, can be identified by the care giver. Laundry, medication, and money management are done by the care giver. The patient can answer the telephone and dial one or two frequent or important numbers. Patients may not relay a message, may not call another person to the telephone, or they may take the receiver off the hook and leave it off.[1-3]

Level 4 is *following*: familiar goal-directed actions are associated with clearly visible cues. The patient can follow a set routine to accomplish vital grooming, dressing, bathing, walking, feeding, and toileting tasks. Departures from the established routine require care giver assistance. Hazards posed by heat, chemical reactions, and electricity are not visible and, thus, may not be recognized. Electrical appliances, such as the stove or iron, may not be turned off, or they may be used when there is a short circuit or exposed wire. Hot food and boiling water may be handled dangerously. Precautions printed on products, such as cleaning and grooming supplies, may be ignored. The safe storage of possessions to avoid theft or destruction may not be considered. Such items as theft of money or a budget for weekly and monthly purchases may not be considered. The driving of a car may result in parking tickets, moving violations, and accidents, with a disregard for fines, insurance, and licenses. Care giver assistance to prevent undesirable consequences is required. The patient, however, may not recognize the presence of any problems and refuse support and treatment.[1-3]

Level 5 is *learning*: exploratory actions are associated with related visible cues. Level 5 seems to be the usual level of functioning for some people (approximately 20% of a control population) and a distressing disability for others (approximately 80%); the difference is associated with social class. Difficulties in planning a course of action and anticipating future events are observed. Some areas of neglect have minor consequences: not preheating the oven; not watering the lawn during a hot spell; not following new, written directions, such as a new recipe; forgetting to buy birthday gifts or stamps, to take clothes to the cleaners, or to get a prescription refilled. Forgetting where the car is parked; being unable to decipher a map, to plan a route to a new location, or to anticipate costs while traveling can be hazardous!

Anticipation of long-term financial security, such as retirement plans, insurance, taxes, or major purchases may require care giver assistance. Level 6 is *anticipating*: planned actions are associated with symbolic cues. Level 6 is designed to describe the absence of a disability, and no care giver support should be required.[1-3]

Upon admission to the hospital most manic patients are functioning at levels 3 and 4. A change in the cognitive level is observed as the lithium takes effect, reaching level 6 about 2 weeks after a therapeutic blood level is reached. Distress over side-effects, with an inability to understand the temporary nature of the discomfort or their own disruptive behavior, occurs at levels 3 and 4. That is the reason for involuntary commitment to a psychiatric hospital.[2,3]

COURSE OF THE DISEASE

The mean age of onset for bipolar affective disorder is 30 years. One manic episode may be the only attack that 50% of the bipolar patients experience. For others the number of episodes, with or without depressive episodes, is variable. The highest risk for another episode is about 12 weeks after recovery; and risk diminishes as the time since the last episode increases. Between episodes in a sample of untreated manic patients, 61% were identified as symptom-free, whereas the rest had detectable symptoms. Those patients who have symptoms, or who have recurrent episodes, can be treated with lower doses of lithium (blood levels range from 0.5 mEq/liter to 1.0 mEq/liter). Lithium can minimize the frequency and intensity of the episodes. Ongoing monitoring of the lithium blood level is essential. When treated, persons with bipolar mood disorder function as well as a comparison group of nonpsychiatric controls.[14]

There are persons who will not take their lithium or who go through several episodes before they agree to take prophylactic lithium. The social consequences of bipolar episodes can effect all aspects of a person's life: divorce, lost custody of children, job loss, lost driver's license, lost license to practice a profession, car accidents, or jail. There are also a number of complications associated with the prolonged use of lithium; fine hand tremors, weight gain, and potential lithium toxicity. The choice can be a difficult one, and at level 6 the patient is able to make the decision.

Lithium does not work for all bipolar patients. Some are nonresponders; their level of function never gets higher than level 4. Others develop lithium toxicity. Toxicity is related to dosage or blood level. Gross bilateral hand tremors that interfere with performance, disorientation, and ataxia are organic signs that suggest toxicity. Fine hand tremors, however, are associated with lithium drug tolerance and are not a cause for concern, but toxicity can cause major organ damage or death. Other medications are usually not as effective as lithium. Currently, carbamazepine, an anticonvulsant medication, is being used with some degree of success.[1,18,25,26,38]

REHABILITATION

The ideal case does not require rehabilitation. The patient comes into the hospital, is treated, and returns to the premorbid level of function. Unfortunately, this disease expresses itself by the use of poor judgment in the management of one's personal affairs. As people return to their premorbid level of function, they frequently discover that they have done serious damage to the quality of their lives. The damages are variable and can include physical disabilities as well as social consequences. Some assistance in appraising the damages, planning restitutions, or coping with a different quality of life may be required.

Patients who refuse to take lithium usually refuse rehabilitation programs as well. They do not think there is anything the matter with them.

Patients who do not respond to lithium or the alternative forms of medical interventions, such as carbamazepine, may participate in a rehabilitation program. Because their functional abilities and the natural course of the disease seem to parallel some schizophrenic disorders, this rehabilitation program is similar, as outlined in the following case studies.

CASE STUDIES

Two cases of bipolar disorders with a fairly long history have been selected to illustrate the differences between taking and not taking prophylactic lithium. To protect the confidentiality of the patient's identities some specific facts have been fictionalized (name, age, and the like). All of the cases in this chapter have some identifying alterations, without, I hope, changing the salient features of the case.

CASE 1   Sarah is a 38-year-old black woman with a 12-year history of a bipolar disorder. She has never had a depressive episode but does have a manic episode about once a year, usually in the fall. Sarah graduated from a private college with a degree in theology and has worked since then as a secretary. Her longest job lasted 10 years, and she has never been fired. She lives alone in an apartment and reports a reasonable number of good friends, contacts with family in the area, and recreational activities.

This is Sarah's tenth psychiatric hospitalization, and it is following her usual pattern. She was brought to the hospital by the police, who found her partly clothed, wandering in the street, and talking incoherently. On admission, she was functioning at level 3. Within 24 to 36 hr she was speaking coherently and reported that she had been taking her prophylactic lithium because "I function better with it." She has called her employer and arranged for a few days of sick leave. The manic episode is clearing quickly and she probably will be discharged within a week. She was functioning at level 2 before admission and usually functions at level 6 at discharge.

CASE 2   Marie, a 43-year-old Chinese woman with a 17-year history of a bipolar disorder, has had at least one depressive episode during her last admission, but the other five admissions were for manic episodes. Six other admissions to psychiatric hospitals have been reported, but the type of episode is unknown. Her mother and a sibling also have bipolar disorders. Marie grew up in Taiwan and came to the United States, by way of Canada, 12 years ago; she is fluent in English and Chinese. She has earned four college degrees, one at the masters level, since coming to the United States (level 6).

After graduating from college, Marie worked in the space industry but was fired three times: twice for talking too much and once for keeping irregular hours (working 80 hr straight and then not showing up for several days). Her last job was 6 years ago when she had a part-time job as a bookkeeper (level 6 or 5). Currently, she is supported by Social Security Insurance for the disabled. Marie lives with a boyfriend, who is a heavy drinker. He brings her to the hospital when she starts staying up all night, talking, and moving things around in the apartment. She bangs on doors, throws things at the boyfriend, empties drawers and cupboards on to the floor, and destroys their property. When this cannot be stopped by the boyfriend, he brings her to the hospital. Before this admission she ran up a 300 dollar long-distance telephone bill in less than a week; she has no money at the present time.

On admission Marie is functioning at level 3, while claiming there is nothing the matter with her. She is hospitalized against her will and seeks legal recourse to obtain her freedom as soon as possible. Lithium is prescribed but therapeutic blood levels are seldom reached before she must be discharged from the hospital (usually 17 days, according to California law). She has been functioning at level 4 when discharged. She reports that she stops taking the lithium as soon as she is released. The boyfriend is unable to give a reliable report about the quality of her functional abilities in between manic episodes, but her education and work histories suggest a functional decline.

Manic episodes are noisy and active. As a result a large number of public servants may be involved: the police or a crisis team may bring the patient to the hospital; the case may be reviewed by a lawyer and a patients' rights advocate; continued hospitalization may involve a public defender; and the decision to discharge may be made by a judge. State laws guide these decisions, with considerable variation between the states. Sarah and Marie illustrate the interrelationships between psychiatry and the law. They also illustrate the importance of recognizing a connection between medication effectiveness and an improvement in functional behavior.

Depressive Mood Disorders and Antidepressants

Numerous attempts have been made to differentiate normal sadness from severe disturbances in mood. The vegetative signs (sleeping, eating, and motor activity disturbances) identify symptoms that respond to the antidepressant medications. A unique sleep disturbance exists: waking up and not being able to go back to sleep. The person may wake up in the middle of the night or wake up too early in the morning. Eating habits may change. Usually there is a loss of appetite, a feeling that it takes too much energy to eat or cook, and loss of weight. The reverse, weight gain, with compulsive overeating, is rare. Motor activity is usually reduced, movements are slow and laborious, and everything seems to require too much energy. Concentration, attention span, ability to think, ability to get things done, ability to take pleasure in activities, and sexual desire are reduced. The difficulties are often worse in the morning. Some people are content to sit in one place for hours, but a few report sudden urge to move (this is not as persistent as the hyperactivity associated with mania).

Chemical compounds with antidepressant characteristics are being developed at a seemingly exponential rate (Table 9-3). At first, it was thought that these drugs had an effect on the availability of norepinephrine and serotonin; these theories now appear to be too simple. The selection of which drug, or combination of drugs, is a part of the ongoing debate in psychiatry. The controversies are complex and probably best left to the sophisticated analysis of the biologic psychiatrist. The rehabilitation professional should be able to recognize the major types of antidepressants and be able to use Table 9-3 as a reference for the compound name and trade name.

TABLE 9-3
Antidepressant Drugs

Generic Name	Trade Name
TRICYCLICS	
Amitriptyline	Amitril, Amitryptyline Elavil, Endep
Clomipramine	Anafranil
Desipramine	Norpramin, Pertofrane
Doxepin	Adapin, Sinequan
Imipramine	Antipress, Imavate Imipramine, Janimine Presamine, SK-Pramine Tofranil
Nortriptyline	Aventyl, Pamelor
Protriptyline	Vivactil, Triptil
Trimipramine	Surmontil
TETRACYCLICS	
Mianserin	
Maprotiline	Ludiomil
BICYCLICS	
Viloxazine	
Zumelidine	
DIBENZEPINES	
Amoxapine	Asendin
Alprazolam	Xanax
UNUSUAL STRUCTURES	
Buproprion	Wellbutrin
Monifensine	Merital
Trazodone	Desyrel
MONOAMINE OXIDASE INHIBITORS (MAOs)	
Isocarboxazid	Marplan
Phenelzine	Nardil
Tranylcypromine	Parnate

The tricyclics have a three-ring nucleus, hence, the name, and are the most frequently prescribed. Originally thought to be antihistamines and then antipsychotics, the discovery of their antidepressant properties was fortuitous. Numerous controlled studies have demonstrated the efficacy of these drugs. "Tricyclics differ mainly in the amount of sedative effect (amitriptyline and doxepin have the highest amount, protriptyline the least) and the amount of anticholinergic effect (amitriptyline and doxepin have the highest amount, desipramine the least)."[15] Selecting the best drug for an individual patient is difficult, clear selection criteria are lacking. Two or three tricyclics may be tried before the psychiatrist decides to try another type of antidepressant.

The monoamine oxidase (MAO) inhibitors are often regarded as a second choice for most depressive episodes. In special cases, such as anxiety, phobia, and hypochondrias associated with depression, the MAOs may be a first choice. Rehabilitation professionals should note the food restrictions: aged foods (cheese, chianti, lox, pickled herring) have a high tyramine content and, therefore, should be avoided.[6]

The remaining drugs listed in Table 9-3 are often lumped into a category called "second generation" drugs. These drugs have various advantages: fewer anticholinergic side-effects, reduced cardiotoxic effects if taken in a suicidal overdose, or quicker production of a clinical response. As psychiatrists gain clinical experience with use of these drugs, they seem to be replacing some of the traditional tricyclics.

Perhaps the most startling aspect of the treatment of depression is that the most effective treatment is electroconvulsive therapy (ECT). The theory of how ECT works is similar to that of the other antidepressants; involving serotonin. Increasing legal restrictions have encouraged a heavier reliance on the antidepressants.[22] If the patient is severely depressed with a high suicide risk, ECT is usually started as soon as possible; a positive ECT response is the quickest and the most reliable. Patients, families, and health professionals have often heard the superstitions about ECT and regard it as a treatment of last resort.[20] The use of ECT raises the question of *risk*; a risk is a chance of encountering harm or loss. Medical treatments incur risks. Currently, the risks associated with ECT are relatively low. It is often used in combination with an antidepressant.[15]

The amphetamines are stimulants that were used to treat depression during the 1930s, but their use declined as more effective drugs were developed. During the 1960s drugs were often used in combination, but unwanted drug synergies developed and the practice declined. Both practices are being reexamined. The use of tricyclics with MAOs and stimulants may be effective with patients who fail to respond or who relapse with the preceding treatments.[12,37] This practice is usually advocated only for exceptionally knowledgeable psychiatrists.

Perserverance may be the key to finding an effective treatment for an individual patient. There are many potential treatments, but finding one that works for an individual can take time; many drugs are tried for 2 or 3 weeks before they are considered a failure. The delay is especially difficult for patients whose presenting symptoms include a sense of hopelessness about their condition. Rehabilitation therapists can be sympathetic about the delay, but they should not succumb to the patient's sense of hopelessness. Phrases like, "When you get better. . .," help to sustain the patient through difficult periods.

Antidepressants can produce unwanted side-effects that are of concern to rehabilitation professionals. The anticholinergic effects include blurred vision, dry mouth, constipation, and urinary hesitancy. Tolerance may develop during the first few weeks of treatment, reducing or eliminating the side-effect. If not, the physician may suggest an alternative. The sedative effects may include fatigue, lassitude, and sleeping at inappropriate times; taking sedative antidepressants at night can reduce these problems. Postural hypotension, tachycardia, and palpitation are frequent cardiovascular effects when there is a rapid increase in the dosage and with the elderly. The patient should be encouraged to rise slowly from a bed or a chair, and the therapist should be ready to steady patients, if they are dizzy. Weight gain is a frequent side-effect, accompanied by a craving for sweets or a search for a relief from the dry mouth. The weight gain is probably related to the metabolic and endocrine effects of the drugs and is very difficult to self-control.[6,15]

COGNITIVE LEVELS

Level 1, with severe depression is seen on rare occasions, usually the patient has not eaten for several days. Therapy with ECT may be started as soon as possible to sustain the person's life. Level 2 is usually accompanied by psychomotor agitation/retardation, disorientation, and confusion. The *DSM–III–R* [10] criteria do not permit a clear differential between dementia and depression at levels 2 and 3. A history of previous depressive episodes may help in making the differential, but if no history is available, the differential is unclear. Many psychiatrists will treat for a possible depression first because depression has a good prognosis; dementia is considered after a failure to respond to antidepressants or to ECT. At level 3 there is usually a profound loss of energy; motor actions are slow and laborious. A simple task that usually would be done in 5 or 10 min may take an hour, and even then the task may not be finished or steps may be skipped. Patients sometimes say that they are too tired to care.

Most people admitted to an acute psychiatric hospital with depression are functioning at level 4. With this population, a clear distinction needs to be made between verbal performance and sensorimotor performance. In the United States most people have had the benefit of a formal education that develops verbal skills (reading, writing, spelling, vocabulary). Verbal skills are often retained, even though the patient is very sick. At level 4 patients frequently sound fine when talking; it is during observations of sensorimotor performance that the disability becomes evident. While working on a task they may be very quiet and slow, completing a 15-min task in 45 min to an hour. A simple mistake seems to produce insurmountable problems for them: they ask for assistance; have difficulty in following demonstrated directions and are overcome by verbal or written directions; refuse to have anything more to do with the difficult activity; or blame other people or objects for their difficulties. At level 4 with depression many people avoid sensorimotor activities, preferring to sit and talk. Activities that are done are usually short, simple, and familiar. New learning, reasoning, and sustained concentration seems to take too much effort.

At level 5 inductive, but not deductive, reasoning occurs. It still takes too much energy to pause to think and plan. They will try new activities and rely on demonstrated directions. Performance at level 6 is usually observed after the change in mood is noted. With affective disorders there may be a 2-week delay in change in functional ability after a change in mood.

COURSE OF THE DISEASE

The average age of onset is about 30, with the majority of patients being younger than patients with bipolar disorders. The average age of onset is somewhat misleading because the age of risk extends throughout the lifespan. Epidemiologically the lifetime risk of having at least one depressive episode is between 15% and 20% of the general population. The length of an episode is variable, a few days to several years; 6 months is often regarded as the average length of an untreated episode. Usually, the antidepressants return people to their premorbid level of function, and antidepressants can be used to prevent recurrent episodes. There are cases of chronic depression that are very difficult for psychiatrists to treat effectively.[14]

Suicide is the ominous complication of this disease; the number of depressed people who eventually die by suicide may be as high as 15%. Criteria that predict who or when are notoriously weak. Increased risk is associated with age over 40, male, and communicating suicidal intent. Alcohol and drug abuse, as forms of self-medication, are associated with depression. In addition, depressed people complicate their lives by making bad decisions, leaving jobs, getting divorces, moving, dropping out of college, or marginally fulfilling work and school responsibilities. Depressed patients are usually advised to avoid major responsibilities and decisions until after the episode is clearly in remission.[14]

REHABILITATION

As with bipolar disorders, most people who have a depressive episode will return to their former lives. Rehabilitation professionals are likely to see two types of depressed patients: people who have injured themselves during a suicide attempt, and people who have a depression secondary to another diagnosis.

Any part of the body can be injured during a suicide attempt. Particularly repugnant are forms of self-mutilation. As a health professional you may find yourself wondering, "How could he do that to himself?" Self-mutilation usually occurs during psychotic episodes for reasons that do not seem logical. Rehabilitation often begins after the psychotic episode has cleared, placing you at a disadvantage because you have not seen the psychotic behavior. You may need to remind yourself that these people can be very different during a psychotic episode.

An amazing number of physical diseases have an association with depression. The symptoms are often severe enough to warrant a diagnosis of a major depression (*DSM–III–R*).[10] Disorders affecting brain function seem to be especially prone to an association with depression. The prevalence of depression in some rehabilitation agencies is high. The question is: Should these depressions be treated with antidepressant medications? The answer is controversial and physicians vary in their use. Psychiatrists are concerned by studies that indicate that antidepressants are often used incorrectly, prescribing too little or not long enough.[15]

One of the most difficult cases that a rehabilitation therapist is likely to encounter is a person who has a chronic depression, functioning at level 4, and has an injury resulting from a suicide attempt. The depression makes the patient feel hopeless and helpless. The cognitive disability impairs new learning, and the reality of a permanent injury may be denied. Attempts at getting the patient to cooperate with your rehabilitation efforts are difficult. When possible, demonstrate what it is you want the patient to do and avoid lengthy discussions about why it is important.

CASE 3   Ernest is an example of a patient who presents treatment dilemmas to psychiatric and rehabilitation professionals. He is a 27-year-old black man who has a history of drug abuse since the age of 12. This is his sixth psychiatric admission after a suicide attempt; he has been hospitalized in Tennessee, Georgia, Texas, Arizona, and California. The suicide attempt made a year ago involved stepping in front of a car, sustaining a spinal cord injury with hemiparesis. He received some rehabilitation at that time but left the program against medical advice (AMA). He says he threw away the leg braces and walker that were given to him. At the present time he uses a wheelchair or walks along the wall with a very unsteady gait.

Three months ago he was admitted to this psychiatric hospital after a suicide attempt. The diagnosis for this patient was difficult to establish, and major depression, personality disorder, and phencyclidine (PCP) abuse were considered. (PCP can mimic the symptoms of depression, mania, and schizophrenia.) Ernest is a difficult patient to manage; he has gotten into fights with other patients; he gouged a nurse on the arm; and he hit a doctor on the back of the head. He has spent days sitting on the floor in a hallway, rocking back and forth and refusing to get up (level 2). Gradually, his behavior improved, without antidepressants; discharge diagnosis was a personality disorder. He was functioning at level 5 when discharged.

A rehabilitation agency accepted Ernest because he has the potential to walk without a walker or a cane. Ernest was supposed to go there after he was discharged from the psychiatric hospital. He did not. He lived on the streets for a few weeks and showed up at his cousin's house.

Ernest is back in the psychiatric hospital after another suicide attempt: he tried to wheel himself onto the freeway and was stopped by the police. This time he admits that he took PCP while he was out of the hospital. His behavior since discharge supports the diagnosis of a personality disorder, and his rehabilitation potential is guarded. The psychiatric staff does not plan to contact the rehabilitation agency to seek reacceptance. This decision is based on a common assumption that people with personality disorders do not cooperate or do not stay long in rehabilitation programs; empirical investigation of this assumption would be helpful in cases like this.

The problem with cases like Ernest is that differential diagnosis in psychiatry is still difficult to make with certainty. The differential is important because it helps to predict the patient's rehabilitation potential: a mood disorder generally has a good rehabilitation potential, but a personality disorder with chronic drug abuse does not. Unfortunately, our ability to predict is limited, and often the decision is made to try the rehabilitation program and see what happens. In this case, Ernest did not even go. Other people with personality disorders do go, but it is my clinical impression that if they refuse to cooperate with the rehabilitation program, they are discharged. Depressed people, in my opinion, have the best potential for a rehabilitation agency when they are functioning at levels 5 and 6 and have enough energy to cooperate with the program. People with personality disorders also function at levels 5 and 6 but fail to cooperate; the differential is often based on the degree of cooperation. The degree of cooperation is, obviously, a questionable criteria on which to base admission to, or termination from, a treatment program. This case exemplifies the difficulty in diagnostic reliability and treatment efficacy that affects psychiatric and rehabilitation professionals. Clearer diagnostic criteria and better medical interventions would be welcomed by all.

SCHIZOPHRENIC DISORDERS AND THE NEUROLEPTICS

Delusions and hallucinations are the predominant symptoms of schizophrenic disorders. Common delusions include a sense of being persecuted or controlled by others or a sense of depersonalization. Hallucinations are usually of voices; one or more voices coming from inside the patient's head or from external sources such as the radio. These symptoms are accompanied by a marked decrease in the patient's previous level of functioning for a duration of at least 6 months.

The diagnosis of schizophrenia has been plagued by the presence of symptoms that are difficult to describe or distinguish from other mental disorders. The flat affect might best be described as an absence of affect. A schizophrenic patient might say the sentence, "You look nice today," with a complete lack of emotional tone. The sentence can have a number of meanings depending on how it is said: You look nice *today*. You look nice today?, and so forth. Said without emotional tone the listener may wonder what the patient means. The flat affect is frequently accompanied by a marked poverty of speech and a failure to establish eye contact with the person being spoken to.

Recent studies have divided schizophrenia into two prognostic groups: relatively good and relatively poor. The good prognostic group seems to have some overlap with affective disorders, commonly referred to as *schizo-affective* disorders. The schizo-affective disorders are often treated with a combination of neuroleptic and an antidepressant or lithium. The poor prognostic group is associated with the symptoms of flat affect and social withdrawal. They are treated with neuroleptic drugs. The neuroleptics are antipsychotic agents that are usually associated with blocking the dopamine receptors in the brain. The neuroleptics often create parkinsonian side-effects and are treated with antiparkinsonian agents (Table 9-4).

The neuroleptics were the first psychotropic agents introduced into psychiatry in the 1950s. The neuroleptics are effective in controlling delusions, hallucinations, and bizarre behavior in a large number of patients. This control has made it possible to reduce the length of hospitalization in a substantial number of cases; some patients used to spend most of their adult lives in psychiatric hospitals. Now, periods of rehospitalization for a few weeks can maintain many people in the community.

COGNITIVE LEVELS

Most patients with a poor prognostic schizophrenic disorder function at level 4. On admission, the hallucinations and delusions can interrupt task performance to such a great extent that the patient functions at level 3. As the neuroleptics take effect, functional performance moves up to level 4 and usually stabilizes there.

TABLE 9-4
Neuroleptic Drugs and Antiparkinsonian Agents

Generic Name	Trade Name
NEUROLEPTICS	
Chlorpromazine	Thorazine
Fluphenazine	Prolixin
Haloperidol	Haldol
Loxapine	Loxitane
Mesoridazine	Serentil, Lidanar
Molindone	Moban, Lidone
Perphenazine	Trilafon
Piperacetazine	Quide
Thioridazine	Mellaril
Thiothixene	Navane
Trifluoperazine	Stelazine
ANTIPARKINSON AGENTS	
Amantadine	Symmetrel
Benztropine	Cogentin
Biperiden	Akineton
Diphenhydramine	Benadryl
Ethopropazine	Parsidol
Orphenadrine	Disipal, Norflex
Procyclidine	Kemadrin
Trihexyphenidyl	Artane

Patients with a good prognostic schizophrenic disorder usually move up to functioning at level 5 or 6. When level 6 is achieved the presence of odd social interaction can usually be detected.

COURSE OF THE DISEASE

The symptoms of a schizophrenic disorder usually appear during the patient's early 20s. Long before the onset of the symptoms, social withdrawal and academic difficulties are common. Researchers are currently investigating genetic, pregnancy, and birth complications that might explain the morphologic abnormalities of the brain that are associated with this disorder.

Good prognostic cases often turn out at follow-up to have the symptoms of a primary mood disorder; the diagnosis is changed. The natural history of the disease then is episodic.

Poor prognostic patients have impairments in all aspects of community living. Education is usually interrupted or terminated by the onset of symptoms. Attempts to work are often characterized by demotions, being fired, quitting, frequent job changes, or financial dependency.[14] The patient is frequently dependent on relatives in the home environment. The patient can usually perform vital tasks, such as eating and dressing, but maintaining a safe and clean living environment usually requires on-site supervision. Many families lack the resources to support these people throughout their adult life, or the patient may reject familial support. Some group homes are available.[14] When group homes are rejected, it is thought that many of these patients become a part of the homeless mentally ill. These people are frequently the victims of injuries, accidents, theft, and violent crime.[21]

REHABILITATION

The rehabilitation of schizophrenic disorders is a controversial topic. The arguments are often based on faith in a treatment philosophy and too infrequently based on controlled, replicated investigations. The psychosocial rehabilitation studies reported often fail to differentiate between poor and good prognosis schizophrenia and, even worse, they often fail to report any diagnosis. Therefore, positive results could be attributed to the presence of a primary mood disorder. Conversely, negative results could be attributed to the presence of dementia. Most psychosocial rehabilitation programs have objectives that would fulfill the needs of good prognostic schizophrenic disorders. The lifelong needs of people with poor prognostic schizophrenic disorders are seldom addressed.

Physical rehabilitation programs will need to modify treatment objectives for the stable level 4 patient with a schizophrenic disorder. Many rehabilitation objectives are fulfilled by teaching the patient a new way of doing things. New learning is severely restricted at level 4. The patient may be able to learn specific, step-by-step procedures if you can demonstrate each step so that it is clearly visible to the patient. It will probably require a lot of your ingenuity, patience, and time. Clearly, the objective should be important to you, other care givers, and the patient. These patients are usually very cooperative and will expend a great amount of energy in trying to follow your instructions. Consultation with care givers outside of the rehabilitation agency may be especially important with these patients because they are frequently unable to clearly communicate their need for assistance.

An illustration of severely psychotic behavior is provided by the following case.

CASE 4   Kim is a 30-year-old white woman who was brought to the hospital by her husband and parents. Both of her parents had been required to restrain her forcefully from using a kitchen knife to "stab the snakes in her stomach." She is 8 months pregnant but denies the pregnancy. This is the third psychiatric hospitalization. At admission she did not answer any questions (mute) and showed no emotional response to the family's concerns or the decision to admit her (flat affect). The family reports that she is unable to care for her basic needs (urinating on self), and they are concerned about the well-being of the unborn child. Involuntary hospitalization with a legal guardian until the delivery is required.

The following occupational therapy observations, made on day 1, were reported to substantiate the presence of a grave disability:

Eating

Patient does not finish meals, gets up and wanders away. She does not follow her diabetic diet and does take and eat sweets from trays of other patients. She did not use utensils and ate with her fingers.

Ambulation

Patient follows others without awareness of destination. She lies in the hallway and refuses to get up when asked by staff; she sits or lies down for hours at a time. Occasionally she wanders around the ward aimlessly. At one point she climbed up on a chair to stare precariously out of a window and had to be assisted down.

Dressing

Patient is in a hospital gown and partially exposed in the dayroom. On one occasion she walked into the dayroom without pajama bottoms on and put the bottoms on in full view of other patients of both sexes. She does not change clothes after urinating or defecating on herself unless directed and provided clothing by the staff.

Bathing

Patient refuses to shower; hair is uncombed and dirty.

Toileting

She wet the bed in the morning and was told to go to the bathroom after meals by staff. While on the toilet she masturbated for 5 minutes. She does not flush the toilet after use. The patient was mute throughout the day. Cognitive level was 2.

Low doses of haloperidol were given to Kim until the baby boy was born. The medicine produced a slight improvement, moving from level 2 to level 3. After the delivery she was functioning at level 4 and discharged when she refused voluntary hospitalization. Kim has another child who is 2 years old. Her parents live close by, and it is hoped that they will constantly monitor her care for the children. Her recent ability to function at level 5 or 6 cannot be established from the available history. She will be followed by an outpatient psychiatrist who has been seeing her for the last 3 years.

The cases presented in this chapter reflect the skewed perspective of rehabilitation professionals. We do not often see the common psychiatric patient who has an episodic illness that responds to medication. We see the nonresponders and the people who suffer the complications of these disorders. Consequently, we need to keep reminding ourselves that our clinical impressions are slanted toward the debilitating aspects of psychiatric diseases. To avoid succumbing to the thought that all psychiatric patients are difficult or have a poor prognosis, a careful distinction between diagnostic categories is helpful. As a rule patients who have a primary mood disorder return to functioning at levels 5 and 6, within the normal range of cognitive function. Most patients seen by psychiatrists have an affective disorder. Persons with a chronic schizophrenic disorder may stabilize at level 4; the number of people who fall within this category appears to be far fewer than often thought, given the revised diagnostic criteria (*DSM–III–R*).[10] Drugs that would effectively treat the personality disorder are unknown, decisions about their care is ambiguous for all health professionals. Recognition of the variability of psychotropic drug efficacy helps in selecting realistic rehabilitation objectives for those persons who have a psychiatric disease.

REFERENCES

1. Allen CK: Independence through activity: The practice of occupational therapy (psychiatry). Am J Occup Ther 36:731–739, 1982
2. Allen CK: Occupational Therapy for Psychiatric Disease: Measurement and Management of Cognitive Disabilities. Boston, Little, Brown & Co, 1985
3. Allen CK, Allen RE: Cognitive disabilities: Measuring the social consequences of mental disorders. J Clin Psychiatry (in press).
4. Andreasen NC et al: Ventricular enlargement in schizophrenia: Relationship to positive and negative symptoms. Am J Psychiatry 139:297–301, 1982
5. Andreasen NC et al: Ventricular enlargement in schizophrenia: Definition and prevalence. Am J Psychiatry 139:292–296, 1982
6. Bassuk EL, Schoonover SC, Gelenberg AJ: The Practitioner's Guide to Psychoactive Drugs, 2nd ed, p 61. New York, Plenum Medical Books, 1983
7. Bernstein JG: Clinical Psychopharmacology, 2nd ed. Boston, John Wright, 1984
8. Brodie JD et al: Patterns of metabolic activity in the treatment of schizophrenia. Ann Neurol. 15(Suppl):5166–5169, 1984
9. Buchsbaum MS, et al: Positron emission tomographic image measurement in schizophrenia and affective disorders. Ann Neurol 15(Suppl):5157–5165, 1984
10. DSM–III–R: Diagnostic and Statistical Manual of Mental Disorders, 3rd ed, revised. Washington, American Psychiatric Association, 1987
11. Fawcett J, Kravetz HM: The long-term management of bipolar disorders and lithium, carbamazepine and antidepressants. J Clin Psychiatry 46:206–209, 1985
12. Feighner JP, Herbstein JH, Damlouji N: Combined MAOI, TCA, and direct stimulant therapy of treatment-resistant depression. J Clin Psychiatry 46:206–209, 1985
13. Golden CG et al: Cerebral ventricular size and neuropsychological impairment in young chronic schizophrenics. Arch Gen Psychiatry 37:725–739, 1979
14. Goodwin DW, Guze SB: Psychiatric Diagnosis, 3rd ed. New York, Oxford University Press, 1984
15. Hollister LE: Clinical Pharmacology of Psychotherapeutic Drugs, 2nd ed, Vol 1, in the Monographs in Clinical Pharmacology series. New York, Churchill-Livingstone, 1983
16. Johnstone EC et al: Cerebral ventricular size and cognitive impairment in chronic schizophrenia. Lancet 2:924–926, 1976
17. Johnstone EC et al: The dementia of dementia praecox. Acta Psychiatry Scand 56:305–324, 1978
18. Kishimoto A et al: Long-term prophylactic effects of carbamazepine in affective disorder. Br J Psychiatry 143:327–331, 1983
19. Klawans HH, Weiner WJ: Textbook of Clinical Neuropharmacology. New York, Raven Press, 1981
20. Janicak PG et al: ECT: An assessment of mental health professionals knowledge and attitudes. J Clin Psychiatry 46:262–266, 1985
21. Lehman AF, Linn LS: Crimes against discharged mental patients in board-and-care homes. Am J Psychiatry 141:271–274, 1984
22. Levy SD, Albrecht E: Electroconvulsive therapy: A survey of use in the private psychiatric hospital. J Clin Psychiatry 46:125–127, 1985
23. Pearlson GD et al: Symptomatic, familiar, perinatal, and social correlates of computerized axial tomography (CAT) changes in schizophrenics and bipolars. J Nerv Ment Dis 173:42–50, 1985
24. Pitts FN, Allen AD, Allen RE: Systemic immunodeficient Epstein-Barr virus syndrome (SIDES) is a major cause of depression (in preparation)

25. Post RM, Uhde TW, Ballenger JC: The efficacy of carbamazepine in affective illness. Adv Biochem Psychopharm 39:421–437, 1984

26. Prien RF et al: Drug therapy in the prevention of recurrences in unipolar and bipolar affective disorders. Arch Gen Psychiatry 41:1096–1104, 1984

27. Reider RO et al: Sulcal prominence in young chronic schizophrenic patients: CT scan findings associated with impairment on neuropsychological tests. Psychiatry Res 1:1–9, 1979

28. Reider RO et al: Computed tomographic scans in patients with schizophrenia, schizoaffective, and bipolar affective disorder. Arch Gen Psychiatry 40:735–739, 1983

29. Research on mental illness and addictive disorders: Progress and prospects. Am J Psychiatry 142(Suppl):9–41, 1985

30. Ross RP, Davis K, Melzar HY: Immunoglobulin studies in patients with psychiatric diseases. Arch Gen Psychiatry 42:124–133, 1985

31. Stevens JR et al: A search for cylomegal virus and herpes viral antigen in brains schizophrenic patients. Arch Gen Psychiatry 41:795–801, 1984

32. Taylor MA, Abrams R: Prediction of treatment response in mania. Arch Gen Psychiatry 38:800–803, 1981

33. Watson CG et al: Schizophrenic birth seasonality in relation to the incidence of infectious diseases and temperature extremes. Arch Gen Psychiatry 41:85–90, 1984

34. Watts CAH: A long-term follow-up of schizophrenic patients: 1946–1983. J Clin Psychiatry 46:210–216, 1985

35. Weinberger DR et al: Poor premorbid adjustment and CT scan abnormalities in chronic schizophrenia. Am J Psychiatry 137:1410–1413, 1980

36. Weinberger DR et al: Lateral cerebral ventricular enlargement in chronic schizophrenia. Arch Gen Psychiatry 36:735–739, 1979

37. White K, Simpson G: Combined MAOI–tricyclic antidepressant treatment: A reevaluation. J Clin Psychopharmacol 1:264–282, 1981

38. Zubenko GS et al: Clonidine in the treatment of mania and mixed bipolar disorder. Am J Psychiatry 141:1617–1618, 1984

The Use of Pharmacologic   10
Agents in the Conservative
Management of the Spinal
Orthopaedic Patient

Trinda F. Metzger
Terry Malone

The nature of orthopaedic medicine precludes this chapter from addressing all aspects of pharmacologic applications to this medical specialty. Hence, the authors were eclectic and have concentrated on the pharmacologic aspects of conservative management of spinal dysfunction. Conservative treatment was selected because these patients are those most likely to be involved with relatively long periods of rehabilitation and pharmacologic treatment.

PHARMACOLOGY AND SPINAL DYSFUNCTION

The area of systemic pharmacology for treatment of patients with back or cervical pain is probably the first, as well as the most popular, treatment of choice. For simplicity we will refer to these patients with back or cervical pain as "back patients"; however, by this designation we imply all back pain including patients with low-back pain, thoracic pain, and cervical pain. Discussion of pharmacology with reference to back pain will have significance for everyone, including your patients and yourselves. This is because it is reported that 75 million Americans suffer back ailments.[3] Back pain is the second leading cause of hospitalization after pregnancy.[59] Eighteen million doctor visits annually are directly in response to back pain.[43,44] It

We would like to thank Dr. Karl Manders, Medical Director, Community Hospitals of Indianapolis, for his helpful review of and recommendations for this chapter.

is stated that back ailments are also more common than any other illness, except headaches or the common cold.[44] Therefore, it is obvious that a significantly large number of Americans suffer, or will suffer, from back pain and that these persons will ultimately end up receiving some type of pharmacologic prescription. These are also the persons whom we will see in our clinics. Consequently, the initial as well as the subsequent pharmacologic management may have considerable positive or negative impact on the patients' prognosis. This can obviously affect the patients' ultimate progress in their total therapeutic management.

Pharmacologic therapy can be the most appropriate or inappropriate treatment, depending on the differential diagnosis, the history, and the type of medication prescribed for the back patient. It is believed by some who treat back patients that the area of systemic pharmacologic therapy is both the most abused and underused therapeutic approach. The abuse of pharmacologic treatment primarily centers around injudicious and excessive use of narcotics, inappropriate withholding of narcotics (immediate after surgery or trauma), and illogical prescribing of muscle-relaxant medications.[30,35,62] The areas of underuse include the use of systemic anti-inflammatory drugs and, less commonly, the anti-neuralgia drugs.[62] Marks and Sachar and Cohen also argue that narcotics are underused for patients with severe acute back pain.[15,36] Psychotropic or antidepressant drugs are also underused or underestimated in their use for back pain patients, especially for those with chronic pain.[37-39,42,52,53] Relatively recent studies suggest analgesic effects of these psychotropic drugs that precede the antidepressant effects.[40,57]

The type of drugs used for back patients varies according to physician and according to the patient's diagnosis. However, the following drug classes are used for back patients: narcotic analgesics, nonnarcotic analgesics, nonsteroidal and steroidal anti-inflammatory agents, antineuralgia agents, psychotropic agents and antidepressants. We will discuss each class individually in the following sections, as well as spinal or nerve blocks that are used for back patients and the types of medications that are used for these blocks. Before we begin the discussion of the various types of drugs that are commonly prescribed for back patients, a case study is presented for review. A drug classification system is then presented followed by a second case study. This format was selected to show how the type of medication prescribed, the timeliness of the prescription, and the preference for solely pharmacologic intervention may alter a patient's ultimate prognosis.

CASE 1   A 37-year-old male mechanic, after lifting a motor out of a forklift by using pulleys and cables, was unable to stand up straight and had excruciating back pain. He was carried to the company physician and given a muscle relaxant acetominophen with chlorzoxazone (Parafon Forte) and an analgesic acetominophen with codeine (Tylenol 3) and sent home for bed rest. The patient continued to have back pain and sometimes the pain radiated down his right leg. Bed rest was continued for 2 weeks and the patient felt relief only while lying down.

Two weeks later the patient visited his family physician, and after explaining his current history while the doctor probed the sore places on his back, the doctor pronounced that he had a severely strained back. The new prescription included a stronger analgesic meperidine (Demerol) and continued use of the Parafon Forte along with more rest at home. Subsequent physician visits involved changes of drugs, different muscle relaxants, and then anti-inflammatory nonsteroidal oral drugs. The patient's questions concerning work, financial matters, and time spans within which he could expect to be cured and be able to return to work at 100% were shrugged off.

After about 4 months without substantial changes in symptoms, the patient was referred to a specialist. It took the patient 2 months to schedule the appointment. After the first examination when no neurologic damage was shown radiologically, he was referred to out-patient physical therapy for moist heat, ultrasound, and massage. The specialist also prescribed her favorite brands of analgesics and anti-inflammatory drugs. The physical therapy referral was for eight sessions and provided only temporary relief. The therapist suggested to the physician that other therapy besides palliative measures might prove more effective. However, the physician felt this was unnecessary.

The specialist decided that the patient needed to be admitted to the hospital for further tests, more intense medications, and bed rest (again). The patient was given parental doses of Demerol and put in bedside traction. Tests revealed (again) normal x-ray findings, and the CT scan showed central bulging of the right lumbar fourth and fifth disks with some bilateral mild facet arthritis at both levels. During the hospitalization, little change of symptoms occurred and a myelogram was performed. The physician felt that the myelogram was indicative of a fifth lumbar disk herniation and suggested surgical intervention. A laminectomy was performed and after the required convalescence, the patient returned to work without any rehabilitation.

During the first few weeks, the patient reported that the back pain was returning, and the physician again prescribed Demerol. Then, into the second month on the job, the patient reinjured his back. He was eventually placed on disability and again turned to the medical model for help. However, now the patient was very depressed, angry, and dependent on his medications. The doctors felt he had some emotional overlay (probably true because he was depressed and narcotics do not improve this problem), and they were frustrated in dealing with this patient. All diagnostic test results were negative, and the patient was eventually referred to a chronic pain clinic. The clinic started a detoxification program for his drug dependencies, psychotherapy for his anger and depression, and intense physical and occupational therapy for treatment of pain, posture, strengthening, endurance, and lumbar dysfunctions.

This particular patient's prognosis might or might not have been different if other medications and approaches were tried first. However, one must wonder about the impact it does have on this type of back patient.

Muscle Relaxants

As a general group, orally prescribed muscle relaxants are not particularly potent. Most of them include muscle relaxation by creating a calming or tranquilizing effect. As mentioned earlier, muscle relaxants are thought to be more useful if a thorough and differential diagnosis is made. However, routine prescribing of these drugs for all back pain is illogical because patients with pure peripheral pain, such as leg or sciatic pain, almost never achieve relief with muscle relaxants. Patients with combined leg and back or arm and neck pain only occasionally obtain relief from these drugs.[62] When it appears that the back pain is more muscular and has little radiation, muscle relaxants may be an excellent choice. However, other medications may still be more effective. Table 10-1 presents common muscle relaxants prescribed for back patients.

For severe acute back pain, most sources feel diazepam (Valium) or other strong narcotic analgesics may be indicated. However, in chronic pain with concurrent depression, the benzodiazepines (minor tranquilizers) that are used as muscle relaxants cause an increase in depression. Recent evidence suggests that benzodiazepines deplete serotonin, often adding to depression and possibly increasing pain perception. The muscle relaxants appear best prescribed for short-term treatment in patients without radicular pain.[66]

Analgesics

Analgesic drugs continue to be the most abused class of drugs.[62] In this section, we will discuss the simple analgesics that, for the most part, are nonnarcotic. These

---

TABLE 10-1
Muscle Relaxants

1. *Diazepam (Valium):* Benzodiazepine tranquilizer, commonly prescribed but causes physical dependence and is a mood depressant; better for postsurgery or acute severe back injury
2. *Methocarbamol (Robaxin):* Has minor tranquilizing effect to muscles
3. *Methocarbamol plus aspirin (Robaxisal):* Combines muscle relaxer effect with anti-inflammatory effect and analgesic effect from the salicylate
4. *Orphenadrine (Disipal):* Longer in duration but similar in effectiveness to methocarbamol
5. *Chlorzoxazone and acetaminophen (Parafon Forte):* Muscle relaxer and mild analgesic; acts centrally and at spinal cord level
6. *Dantrolene sodium (Dantrium):* Extremely potent, produces rapid muscle relaxation and begins to produce muscle weakness; useful in severe cases with visible palpable muscle spasms; acts directly on muscle
7. *Chlorzoxazone (Paraflex):* Inhibits muscle spasm at the spinal cord level
8. *Cyclobenzaprine (Flexeril):* Relieves skeletal muscle spasm of local origin without interfering with muscle function; not effective with centrally produced muscle spasms
9. *Baclofen (Lioresal):* Produces same effects as diazepam but is less likely to produce sedation or to reduce voluntary power or residual muscle weakness; thought to work at spinal cord level and possibly supraspinally

drugs are prescribed inordinately for back pain patients when other drugs may be more appropriate. One important note to remember with simple analgesics is that they only relieve pain, whereas anti-inflammatory drugs can act peripherally to alter inflamed tissue.[62] Although frequently divided into analgesic and anti-inflammatory agents, it is difficult, but important, to distinguish among these drugs because some of them have both properties. Aspirin is both an analgesic and an anti-inflammatory. If taken on an as-needed basis, aspirin is an analgesic; if taken regularly at higher levels it acts both as an anti-inflammatory and an analgesic. Simple nonnarcotic analgesics usually act centrally, as well as peripherally on pain. Codeine is actually a narcotic analgesic, which occurs naturally in opium and is structurally related to morphine. Codeine and other similar morphinelike drugs are still considered in the category of simple analgesics because of their moderate analgesic effect. A dangerous aspect of simple analgesics, such as codeine or propoxyphene (Darvon), is that because they are not considered to be strong narcotics, physicians may prescribe them on a long-term basis. Any long-term use of weak or strong narcotics can exacerbate depression.[21,58,61] Depression changes the patient's perception of pain for the worse. Table 10-2 presents some simple analgesics commonly prescribed for back pain patients.

Indication for the use of simple analgesics include conditions in which pain is intermittent and the drugs can, therefore, be taken on demand. Long-term use of non-steroidal anti-inflammatory drugs (NSAIDs) can lead to gastric bleeding and other gastrointestinal problems. Long-term use of morphinelike drugs, such as propoxyphene can lead to addiction and exacerbate depression and pain.[20] Aspirin is still one of the most effective analgesics. However, if gastric irritation is a problem, there are other very effective analgesics to substitute for aspirin. The greatest limitaton to the simple analgesics, if they are not NSAIDs, is that they only relieve pain and do not change or reach the cause of the problem.

Narcotic Analgesics

Narcotic analgesics are the opiates derived from the poppy plant. This use of the poppy as a sedative anodyne has been traced back to the 16th century B.C. Opium is the older form of the drug, and morphine was isolated in 1803 by Seturner.[1] Narcotics, or the opiates, and the synthetic compounds similar to the opiates, are classified according to their relationship to morphine. They act on the endorphin system in the central nervous system (CNS), and tend to cause physical as well as psychologic addiction.[20,39] Opioids also act on the CNS to alter the patient's emotional response to pain, but actually neither the opiates nor the opioids block the transmission of pain impulses nor reduce the input of impulses at the site of damage or pain.[58] Opiates are the treatment of choice for severe acute pain or chronic cancer pain. However, most back pain patients are not in the severe acute category. The physician who decides to prescribe narcotics for back pain patient must do so with extreme caution. Physical and psychologic dependence must be considered, especially for relief of chronic back pain. Also, the depressing effect that narcotics have on the CNS must be a factor.[1,59] Most chronic back patients are commonly depressed from being off work, from being unable to complete family obligations, and from the length of their convalescence. Long-term use of narcotics can further add to this depressed state and further increase pain.[1,58,62] As mentioned

TABLE 10-2
Simple Analgesics

A. *Morphinelike drugs:* central action
   1. *Codeine:* orally or parentally, commonly combined with aspirin or acetaminophen (seldom used alone as analgesic) (APC with Codeine No. 3 and 4)
   2. *Oxycodone:* semisynthetic morphine narcotic agonist
      Percodan: oxycodone and aspirin
      Percocet: oxycodone and acetaminophen
B. *Agonist-antagonist:* centrally acting, does not synergize well with opium derivatives
   1. *Pentazocine (Talwin):* potent analgesic administered orally or parenterally, has frequent side-effects such as nausea, dizziness, mental changes.
   2. *Propoxyphene (Darvon):* Available alone orally or compounded with aspirin or acetaminophen, (*Darvocet:* is propoxyphene and acetaminophen)
C. *Not morphinelike:* central action
   1. *Nalbuphine (Nubain):* most potent of synthetic narcotic pain relievers; only available parenterally; has decreased addiction potential and decreased respiratory depression potential
   2. *Methotrimeprazine (Levoprome):* potent, nonaddictive compares favorably with morphine, only available parenterally–intramuscular; actually a phenothiazine that is thought to affect the histamine and kinin systems of the inflammatory process

D. *Peripherally acting analgesics*

   NSAIDs: affect prostaglandin synthesis, have analgesic and anti-inflammatory properties
   1. *Aspirin:* most effective but has gastric side-effects; is less of a problem when used as an analgesic
   2. *Diflunisal (Dolobid):* also promotes GI irritation
   3. *Ibuprofen (Motrin):* GI irritation
   4. *Naproxen (Naprosyn):* GI irritation

   Non-NSAID: pure analgesic no anti-inflammatory effects/Acetaminophen (paracetamol; Tylenol): synergizes well with opium derivatives

---

earlier in this chapter, the mechanism for increase of pain with depression occurs from changes in the brain's biogenic amines and how they affect endorphins.[34] Depression of the CNS alters the brain's serotonin and norepinephrine levels causing an increase in the perception of pain.[20,58] Narcotics are grouped according to their strength and relationship to morphine in terms of agonist and antagonist properties. Table 10-3 outlines some narcotic analgesics.

A frequent problem is the underuse of narcotics after back surgery. Physicians and patients may resist narcotics because of their abuse potential in most situations.[62] It is believed that postoperative pain is very distressing and if these patients are denied adequate relief in this early period, they quickly begin to fear and dread their pain. This can actually cause them to demand more and more pain-relieving medications. This pattern can be difficult to break once it is established. It is better to give sufficiently strong opioids upon a patient's required request, rather than on a set schedule, and switch or alternate parenteral and oral applications.[30,62] Thus, the most appropriate use of strong narcotics for back patients may be suggested as follows: after back surgery, for acute injury, and for severe acute back pain if hospitalized.[62]

Anti-Inflammatory Agents

Anti-inflammatory drugs are one of the most effective, yet underused noninvasive therapies available for back patients.[62] Back pain specialists find it discouraging to repeatedly accept referrals of patients with chronic pain who have never had a trial or anti-inflammatory therapy. These patients often respond dramatically to this relatively simple therapeutic measure.[62]

The best candidates for anti-inflammatory therapy include any new back pain patient, including those with sciatica.[12] However, sciatica patients, especially those with burning or tingling, may better benefit from antineuralgia drugs or from direct blocks with steroid drugs.[50,51,62] The best results reported for the use of anti-inflammatory drugs are in patients who have chronic aching, especially those with the "double peak" characteristic of "arthritislike" pain. Patients with chronic lumbago, who have not responded to inactivity, frequently do well with these medications.[62]

Physicians prescribing anti-inflammatory drugs for back patients must be cognizant of their substantial analgesic properties. When NSAIDs are given in a single dose they act as analgesics, and when given regularly they have additional effects on inflamed tissues. Thus, in addition to relieving pain they reduce the cardinal signs of inflammation: swelling, warmth, tenderness, and stiffness.[26]

Aspirin is the basic standard against which all other anti-inflammatory drugs are judged. Most back patients may, or may not, have tried aspirin before seeing their physician. Most, even if they had taken aspirin, would not have taken it in a manner conducive to promote an anti-inflammatory effect. Nonetheless, physicians do prescribe systemic analgesics that include aspirin as a secondary compound. It would seem appropriate to prescribe an analgesic with aspirin as a secondary compound, if the patient has no history of gastrointestinal problems or to prescribe large regular doses of aspirin, thus inducing analgesic and anti-inflammatory properties. However, the patient may feel the doctor is not taking his pain or problem seriously. Patients have underestimated the effects of aspirin because it is available over-the-counter. Clinical evidence suggests, however, that 650 mg of aspirin is equianalgesic to 60 mg of codeine.[1] Aaronoff feels that it has yet to be conclusively proved that the nonsteroidal drugs offer any major advantage over aspirin, except for those patients unable to tolerate the effects of the acetylsalicyclic acid![1]

TABLE 10-3
Narcotic Analgesics

1. *Morphine:* Strong analgesic, effects mediated from opiate receptors in the brain and CNS; given orally, parentally
2. *Hydromorphone (Dilaudid):* Most potent opoid in general use; narcotic agonist
3. *Methodone:* Morphinelike, synthetic narcotic agonist; minor withdrawal; used only occasionally used for failed back patients
4. *Merperidine (Demerol):* Narcotic analgesic and antispasmodic; can produce physical and psychologic dependence
5. *Buprenorphine (Buprenex):* Morphine-type; narcotic agonist–antagonist
6. *Nalbuphine (Nubain):* Narcotic agonist–antagonist, nalorphine-type
7. *Butorphanol (Stadol):* Narcotic agonist–antagonist

The NSAIDs, whose primary action is the inhibition of prostaglandin synthesis, are increasing in number and importance. There are four general groups: indomethacin, fenamates, tolmetin, and the propionic acid derivatives.[1] The arrival of phenylbutazone and indomethacin was regarded as presenting alternatives to aspirin. But the propionic derivatives introduced an entirely new order of tolerance and, certainly, displaced aspirin from its central position.[25,26] These drugs are all said to have diminished likelihood of causing gastrointestinal irritation and bleeding when compared with aspirin, but each may be poorly tolerated by some patients.[62] The propionic acid derivatives, represented by ibuprofen, naproxen, and fenoprofen, are the most widely used NSAIDs in American clinical practice. In addition to their effect on prostaglandin synthesis, they are thought to affect the histamine and kinin systems of inflammation.[1] Table 10-4 presents the common NSAIDs used with back patients.

Most of the propionic acid-type anti-inflammatory drugs have some analgesic properties as well as anti-inflammatory properties. Although a characteristic of these drugs is their gastric side-effects, including indigestion, nausea, headaches, and allergic rashes, they are considered very safe.[26]

Steroidal Anti-Inflammatory Agents

Adrenal corticosteroids remain the most effective of the anti-inflammatory drugs and are often considered wonder drugs of the 20th century.[20] Among these, prednisone, dexamethasone, and methylprednisolone are probably the most popular.[62] The panorama of potential side-effects of corticosteroids is lengthy and is most frequently associated with long-term treatment. Ideally, these drugs are used in modest doses for back patients with specific indications.[26] Dangerous side-effects include Cushing's syndrome, fluid retention, hormonal system disturbances, hypertension, myopathic weakness, osteoporosis, and psychiatric disturbances. Although long-term use is dangerous and, therefore, of limited usefulness for chronic back pain patients, local depository injections and short-course therapy are extremely helpful for these patients. (Local injection will be discussed in a later section.)[20,62,63,64] Short-course, high-dose, systemic steroid therapy was advocated by British clinicians, who reported spectacular results in back patients.[62,64] Wilkinson reported that his success with this method of dexamethasone beginning with 64 mg/day and tapering over 1 to 2 weeks was rather modest. He continues to use this method, but only with hospitalization, for patients with acute or subacute episodes of lumbago, sciatica, or both, who have limited or stable neurologic deficits. He prefers to use dexamethasone (Decadron) or methylprednisolone (Medrol). These two drugs seem to have less psychologic complication, and caused less fluid retention than other corticosteroids.[62] Small doses of prednisolone (5 mg to 7.5 mg) are reported to be comparable in effectiveness with a large dose of indomethacin.[40] A number of patients with acute back pain and sciatic pain syndromes will benefit from either systemic or local use of corticosteroids. Approximately half of those treated will consider themselves "cured." The other half will improve for a short period and then require alternative therapy or surgery.[20]

Corticosteroids are available in many forms; hence, the physician must decide whether to administer the drug systemically, locally, intrathecally, epidurally, or into the facets or disk.[20,62-64] Local injections or blocks would seem preferable to

---

TABLE 10-4
NSAIDs

1. *Aspirin:* A salicylate, 600–1000 mg daily, commonly combined with centrally acting analgesics, such as codeine and propoxyphene (Darvon).
2. *Indomethacin (Indocin):* An indene derivative, 25–50 mg three to four times a day; strong anti-inflammatory activities that compares with salicylates; reported to be reliable for back patients, but long-term use leads to accommodation to drug
3. *Phenylbutazone (Butazolidin):* A pyrazole, produces bone marrow suppression, but this was recently found to be dose-related; given in loading doses to back patients; 400–800 mg for 1–2 days and then reduced to 100 mg daily for an addition 4–6 days
4. *Ibuprofen (Motrin):* A propionic acid derivative, weaker anti-inflammatory when compared to aspirin or phenylbutazone; has wide acceptance because of infrequent side-effects; given orally in 300–400 mg; give to back patients t.i.d. or q.i.d.
5. *Naproxen (Naprosyn):* A propionic acid derivative; has high incidence of GI reactions, nausea, and abdominal pain; b.i.d. is recommended for back pain
6. *Fenoprofen calcium (Nalfon):* A propionic acid derivative; has short plasma half-life; works quickly but must be taken frequently; food decreases the drug blood level; causes headaches, somnolence, tinnitus, dyspepsia; commonly given in dosages of 600 mg q.i.d.
7. *Sulindac (Clinoril):* An indene derivative, relative of indomethacin but behaves like a propionic acid derivative like naproxen; has long duration that permits effective medication for 3 hr
8. *Tolmetin (Tolectin):* An indene derivative, but clinically similar to indomethacin; also has similar GI effects and headaches as side effects; 200 mg tablets with recommended dosage of 400 mg t.i.d.
9. *Diflunisal (Dolobid):* A salicylate; has a plasma half-life of 8–10 hr, and this decreases frequency of administration to two to three times a day; back patients are commonly given 500 mg stat and then 250–500 mg b.i.d. (250 mg oral diflunisal is equianalgesic to 650 mg aspirin or 60 mg of codeine)

---

minimize the adverse effects associated with systemic administration. Because of the dangers of adhesive arachnoiditis, intrathecal injection of steroids is no longer recommended; epidural blocks with the instillation of steroids are favored,[20] if steroids are to be used with the block. Patients experiencing acute episodes of pain are frequently treated with short courses of systemic therapy of 2 weeks. This is often followed by local injection.[20] Thus, it appears that steroids are reserved for the management of isolated, acutely painful back pain episodes or for carefully selected chronic pain patients. They are not normally a long-term solution for chronic back pain; however, short trials of systemic or local blocks may be indicated. Possibly, the use of steroids through blocks, local injections, or short-term systemic trials may reduce the need for hospitalization, the length of hospitalization, or the need for surgery.[20,62] It is believed by some that the local injections of cortisone for back pain is the most effective use of steroids for back patients, especially in the early stage. Table 10-5 outlines the most common steroids used for back patients.

An additional anti-inflammatory agent that may be useful in treating back pain is colchicine. Rask has published studies showing a 90% success rate; however, this treatment remains controversial.

In summarizing the use of anti-inflammatory drugs, the delay in administration of these drugs is not advisable. The exclusive reliance on analgesic medications

TABLE 10-5
Corticosteroids

1. *Methylprednisolone (Medrol):* Glucocorticoid available in tablets and in liquid suspensions
2. *Dexamethasone (Decadron):* Synthetic adrenocortical steroid available in tablets and with phosphate for injections
3. *Prednisone (Deltasone):* available in tablet or in liquid suspension for injection
4. *Adrenocorticotropic hormone (ACTH):* 40 or 80 units in ACTH for injection
5. *Hydrocortisone:* Available in tablets, creams, or in liquid suspensions

before switching to anti-inflammatory drugs may decrease the ability of the anti-inflammatory to help the patient.[20] Anti-inflammatory drug therapy is complicated by the large array of available drugs, especially in the nonsteroidal category. It is too easy for surgeons to become trapped into performing surgery and to be reluctant to work patients through an effective anti-inflammatory drug program.

Antineuralgia

Back patients who principally have burning, tingling, radiating, sciatica, or lancinating pains are thought to have neural pain. Several investigators have reported that the antineuralgia drugs can be used to treat back pain if it is thought to be nerve related.[1,55,62] Most useful among the neuralgia drugs are the anticonvulsant drugs. Phenytoin (Dilantin) and carbamazepine (Tegretol) are widely known in the treatment of multiple sclerosis or tic douloureux, but their effectiveness in treating chronic sciatica is often overlooked.[62] Wilkinson also reported success with specific vitamin therapy, usually used in adjunct with an antineuralgia drug.[62] Aronoff and Evans suggest the following drugs to be tried first; carbamazepine, then if no response, clonazepam; then phenytoin; and finally valproate.[1,56,57] These drugs do not help mechanical irritation, but rather non-mechanical sciatica such as diabetic neuropathy, metabolic neuropathy, and shingles. Treatment of peripheral neuropathies are discussed by Panis and Aronoff.[45] The use of vitamin therapy for neuralgia has

TABLE 10-6
Antineuralgic Drugs

1. *Carbamazepin (Tegretol):* Used most commonly for nerve pain; thought to be the most effective antineuralgic; has long half-life but falls at 6–8 hr; long-term use may cause mental slowing, which is considered to be one of its hazards
2. *Phenytoin (Dilantin):* Causes skin rashes or ataxia with chronic buildup; also has a long half-life
3. *Clonazepam (Clonopin):* A newer anticonvulsant that has considerable antineuralgic properties; causes drowsiness initially; useful for patients with acute sciatica
4. *Valproic acid (Depakene):* Last choice of the anticonvulsant drugs for neuralgic pain

questionable scientific validity; however, it is reported to be useful clinically both alone or as an adjunct with an anticonvulsant drug. Thiamine hydrochloride (vitamin B_2), 200 mg to 400 mg daily, is used, with full awareness that a considerable amount is excreted in the urine at that dose level. It has clearly been shown that nervous tissue biochemically depends heavily on thiamine, and that damage and regenerating tissue requires larger amounts.[62] Thus, even if the effect is placebo, it is safe, effective, and it may be dietically beneficial. Table 10-6 presents the antineuralgic drugs that have been suggested for neuralgic pain.

The literature discussing the use of antineuralgia drugs is still sparse compared with that for analgesics or anti-inflammatory drugs. Yet, for specific types of back pain, these drugs may be the pharmacologic treatment of choice.

Psychotropic Drugs

The various psychotropic drugs, which include the antidepressants and the tranquilizers, are often useful in the management of back pain (especially chronic back pain).[18,24,62] Human pain is an experience with an affective element. Therefore, it is not surprising that psychotropic drugs are used to treat the back patients because subjective pain can be modified with psychic factors.[62] Patients who suffer long-term pain with home and job anxieties will most certainly exhibit some emotional depression. Also, these patients may have been on long-term narcotic therapy, by which the drugs themselves can lead to emotional and reactive depression, exacerbating the patient's perception of pain, as discussed by Hendler.[24] Hendler suggests the following information on how depression increases pain perception: Depression leads to abnormalities in the levels of central nervous system biogenic amines, specifically, norepinephrine, serotonin, and dopamine. Ninety percent of biogenic amine receptors are in the limbic system, thus, it is rich in endorphins, which acts as neurotransmitters in modulating pain perception.[1,24] Research indicates that (1) serotonin potentiates the analgesic action of endorphins, raising pain thresholds; (2) norepinephrine inhibits endorphin analgesia and lowers pain thresholds; (3) it is likely that depressive illness alters the serotonin/norepinephrine ratio in the brain, increasing the perception of pain.[1,24] The antidepressants have been shown to affect levels of biogenic amines in the CNS. Clomipramine, doxepin, and amitriptyline have been found to block synaptic reuptake of serotonin.[16,24] This results in higher concentrations of serotonin versus norepinephrine at the synaptic cleft. Because serotonin potentiates the analgesic action of endorphins and norepinephrine inhibits the analgesic action of endorphins, this balance alteration could explain how antidepressants lower pain perception.[1,24] Monks and Merskey also discuss the many possibilities for why these psychotrophic drugs produce an analgesic effect independent of their psychologic effects.[39] The most impressive example is revealed by research that illustrates that the analgesic actions of antidepressants are not mediated by antidepressant action.[17,18,31,33,37,39] The two main types of antidepressants used to treat chronic back pain are the tricyclic antidepressants (TCAD) and the monamine oxidase inhibitors (MAOI).[1,17,33,39,62] The onset of analgesia with the tricyclic antidepressants in chronic pain states is more rapid than the usual onset of an antidepressant in clinically depressed patients (3 to 7 days versus 14 to 21 days).[39,40] Also, chronic pain relief with the TCADs and MAOIs has been reported despite lack of antidepressant response. Similar improvement was obtained in patients without detectable depression.[39,61] There is little evidence to support the use of one TCAD over any other. There is slight evidence that low back pain patients respond better to clomipramine and impramine.[53] Imipramine, desipramine, and amitriptyline have also been suggested as being effective with back patients.[53,62] These drugs also seem to be especially effective in relieving pain of neuralgic origin.[62] The MAOI phenelzine has been used for patients with back pain.[39] Side-effect of MAOIs include urinary retention, orthostatic hypotension, CNS effects, severe parenchymal hepatotoxic reactions, hypertensive crises, and drug interactions. Fortunately, serious side-effects are rare if medications, foods, and beverages with sympathomimetic activities are strictly avoided. The TCAD adverse effects include anticholinergic effects (dry mouth, palpitations, decreased visual accommodation, constipation, edema); sometimes, serious side-effects such as postural hypertension, loss of consciousness, urinary retention, and paralytic ileus occur.[39] It has been suggested that if a treatment fails with one TCAD it may be successful with another that has different pharmacologic properties.[39]

The minor tranquilizers include the benzodiazepines and the phenothiazines. These tranquilizers have also proved to be helpful with some pain sufferers. These drugs have been used in an attempt to diminish anxiety, excessive muscle tension, and insomnia caused by acute and chronic pain states.[1,15,17,40] However, it has been suggested that benzodiazepines may diminish brain serotonin turnover.[39] Serotonin potentiates the analgesic action of endorphins and, if this is true, the benzodiazepines may actually increase the perception of pain.[24] There is also reason to believe that muscle tension has been an overstated cause of chronic pain.[37] A small number of studies have reported on the treatment of chronic pain with the benzodiazepines.[39,40] The results also showed that the benzodiazepines were inferior to the tricyclic antidepressants.[39,40] Several authors have reservations in using the benzodiazepines or phenothiazines for chronic pain. These drugs may be a source of additional confusion, drowsiness, and dysphoria.[1,39] Phenothiazines also have troublesome side-effects including dry mouth, blurred vision, postural hypertension, weight gain, constipation, and urine retention. Benzodiazepines are also addictive (when given for longer than 6 weeks). They produce daytime sedation and impair coordination and judgment and other forms of cognitive judgment.[16,17,36] However, in five papers reporting on short-term benzodiazepine use in chronic pain, no severe adverse effects were reported.[39,40] Another study reported that global measures of cognitive function and EEG findings were more disturbed in patients taking benzodiazepines than in those taking only narcotics.[24,39] Table 10-7 includes psychotropic drugs used with pain patients.

Pharmacologic agents such as these psychotrophic drugs can be very effective in treating back patients. Back patients with chronic pain and emotional or reactive depression benefit in particular. However, these drugs will not treat underlying conflicts, solve family problems, or resolve motivational issues. Thus, the pain must also be treated multidimensionally with a variety of other medical, psychotherapeutic interventions.[1]

Regional Blocks and Local Anesthesia

Analgesic blocks may be performed utilizing a local anesthetic only, or they may combine the anesthetic with a corticosteroid. Epidural blocks that use the com-

TABLE 10-7
Psychotropic Drugs

ANTIDEPRESSANTS
1. *Imipramine (Tofranil):*   TCAD
2. *Desipramine (Pertofrane):*   TCAD, fewer anticholinergic effects
3. *Amitriptyline (Elavil):*   TCAD, more-sedating effects
4. *Doxepin (Adapin):*   TCAD, more sedating, lack of addicting potential, anti-anxiety
5. *Phenelzine (Nardil):*   MAOI; insomnia common side-effect; generally useful if TCAD has failed, not first choice and requires strict dietary control
6. *Tranylcypromine (Parnate):*   MAOI; generally useful if TCAD has failed; also requires strict dietary control

TRANQUILIZERS
1. *Diazepam (Valium):*   Benzodiazepine; also commonly prescribed as a muscle relaxant
2. *Meprobamate (Equanil):*   Benzodiazepine; discussed in section on muscle relaxants
3. *Flurazepam (Dalmane):*   Benzodiazepine; commonly prescribed
4. *Chloridazepoxide (Librium):*   Benzodiazepine; commonly prescribed
5. *Methotrimeprazine (levomepromazine; Levoprome):*   Phenothiazine; high doses lead to somnolence and delirium
6. *Chlorporthixene (Taractan):*   Phenothiazine; high doses can lead to somnolence and delirium
7. *Haloperidol (Haldol):*   Phenothiazine; less sedation effect and fewer anticholinergic effects
8. *Lorazepam (Ativan):*   Benzodiazepine; antianxiety agent

bination of steroids and anesthetic are still favored for back pain.[20] However, increasingly blocks using only anesthetics are being used. Blocks utilizing steroids are preferred to systemic applications of this drug. Areas of back pain treated with local blocks include

1. *Myofascial pain syndromes:* 5–10 mL dilute of long-lasting anesthetic such as bupivacaine (0.25%) is used.[7,9,57]
2. *Muscular pain:* intramuscular injections for severe muscle spasm.[7,9,20]
3. *Ligamentous sprains:* local anesthetic used for painful ligaments of the lumbosacral, sacroiliac, sacrococcygeal, and interspinous ligaments of the whole spine.[10]
4. *Facet synovitis or arthritis:* intra-articular injections of facets, using local anesthetic alone or with steroid. Useful also as a prognostic procedure in facet syndrome.
5. *Postoperative scars:* local anesthetic is utilized in a series of 6 to 8 injections.
6. *Paravertebral blocks:* for cervical, thoracic, or lumbar pain. Good for low back and neck area to determine diagnostically the levels of root irritation.
7. *Spinal blocks:* local anesthetic to any level including brachial plexus to block pain in whole area.[10]
8. *Sciatic nerve blocks:* to temporarily control severe or acute pain from sciatica.

The basic indications for blocks include diagnostic, prognostic, and therapeutic pain-relieving purposes. The patient selection includes lumbar, cervical, or thoracic disk; facet, ligamentous, or muscular pain. The patient with the disk syndrome and a normal myelogram is also a good candidate, especially if other measures have been tried. Also, patients with any back pain with multiple myelographic defects and the absence of specific neurologic damage is a candidate. Facet syndrome and sacroiliac syndromes are especially responsive to blocks.[20] Some common local anesthetics used include[10]

1. *Bupivacaine (Marcaine)*: fast onset, long duration, moderate penetrance (diffusibility)
2. *Lidocaine (Xylocaine)*: fast onset, moderate duration, marked penetrance
3. *Etidocaine (Duranest)*: very fast onset, moderate penetrance, long duration
4. *Mepivacaine (Carbocaine)*: moderate onset, penetrance, and duration
5. *Procaine (Novocain)*: moderate onset and penetrance, short duration

Side-effects include several reactions: systemic toxic reactions; very high or total spinal anesthesia; pneumothorax; and neurologic complications. The systemic toxic reactions result from an excessive dose, and accidental intravenous injection of a therapeutic dose, or an abnormal rate of absorption. Very high or total anesthesia and consequent respiratory paralysis and hypotension may develop from subarachnoid attempts of paravertebral blocks. Within a few minutes the patient will develop bilateral analgesia. If the solution is more than 3 ml to 4 ml, in the latter case, it will ascend rapidly and involve the cranial and cervical nerves. The patient may become drowsy, dyspneic, unable to speak, develop apnea, and may lose consciousness. Pneumothorax occurs from injecting the needle too deeply in the thoracic region.[10] These problems occur very infrequently, but the physician must be ready to react quickly if something unusual does occur. The physician must select a practitioner who has, or must himself have, a thorough knowledge of the structure, anatomy, technique, and proper selection of patients for blocks to be safe and effective.

The techniques for using these various medications for back pain are also varied and sometimes complicated. However, we will review another case study of possibly more ideal use of pharmacologic intervention for the treatment of back pain.

CASE 2   A 29-year-old female nurse injured her lower and upper back while lifting a patient. She complained of severe pain with some radiation up through the shoulders and down into one hip. She was sent to the emergency room and the covering physician sent her home with an analgesic (acetaminophen/propoxyphene; Darvocet) and instructions to use cold packs or heat with bed rest for 24 to 48 hr, depending on the severity of pain, and then to visit her family physician. The patient stayed with bed rest for 24 hr and used ice packs and hot showers. The symptoms were about the same, except now the patient was more stiff, and she noticed that gentle activity such as walking felt better than sitting or bending forward. She visited her physician who prescribed an anti-inflammatory (indomethacin; Indocin) four times a day for 3 to 4 weeks and an analgesic (pentazocine; Talwin) on an as-needed basis. She was also instructed to keep moving at home with frequent rest periods and to avoid prolonged postures such as sitting.

The patient was able to return to work in 2 weeks with minimal pain but still continued her medications. After 4 weeks the patient discontinued her medications. Six months later she again injured her back while lifting a heavy patient by herself. This time the low back pain predominated, and she had more leg pain. A repeat of the same medications and home rest did not alleviate the pain. The family doctor changed the anti-inflammatory medications and initiated a stronger analgesic without avail. The physicain then admitted the patient to the hospital for testing and more extensive therapy. All of the diagnostic test results were negative, except for a slight bulge of her L4-5 disk on the opposite side of her back and leg pain. Her physician decided to try local injection of steroid into the hip and sent her to physical therapy for ice massage, soft-tissue techniques, and possibly traction if tolerated. The physician also asked for patient education on posture, positioning, and especially body mechanics because the patient had a history of problems with lifting. The traction made her worse and was discontinued; however, the soft-tissue techniques, positioning, and modalities, along with her steroid therapy caused a dramatic decrease in the pain. The patient was discharged and continued her pharmacologic therapy and her physical therapy for continued education and gradual exercise to prepare her for return to work. Three and a half weeks after discharge the patient returned to work and has remained asymptomatic for 2 years.

In reviewing all the pharmacologic categories prescribed for back pain, it becomes obvious there are many possibilities for types of drugs and for the method of administration. There are also many ways in which these drugs can be misused including (1) overuse or underuse, (2) inappropriate prescription for the type of pain or patient situation, (3) inappropriate withholding of drugs, (4) lack of flexibility in utilizing various drug types or in alternating drugs of the same category when problems occur, and (5) preference for only pharmacologic intervention. This latter activity also may hinder the patient's prognosis because the physician's firm reliance on pharmacologic management may deprive the patient of other effective therapies. Additional therapies may serve to further augment the effects of the medications. Rarely, will patients recuperate with the medication alone, unless an arthritic or acutely inflamed ailment is present. Here, anti-inflammatory medications can make a huge difference.[62] Consideration must also be given to why the patient has the pain in the first place. Modifications of job, home, and leisure activities should be initiated. Additional therapeutic services can be especially helpful if used in a timely and appropriate manner. Pharmacologic therapy should be tailored to the patients disorder. Prescribing muscle relaxants for a patient whose back pain stems from a nerve or arthritis is illogical (unless that pain has elicited a true visible muscle spasm). It is easy for neurosurgeons and orthopaedic surgeons to become more interested in surgery than in conservative pharmacologic therapy.[62] Therefore, they may be reluctant to spend the necessary time with back patients to work through an effective program. General practitioners, rheumatologists, internists, and clinical pharmacologists can perform this role admirably.[62] Finally, the patients should be made a part of the decision-making and therapeutic process. They should be educated in the goals, alternatives, and risks of their therapeutic process. Medicines left in a bottle do little good, improperly performed exercises may do harm, and patients with unrealistic expectations, or no expectations, are difficult to treat successfully.[62]

REFERENCES

1. Aronoff GM, Evans WO: Pharmacological management of chronic pain. In Aronoff GM (ed): Evaluation and Treatment of Chronic Pain, pp 435–449. Baltimore, Schwarzenberg, 1985
2. Antonakes JA: Claims cost of back pain. Best's Rev Sept 1981
3. Back pain monitor: Disability Stat 3(1):4, 1985
4. Behar M, Magora F, Olshwang D et al: Epidural morphine in treatment of pain. Lancet 1:527–528, 1979
5. Blumer D, Heilbronn M: Second-year follow-up study on systematic treatment of chronic pain with antidepressants. Henry Ford Hosp Med J 29:67–68, 1981
6. Boas RA: Facette joint injections. In Staton-Hicks M, Boas RA (eds): Chronic Low Back Pain, pp 199–211. New York, Raven Press, 1982
7. Bonica JJ: Clinical Applications of Diagnostic and Therapeutic Nerve Blocks. Springfield, Charles C Thomas, 1959
8. Bonica JJ: Basic principles in managing chronic pain. Arch Surg 112:783–788, 1977
9. Bonica JJ: The Management of Pain. Philadelphia, Lea & Febiger, 1953
10. Bonica JJ: Local anesthesia and regional blocks. In Wall PD and Melzack R (eds): Textbook of Pain, pp 541–557. New York, Churchill-Livingston, 1984
11. Braun W: Intradisc injection of Trasylol in lumbar intervertebral disc syndrome. Neurosurg Rev 1:21–24, 1979
12. Cantor G: Anti-inflammatory drug therapy for low back pain. In Stanton-Hicks M, Boas RA (eds): Chronic Low Back Pain, pp 157–169. New York, Raven Press, 1982
13. Carron H, Toomey TC: Epidural steroid therapy for low back pain. In Stanton-Hicks M, Boas RA (eds): Chronic Low Back Pain, pp 193–198. New York, Raven Press, 1982
14. Churcher M: Peripheral nerve blocks in relief of Intractable Pain. Amsterdam, Excerpta Medica, 1978
15. Cohen FL: Post surgical pain relief; patient's status and nurses' medication and choices. Pain 9:265–274, 1980
16. Committee on the Review of Medicine: Systematic review of the benzodiazepines. Guidelines for data sheets on diazepam, chlordiazepoxide, medazepam, clorazepate, lorazepam, oxazepam, temazepam, triazolam, nitrazepam and flurazepam. Br Med J 280:910–912, 1980
17. Duthie AM: The use of phenothiazines and triccyclic antidepressants in the treatment of intractable pain. S Afr Med J 51:246–247, 1977
18. Evans W, Gensler F, Blackwell B et al: The effects of antidepressants on pain relief and mood in the chronically ill. Psychosomatics 14:214–219, 1973
19. Feffer HL: Regional use of steroids in the management of lumbar intervertebral disc disease. Orthop Clin N Am 6:249–253, 1975
20. Finneson BE: Low Back Pain, pp 211–219. Philadelphia, JB Lippincott, 1980
21. Fuentes JA, Garzon J, Del Rio J: Potentiation of morphine analgesia in mice after inhibition of brain type B monoamine oxidase. Neuropharmacology 16:857–862, 1977
22. Gessel AH: Electromyographic biofeedback and tricyclic antidepressant in myofascial pain-dysfunction syndrome: Psychological predictors of outcome. J Am Dent Assoc 91:1048–1052, 1975
23. Hannington-Kiff JG: Treatment of intractable pain by bupivacaine nerve block. Lancet 2:1392–1394, 1971
24. Hendler N: The anatomy and psychopharmacology of chronic pain. J Clin Psychiatry 43:8, (sec 2), 15–20, 1982
25. Huskisson EC, Woolf DL, Balme H et al: Four new anti-inflammatory drugs: Responses and variations. Br Med J 1:1048–1049, 1976

26. Huskisson EC: Non-narcotic analgesics. In Wall PD and Melzack R (eds): Textbook of Pain, pp 505–513. New York, Churchhill Livingston, 1984
27. Johansson F, Von Knorring L, Sedvall G et al: A double-blind controlled study of a serotonin uptake inhibitor (zimelidine) versus placebo in chronic pain patients. Pain 7:69–78, 1979
28. Johansson F, Von Knorring L, Sedvall G et al: Changes in endorphins and 5-hydroxyindoleacetic acid in cerebrospinal fluid as a result of treatment with a serotonin uptake inhibitor (zimelidine) in chronic pain patients. Psychiatry Res 2:167–172, 1980
29. Judd AT, Tempest SM, Clarke IMC: The anesthetist and the pain clinic: Destromoramide analgesia. Br Med J 282:75–76, 1981
30. Kay B: A study of strong oral analgesics; the relief of postoperative pain using dextro-moramide, pentazocine and bezitranide. Br J Anaesth 45:623–628, 1973
31. Kocher R: Use of psychotropic drugs for treatment of chronic severe pain. In Bonica JJ, Albe Fessard D (eds): Advances in Pain Research and Therapy 1, pp 579–582. New York, Raven Press, 1976
32. Kraus H: Clinical Treatment of Back and Neck Pain. New York, McGraw-Hill, 1970
33. Lee R, Spencer PSJ: Antidepressants and pain: A review of the pharmacologic data supporting the use of certain tricyclics in chronic pain. J Int Med Res 5(Suppl 1):146–156, 1977
34. Liberty Mutual Insurance Company, Research Center, Hopkinton, MA (unpublished data).
35. Long DM: Use and Misuse of Drug Therapy in Chronic Pain, pp 226–227. First World Congress on Pain, Florence, 1975
36. Marks RM, Sachar EJ: Undertreatment of medical inpatients with narcotic and analgesics. Ann Intern Med 78:173–181, 1973
37. Merskey H, Hester RN: The treatment of chronic pain with psychotrophic drugs. Postgrad Med J 48:594–598, 1972
38. Messing R, Lytle LD: Serotonin-containing neurons: Their possible role in pain and analgesia. Pain 4:1–21, 1977
39. Monks R, Merskey H: Psychotropic drugs. In Wall and Melzack (eds): Textbook of Pain, pp 526–537. New York, Churchill Livingston, 1984
40. Monks RC: The use of psychotropic drugs in human chronic pain: A review. 6th World Congress of the International College of Psychosomatic Medicine. Montreal, Canada, September 15, 1981
41. Montilla E, Fredrik WS, Cass LJ: Analgesic effect of methotrimeprazine and morphine. Arch Intern Med 111:91–94, 1963
42. Murphy DL, Campbell I, Costa JL: Status of the indoleamine hypothesis of the effective disorders. In Lipton MZ, Mascio AD, Killam KF (eds): Psychopharmacology: a Generation of Progress, pp 1235–1247. New York, Raven Press, 1978
43. NCCI Low Back Study: Unpublished report, National Council on Compensation Insurance, New York, 1984
44. Palmer B: Firms try to crack back problems. USA Today July 22, 1985
45. Panis W, Aamoff GM: Painful peripheral neuropathies. In Mediguide to Pain, Vol 5, 1. New York, Lawrence Dellacorte Publications, 1984
46. Peterson TH: Injection treatment for back pain. Am J Orthop 5:320–325, 1963
47. Rask M: Persistent back pain? Old cure urged. PT Bull p 3, February 26, 1986
48. Rowe ML: Low back disability in industry. Updated position. J Occup Med 12:476–478, 1971
49. Schildkraut JN: Current status on the catecholamine hypotheses of affective disorders. In Lipton MA, Mascio AD, Killam KF (eds): psychopharmacology: A Generation of Progress, pp 1223–1234. New York, Raven Press, 1978
50. Schutz H, Longheed WH, Wortzman G et al: Intervertebral nerve root block in investigation of chronic lumbar disc disease. Can J Surg 16:217–221, 1973
51. Sedzimir CB: Lumbosacral root pain. In Lipton S (ed): Persistent Pain: Modern Methods of Treatment, Vol 2. London, Academic Press, 1980

52. Singh G: Drug treatment of chronic intractable pain in patients referred to a psychiatry clinic. J Indian Med Assoc 56:341–345, 1971
53. Sternback RA, Janowsky DS, Huey IY et al: Effects of altering brain serotonin activity on human chronic pain. In Bonica JJ, Albe Fessard D (eds): Advances in Pain Research and Therapy, pp 601–606. New York, Raven Press, 1976
54. Sternback RA, Murphy RW, Akeson WH et al: Chronic low back pain, the "low back loser." Postgrad Med J 53:135–138, 1973
55. Sweet WH, Poletti CE: Treatment of trigeminal neuralgia: Comparisons between carbamazepine, retrogasserian and radiofrequency lesions, retrogasserian glycerol. Presentation at the American Pain Society, Chicago, Nov, 1983.
56. Swerdlow M: The treatment of shooting pain. Postgrad Med J 56:159–161, 1980
57. Travell J: Myofascial trigger points. In Bonica JJ, Albe Fessard DG (eds): Advances in Pain Research and Therapy, pp 601–606. New York, Raven Press, 1976
58. Twycross RB: Narcotics. In Wall PD and Melzack R (eds): Textbook of Pain, pp 514–525. New York, Churchhill Livingston, 1984
59. U.S. Dept. of Health and Human Services: Prevalence of Selected Impairments. United States 1977. DHHS Publ (PHS) 81–1562, 1982
60. U.S. Dept. of Labor, Bureau of Labor Statistics: Back Injuries Associated with Lifting. Bulletin 2144, August 1982
61. Watson CP et al: Amitriptyline versus placebo in postherpetic neuralgia. Neurology 32:671–673, 1982
62. Wilkinson HA: The Failed Back Syndrome, pp 1–3, 166–183. Philadelphia, Harper & Row, 1983
63. Wilkinson HA, Mark VH, White JC: Further experiences with intrathecal phenol for the relief of pain. J Chronic Dis 17:1055–1059, 1964
64. Wilkinson HA, Schuman N: Intradiscal corticosteroids in the treatment of lumbar and cervical disc problems. Spine 5:385–389, 1980
65. Wyant GM: Chronic pain syndromes and their treatment: II The piriformis syndrome. Can Anaesth Soc J 26:305–308, 1979
66. Young RR, Delwade PM: Spasticity, Part I and II. N Engl J Med 304:28–33, 96–99, 1981
67. Zweifach B, Grant L, McCloskey R: Inflammatory Process, Vol. III, p 173. New York, Academic Press, 1973

Renal Rehabilitation   11

Christina M. Sokolek
George R. Aronoff

The recognition of interrelationships between all organ systems has forced the re-habilitation professional to take a holistic approach to the evaluation and treatment of patients. However, to gain a clear understanding of the patient we categorize diseases into separate entities. Many therapy departments have established a classification system of patients treated. Typically, patients are divided into services such as: general surgery, orthopaedics, cardiology, neurology, pulmonary, pediatrics, geriatrics, rheumatology, and oncology. Patients with renal disease fit into these categories based on their primary diagnosis, the manifestations of the underlying disease, or the complications of drug therapy. This chapter identifies some of the common problems seen in patients with compromised renal function and discusses the ramifications of drug intervention.

The kidneys work in conjunction with the circulatory, digestive, respiratory, endocrine, musculoskeletal, central and peripheral nervous systems to maintain a homeostasis of the internal environment. Renal dysfunction may result from primary disease processes, such as polycystic kidney disease and rapidly progressive glomerulonephritis, or it may be secondary to systemic diseases, such as diabetes mellitus, systemic lupus erythmatosus, and scleroderma. The rehabilitation therapist plays an active role in helping the patient minimize complications of their renal disease as it affects the other systems.

The kidneys have a direct effect on drug disposition. Renal dysfunction affects drug absorption, distribution, metabolism, and excretion. Patients with renal disease treated by a therapist have responses different from similar patients without renal dysfunction. The therapist needs to be aware of the patient's overall status and his renal function.

247

ACUTE RENAL FAILURE

Renal insufficiency is defined by the duration and the amount of insufficiency. "Acute renal failure (ARF) is characterized by an abrupt, frequently reversible decline in renal function which is attended by the inability of the kidneys to maintain the internal physiologic environment of the body."[7] Acute renal failure can be classified by whether the insult is a vascular disorder, a tubular lesion, or an obstructive lesion:

1. "*Vascular disorders*, which may be (a) pre-glomerular, including decreased cardiac output from any cause, or arterial disease, i.e., thrombosis, emboli, vasculitis or hypertension, or (b) glomerular diseases, which are essentially capillary vasculitides at the glomerular level, encompassing poststreptococcal glomerulonephritis, connective tissue disorders, hypersensitivity, angiitis, and rapidly progressive glomerulonephritis, to name just a few.
2. *Tubular lesions* are the most common cause of acute renal failure. Often referred to as *acute tubular necrosis*, this is a diverse group of kidney disorders secondary to toxins, hypotension, hemolysis, or intratubular obstruction.
3. *Obstructive lesions*, which consist of ureteral obstruction, either intrinsic or extrinsic, bladder outlet obstruction, prostatic or urethral obstruction."[7]

When patients suffer ARF, recovery is expected within 4 to 6 weeks. The rehabilitative health professional may be asked to help preserve muscular function during the interval until normal renal function returns. Usually, with the resolution of ARF, the organ systems involved return to normal function. When consulted about a patient with renal failure as a secondary diagnosis or as a complication of surgery the required time reference set for rehabilitation may be extended. This observation can clearly be seen for the patients on a cardiac rehabilitation program after coronary bypass grafting or any cardiovascular surgery. Fatigue remains an important factor after the initial crisis has passed.

CHRONIC RENAL FAILURE

"Chronic renal disease may be viewed as a progressive, relentless decline in the nephron population. A continually smaller population of nephrons are faced with the task of maintaining the internal environment that previously was distributed among many more nephrons."[6]

"Renal function deterioration may be classified according to several successive stages as follows:

1. *Diminished renal reserve.* Kidney function is mildly reduced, but excretory and regulatory functions are sufficiently intact to maintain a normal internal environment.
2. *Renal insufficiency.* At this stage, some evidence of impaired capacity to maintain the internal environment may appear. There may be a mild azotemia, slightly impaired concentrating ability, and some anemia. If the patient is stressed by dehydration, infection, heart failure, etc., renal abnormalities may become much more prominent.

3. *Renal failure.* Kidney function has deteriorated to the point of chronic and persistent abnormalities in the internal environment. This situation generally occurs when the creatinine clearance (C_{Cr}) has declined to less than 20 ml/min.
4. *The uremic syndrome.* A constellation of clinical signs and symptoms may appear in the patient with chronic renal failure. The point at which these become manifest is variable, but they generally become evident at clearances less than 15 ml/min. However, it is not uncommon to see patients with definite, severe renal failure who are essentially asymptomatic."[5]

UREMIA

The uremic syndrome, seen in patients with severe chronic renal failure, affects every organ system.[2,4] The extent of involvement is dependent on how well the internal environment is controlled. Many of the symptoms will resolve with improvement in renal function. Neurologic impairment may involve the central nervous system and cause changes in the attention span, personality, sleep patterns, and habits. Tremor, asterixis, muscle twitching, ataxia, nystagmus, vertigo, or hemiplegia may develop. Peripheral neuropathies and prolonged conduction nerve times may occur. Neurologic changes should be noted by any therapist working with the patients and brought to the attention of the physician. "General strengthening" programs may need to be tailored in the presence of central nervous system changes. In the presence of peripheral changes, setting of goals may have to be modified temporarily, if the problem is acute, and on a more permanent basis if the renal failure develops to a chronic state.

Hypertension, congestive heart failure, pericarditis, coronary artery disease, and arrhythmias are possible cardiovascular sequelae in chronic renal failure.[1,2] Vigorous exercise should be totally withdrawn if severe hypertension is present. As the blood pressure reaches a steady state, monitored exercise with specified cardiac guidelines can be pursued.

Weakness or osteodystrophy affects the musculoskeletal system. The therapist can play an important role in maintaining joint structures. Soft-tissue integrity should be preserved with well-defined and monitored exercise programs at the onset of uremic crisis.

The therapist can document manifestations of cutaneous involvement which include pigmentation, purpura, "frost," pruritus, and nail changes. The therapist should realize that diphenhydramine (Benadryl) and other medications given to relieve the itching cause sedation.

Uremic disturbance of endocrine function may lead to changes in menstruation, potency, libido, nocturia, polyuria, and diurnal rhythm. Hormonal changes also cause psychologic effects directly or by the changes placed on the patient's physical being.

Gastrointestinal signs of uremia include nausea, emesis, bleeding, diarrhea, parotitis, pancreatitis, and peptic ulcers. Patients with gastrointestinal complaints do not feel like working. The therapist needs to be compassionate and not push the patients beyond their tolerance. The therapist should remain supportive when these patients try to continue their rehabilitation programs.

Patients with chronic renal failure develop conjunctivitis, ocular calcium desposition, elevated intraocular pressure, diabetic and hypertensive retinopathy. Patients with elevated intraocular pressure should be prevented from performing activities that increase their blood pressure. These patients should be monitored and their programs supervised at all times. Elevated intraocular pressure can irreparably damage vision.

Patients become anemic and develop bleeding tendencies, platelet abnormalities, and hemolysis. When platelet abnormalities affect bleeding time, the outlined program must be modified. Active assistive range-of-motion diminishes the chances of hemorrhage. When platelet abnormalities or coagulopathies are noted, the therapist should discuss the rehabilitation program with the patient's physician.

Uremia-induced alterations of intermediary metabolism result in impairment of carbohydrate tolerance and protein synthesis, in abnormal enzyme function, and in fat wasting.[1] Muscle building is not possible during this stage. The patient is incapable of metabolizing nutrients to their proper constituents. It is hoped that fat and tissue wasting can be limited. A vigorous, restorative program will be needed when the patient improves.

Psychologic changes from the uremic syndrome include depression, agitation, suicidal behavior, anxiety, fear, denial, and psychosis. These must be identified and monitored carefully.

Therapists work with renal failure patients because of the manifestations of their renal disease, complications of their renal dysfunction, or complications of drug therapy. The disciplines within the core of the rehabilitation professions need a broad view of how the patient with renal failure will benefit from a multidisciplinary approach. In addition to knowing the signs of the uremic syndrome, the therapist needs to have an understanding of treatment procedures available to the patient with progressive deterioration of kidney function.

DIALYSIS

Most patients with renal failure need dialysis during their treatment. An arteriovenous access is used for hemodialysis and can be either an external shunt or an internal fistula. Complications of external shunts including thrombosis, infection, accidental dislodgement of the catheter, and erosion of the skin can necessitate multiple surgeries to maintain the device. Some of the complications of an internal arteriovenous fistula include thrombosis, venous hypertension, arterial insufficiency, aneurysms, and pseudoaneurysms.[2] After surgery the therapist should be cautioned against maintaining full flexion at the elbow because this impedes venous return and can cause a clot in the venous portion of an arm access. After surgery the involved limb should be exercised only in a pain-free range, active or even active assistively. When the surgical site has healed, vigorous exercise should be incorporated to increase the muscle mass, which will protect and aid the access.

Patients receiving hemodialysis inherently have a defined proportion of their schedule that is sedentary, which leads to weakness, loss of endurance, and a change in life-style. The role of the rehabilitation professional team is to counteract this tendency and to enable the patient to maintain a life-style compatible with his expectations and potential.[3,9]

Peritoneal dialysis is another form of dialysis that is especially indicated for active patients, patients with severe cardiovascular disease, or patients with difficult vascular accesses. Chronic ambulatory peritoneal dialysis (CAPD) allows increased mobility, an advantage over hemodialysis.

RENAL TRANSPLANTS

Kidney transplantation is an alternative to dialysis for younger patients with end-stage renal disease. The risks of dialysis or transplantations and the psychosocial aspects of both need to be addressed before initiating either regimen. Renal transplants are the most successful when the organ compatibility is near that of an identical twin and when an appropriate regimen of immunosuppression is incorporated. There are many possible complications of renal transplantation. These problems relate to the quality of the donor kidneys, complications of rejection, and complications of immunosuppressive therapy. One of the major concerns of immunosuppression is extreme susceptibility to infections and a simultaneous inability to fight the infecting organism once it is present. Immediately after surgery, the patient receives very large doses of immunosuppressive medication and is kept in isolation. Steroid doses are slowly tapered, but the patients are kept on low doses as long as the transplanted kidney functions. They are cautioned about being in crowds and are urged to minimize exposure to possible carriers. Therapists need to practice reverse isolation as well as aseptic technique. The therapist probably should not work on a transplant unit when ill with a cold, flu, or any other infectious illness.

Corticosteroids affect the musuloskeletal system. In children, steroids block growth stimulating hormones. The child with a transplant has limited growth in stature and bone structure. In the child as well as the adult, avascular joint necrosis is a possible sequel of steroid therapy. Pain and deformity can occur in children with a resultant growth decrease.

Long-term steroid use also leads to proximal muscle weakness. This weakness, often illustrated in quadriceps dysfunction, leads to difficulty with any gross motor movement involving the legs, including stair climbing, standing up from low surfaces, and getting out of bathtubs. Arthralgias and myalgias also may occur, but they usually abate. During the painful stage, disuse occurs and muscle wasting develops. Because the patient is receiving steroids, muscle building is difficult. The development of an exercise program that will maintain muscle strength, improve collateral circulation, and provide normal weight-bearing and non–weight-bearing stresses to the bones and the joints can be potentially prophylactic.[1]

Osteoporosis is also a frequent complication. In the presence of long-term steroid use in a person with known steroid-induced weakness, a vigorous exercise program should not be initiated before the bone status is determined. If that is not possible, a very conservative, slowly graded, progressive exercise program should be developed. The primary goal is functional improvement rather than specified muscle strength changes. The use of pool therapy is frequently indicated in these patients.

There are other complications of importance to the rehabilitation professional. Pulmonary problems can affect the patient's endurance and subsequent amount of energy. His life-style can be assessed and tailored to his abilities by the occupational therapist. Cataracts and infections can directly affect the patient's level of activity. Dermatologic changes including loss of hair and increased bruisability, infections, and cushingoid features will require that the patient redefine his self-image. A social worker may be able to help. Diabetes can be better managed with patient education from the nurse educator.

There are significant ramifications of initiating immunosuppressive therapy to counteract rejection of the transplanted kidney. Each should be dealt with to enable the patient to live his life fully.

MEDICATIONS

Other than the immunosuppressive agents, primarily methylprednisolone (Medrol), prednisone, and azathioprine (Imuran), many drugs are commonly used in patients with renal impairment. Each has its own side-effects that are present when used in healthy individuals, but some have different effects in patients with renal dysfunction.

The analgesics include acetaminophen, aspirin, and the narcotics. Acetaminophen has very few side-effects. The problem with aspirin in the renally impaired patient is that the gastrointestinal effects are greatly exacerbated, especially the tendency toward bleeding. With bleeding, anemia may develop, and the therapist should know that the patient will be weaker and have poor endurance. The normal mental changes associated with narcotics are enhanced. Narcotics can cause sedation of the respiratory, cardiovascular, and reflex systems. Endurance and tolerance to activities will be directly influenced.

Magnesium-containing antacids are usually avoided in patients with renal disease secondary to their tendency toward central nervous system depression including muscular weakness and paralysis. These antacids also tend to act as a laxative. Alternatively, non-magnesium antacids tend to constipate. Cimetidine can lead to mental confusion. An approach of consistency in scheduling, and a simple and well-defined program, may help decrease the amplitude of the confusion.

Anticoagulants offer no really important changes for the patient with impaired renal function, but they do have the adverse side-effects of hemorrhage, local irritation, hematoma, and tissue sloughing. Heparin and warfarin (Coumadin) are two of the drugs used with dialysis to keep an access patent. All efforts should be taken to keep these patients from bruising themselves, and any injury needs to be reported.

Increased sedation is a side-effect of antihistamines in these patients. Diphenhydramine (Benadryl), trimeprazine (Temaril), and hydroxyzine (Vistaril) are commonly used, when needed, to treat the pruritus associated with the uremic syndrome and with antibiotic therapy. A sedated person will need supervision in their program for maintaining motivation and as a safety measure if they are working with hazardous equipment.

Antihypertensive agents [reserpine, atenolol (Tenormin), hydralazine, clonidine] have many potential side-effects including depression of the sympathetic nervous system, fatigue, headaches, dizziness, sexual dysfunction, and cardiovascular changes. Hypotension and bradycardia are two of the common cardiac changes. If a patient is taking one of these drugs, then assessment of vital signs is important with the changing of positions and with the initiation of any exercise or activity program. The clinical variables specified by the physicians should be followed. They should be notified in the presence of any unwanted or adverse response. The most significant concern with renal dysfunction is the sedation and fatigue factor. β-Blockers and diuretics are not often used in this group of patients because they have decreased effectiveness in parallel with the decreased renal function. They can also be "too effective" in the instance of marked improvement in renal function.

Except for the coricosteroids and azathioprine, the antineoplastic agents [cyclophosphamide (Cytoxan), methotrexate, cisplatin, vincristine] are not frequently used with renal patients. Patients with unresponsive tumors do not remain on hemodialysis.

The cardiac drugs, divided as antiarrhythmic agents [disopyramide (Norpace), lidocaine, procainamide, propranolol, quinidine] and glycosides (digoxin and digitoxin) have many cardiovascular effects, primarily hypotension and bradycardia. They can also give patients problems of vertigo, syncope, headaches, dizziness, diaphoresis, shortness of breath, and nausea. The side-effects are not different for the patient with renal disease, but they are definitely increased, secondary to increased activity of the metabolite and decreased ability to excrete it. An example would be procainamide and its metabolite, N-acetylprocainamide (NAPA), which causes hypotension and cardiovascular changes.

Barbiturates, benzodiazepines, phenothiazines, and tricyclic antidepressants, all may lead to weakness, fatigue, and a decreased sense of well-being. It may be very difficult with patients taking one of these drugs to differentiate between the weakness and fatigue of their primary illness and that caused by the drugs used to treat them. These patients need to be closely monitored. They need to be given attainable short-term goals to keep from feeding into the depression. It will be most difficult to motivate a patient to be enthusiastic about therapy if they are fatigued, weak, and feeling despondent. In addition, the first two groups of CNS depressants have more pronounced effects because of accumulation of the drugs and their metabolites in renal failure. They can be present for several days before their excretion and the resolution of symptoms. A therapist needs to be aware that even though one of the drugs has been stopped it may take days before it is cleared from the patient's system. Diazepam and N-methyldiazepam, the metabolite, have sedative and hypnotic effects and have a very long half-life.

Insulin, a hypoglycemic agent, has specific side-effects if administered in excess of the requirement. Insulin requirements are significantly less because insulin excretion decreases with worsening renal function. The patient with diabetes who is receiving insulin and develops renal failure will actually require less insulin! Patients taking insulin need to have monitored activity programs to help regulate serum glucose concentrations by coordinating exercise with the serum glucose cycles and insulin doses. You want to have patients exercise during the peak phase of their glucose cycle, which is approximately 2 to 3 hr after eating. They will need to adjust their insulin dosages. They will not need as much insulin to control the serum glucose concentrations if they burn off the sugar with exercise. You do not want to have a patient exercise just before a meal when their serum glucose is very low because the exercise may create a hypoglycemic reaction. A regular schedule of exercise would be beneficial in managing the diabetes.

Drugs used to treat gout (probenecid, colchicine, and allopurinol) and arthritis (nonsteroidal anti-inflammatory agents, antimalarials, and immunosuppressive agents) commonly have side-effects including nausea, vomiting, anorexia, gastrointestinal bleeding, headaches, tinnitus, and some cardiovascular changes such as edema, palpitations, and tachycardia. If you find that your patient is not tolerating exercise or activity well, you must try to have the patient identify the cause and then assess vital signs. The significant difference for the renal patient, especially with the nonsteroidal anti-inflammatory agents, is that the gastrointestinal symptoms can be exacerbated, similar to the effects seen with aspirin-containing analgesics.

Neurologic agents, including phenytoin (Dilantin), levodopa (antiparkinsonism agent), neostigmine, and primidone, need to be supervised in the event of side-effects involving the cardiovascular system, the CNS, and the gastrointestinal system, with no real change for the patient with renal disease, except that primidone is removed by hemodialysis. Phenytoin can induce such CNS changes as postural disturbances, incoordination, dizziness, as well as extrapyramidal signs. Grimacing, bruxism, and twisting of the tongue are some of the adverse effects occasionally seen with L-dopa. Patients taking neostigmine (cholinergic) may have parasympathetic responses as a side-effect including hypotension, bradycardia, asthma attacks, flushing, and sweating. These patients must be closely monitored. Exercise should be stopped until the medication and its side-effects can be controlled.

The last group of drugs, the antimicrobials, is of major significance for the patient with renal disease. Many renal patients develop infections either as a result of their disease state or because of their low tolerance to fighting infections related to their immunosuppressive therapies.

Many of the antimicrobials, including the antifungal agents (amphotericin), antituberculous agents (isoniazid) and the cephalosporins affect the gastrointestinal system (anorexia, nausea, vomiting, malaise). The antifungal agents may cause transitory vestibular changes, but the antitubercular and aminoglycosides can have irreversible vestibular and auditory toxicity. Most of the agents also lead to a transitory muscular weakness.[8]

Strengthening is very difficult with an antimicrobial regimen for two reasons. The infecting organisms may cause fevers, pain, discomfort, or nausea; the drugs used in treatment may also cause these effects. When patients are sick, their bodies are using a great deal of energy fighting the organism. In the beginning, a therapy program may have to deal primarily with issues of preserving range-of-motion and joint function. Strengthening and endurance would be goals in the later stages.

Patients with renal disease must deal with the disease entity itself, the many complications involving other organ systems and the altered effects of the drugs being used to treat the disease. Therapists need to take a holistic approach to the evaluation and treatment of the patients with renal disease. They need to be fully aware of the diagnosis for each patient and to have an understanding of the interaction that exists between the organ systems and the potential problems. Finally, the patient will benefit from the therapist who has a knowledge of the medications being used to treat the different aspects of the disease and the side-effects of the drug intervention.

CASE 1   The patient is a 27-year-old white female nurse with chronic renal failure. Her renal disease started in 1985 with postinfectious chronic glomerulonephritis. She has been on CAPD since 1986 and had been taking propranolol (Inderal) for blood pressure control. She was admitted February 1989, for an elective cadaveric renal transplant. The patient was initially placed on a regimen of high doses of azathioprine (Imuran) and methyprednisolone (Medrol), and the two drugs were then slowly tapered. Reverse isolation was utilized. The staff wore masks and gowns. Hand-washing was practiced. The patient wore a mask whenever she left the room. Six days after surgery, the patient was referred to physical therapy for evaluation and treatment to establish an exercise program that would improve her cardiovascular fitness and limit the complications of immunosuppressive treatment.

The patient reported that she had been very active before the onset of her kidney disease and enjoyed playing volleyball and tennis. She had been able to work as a nurse, but was very fatigued by the end of each day and unable to continue being active in sports. She denied any specific musculoskeletal complaints, other than the fatigue. Her primary reason for wanting to transplant was to be able to resume a normal and active life-style. The patient also expressed concerns about the medications she had been taking. Because she was a nurse, she understood that there would be weight gain from the drugs and that there was a potential for decreased muscular strength and joint problems with long-term use. She also expressed concern about the possibilities of myalgias and arthralgias developing as the medications were being tapered.

Initial evaluation revealed a medium-build woman with general muscle weakness. Strength was assessed to be "good." Joint examination, especially of the knees, showed normal function. A submaximal exercise stress test by bicycle ergometry revealed no cardiac arrhythmias and a fitness level of "fair." Her heart rate rose from 115 to 170, but her blood pressure remained fairly stable at 110/86 to 130/85, because of the Inderal.

The patient was placed on a general strengthening program using free weights and also on an aerobic exercise program using a stationary bike. She was to ride for a minimum of 15 min and work up to 45 min, three to five times a week with a target heart rate of 125 to 165. Both programs were to be continued until the patient was able to return to work and to engage in sports activities.

One week after beginning the program, she developed hip and knee pain. At that point she was independent with her program and riding the bike for 10 min at a heart rate of 130 bpm. She notified the physician. He gave her acetaminophen with codeine (Tylenol #3) for pain and requested physical therapy to reevaluate the program. The therapist treated her with heat modalities to relieve the pain after determining that she had joint pain but no identified bursitis or tendonitis. Bike riding was discontinued for 3 days. It was then resumed without the HR assessments until she could ride for 15 min without pain. This took 6 additional days, at which time she continued the regimen as previously outlined. She was discharged 24 days after her transplant. At that point she was riding 20 to 25 min, with a sustained HR of 130.

She returned for reevaluation 3 months later. Her biking program included riding five times a week for 30 min at a sustained HR of 140 and a upper extremity strengthening program using 5 to 10 lb of weight. She reported feeling very well, and felt ready to return to work and to begin playing sports. The evaluation revealed good/good-plus strength and a fitness level of good. She was given clearance by her physician to return to work and to begin noncontact sports as tolerated.

CASE 2   The patient, a 67-year-old white woman with a history of severe coronary artery disease, including a myocardial infarction in 1986, was placed on a regimen of propranolol and sublingual nitroglycerin p.r.n. She was controlled fairly well and was experiencing angina only with overexertion. She presented in May 1988, with an increase in angina and with episodes of pain at rest. Cardiac catheterization showed 90% stenosis of the left coronary artery, 50% to 60% narrowing of the right coronary artery, and 60% to 70% stenosis of the left circumflex artery. Coronary artery bypass grafting of these vessels was performed May 25, 1988. Postoperatively, she developed mediastinal bleeding and was taken back to surgery May 26, for cauterization of the offending vessels. She subsequently developed acute renal failure with an increase in weight, a decrease in urine output, and significant change in BUN and creatinine levels. The patient was treated with furosemide (Lasix) and digitoxin, and renal function began to return. The patient remained in ICU until June 8 or POD 14.

At this facility, open heart surgery patients are followed by physical therapy per a protocol that begins with pre-pump instructions in quad sets, ankle pumps, diaphragmatic breathing, and coughing. The patients are seen in ICU POD 2 for active or active assistive ROM for 5 to 10 repetitions and review of the leg exercises. A walking or biking program with monitoring of heart rate and blood pressure is initiated after transfer to the ward. The patients are instructed in the program to be continued at home. Patients are usually discharged POD 7 to 8 and are walking 1/4 to 1/2 mile.

Because of the development of the renal failure and an unstable medical status, physical therapy was not resumed until POD 7. The patient initially tolerated active-assistive ROM times 5 reps with minimal change in HR and BP and progressed to active ROM times 10 reps by POD 14.

At the time of transfer, the patient was taking atenolol (Tenormin), digitoxin, and Lasix and had orders to be ambulated BID as tolerated. Her supine resting HR was 72 and BP was 110/70, and seated they were 76 and 105/72, and standing they were 84 and 95/65. She complained of being light-headed during the standing evaluation and was returning to bed. Her vital signs returned to 74 and 115/70 respectively. That day, walking was not attempted. Exercises were continued. They were conducted in a sitting position to increase tolerance to the upright positions. On the second day, her HR went from 64 to 68 and BP from 100/65 to 80/55 with the changing of positions.

The physician was notified. He felt that the lower heart rates and blood pressures were due to a combination of the Tenormin and orthostatic hypotension, and he ordered nursing to hold the next dose and then lower subsequent doses. He requested ambulation to be withheld until the next day. On POD 16, she tolerated ambulating 50 ft with minimal assistance of 1. Her vital signs remained stable.

She was discharged POD 26, ambulating 450 ft (or less than 0.1 mile) using a cane. She was independent with the program, understanding the cardiac signs/symptoms and was able to monitor her HR and response to activity. She was placed on a walking program with instructions to increase distance as tolerated, rather than by the set standard (approximately 1/4 mile every 6 to 8 days) because fatigue remained a significant factor for her even though her renal function had returned to baseline.

CASE 3   The patient is a 62-year-old black man who has chronic renal failure from long-standing, poorly controlled hypertension. He is on chronic hemodialysis and was admitted for repair of his right arteriovenous fistula, which has developed an aneurysm. His medications included warfarin (Coumadin). He went into surgery on 7/13/88, for the repair. He was referred to physical therapy postoperatively to be instructed in exercises for the right arm.

The patient related that he was being transported to a dialysis unit Monday, Wednesday, Friday for 4 hr each day. He reported that he has not been doing very well at home. He has been having trouble with taking care of himself, including dressing, fixing meals, and getting out of chairs. He feels it is because he does not have adequate strength. He lives alone, and has friends at the apartment complex that help with shopping and driving.

Evaluation revealed an obese, black man, appearing older than stated age, who was diffusely weak. He had multiple surgical scars on both forearms. His right arm had "fair-plus" proximal strength, and "fair" distal strength. His left arm had "good-minus" proximal strength and "fair-plus," distally. His legs were generally "good," but the quadriceps were slightly weaker. Vital signs included a HR of 84 and BP of 150/90. Because of his general weakness, he was tested on a bike, riding without resistance, and could ride for 5 min without resistance before becoming fatigued.

He was placed on a general exercise program that involved

1. Using 2 lb cuff weights for his left arm
2. Active ROM for his right arm because he was only a few days postoperative. Also included in the program was the use of a nerf ball and putty to begin increasing muscle bulk of the finger flexors to facilitate venous return and maturation of the fistula.
3. Using 3 lb cuff weights for his legs, working on strengthening as well as endurance.

He needed instructions in precautions for his right AVF to extend the life at the fistula. Some of the considerations were to avoid prolonged flexion of the elbow and shoulder, which can impede venous return. It was found that he frequently slept on his right side with his right arm tucked under him and that he would fall asleep in a chair with his head propped with his arm.

Also included in the program were instructions to be careful with the right hand functions. The previous multiple surgeries had led to compromised circulation to his hand. Coumadin was being used to maintain his fistula, but it was increased to assist the perfusion of circulation to his hand. He needed to be educated to protect the hand, as well as all of his extremities against injury, which could cause excessive bleeding.

REFERENCES

1. Bandel-Walcer R: Physical therapy and exercise: An under-utilized patient service. Nephrol Nurse S(3):16–20, 1983
2. Friedman EA (ed): Strategy in Renal Failure. New York, John Wiley & Sons, 1978
3. Goldberg AP, Geltman EM, Hasberg JM et al: Therapeutic benefits of exercise training for hemodialysis patients. Kidney Int 16:S303–S309, 1983
4. Gray PJ: Management of patients with chronic renal failure. Role of physical therapy. Phys Ther 62:173–176, 1982
5. Kleit SA (ed): Sophomore Introduction to Clinical Medicine. Renal Section, p 19. Medical Educational Resources Program. Indiana University School of Medicine, Indianapolis, 1983
6. Kleit SA (ed): Sophomore Introduction to Clinical Medicine. Renal Section, p 21. Medical Educational Resources Program. Indiana University School of Medicine, Indianapolis, 1983
7. Kleit SA (ed): Sophomore Introduction to Clinical Medicine. Renal Section, p 43. Medical Educational Resources Program. Indiana University School of Medicine, Indianapolis, 1983
8. Loebl S, Spratto G, Heckheimer E: The Nurse's Drug Handbook, 3rd ed. New York, John Wiley & Sons, 1983
9. Underwood HC, Cardenas DD, Kutner NG: Effects of low-risk exercise therapy for chronic dialysis patients. Dial Transplant 14:688–695, 1985

BIBLIOGRAPHY

Brundage DJ: Nursing Management of Renal Problems, 2nd ed. St Louis, CV Mosby, 1980
Churg J, Sobin LH: Renal Disease Classification and Atlas of Glomerular Diseases. Igaku-Shoin, Tokyo and New York, 1982
Levine DZ: Care of the Renal Patient. Philadelphia, WB Saunders, 1983
Loebl S, Spratto G, Heckheimer E: The Nurse's Drug Handbook, 3rd ed. New York, John Wiley & Sons, 1983

Pharmacologic Considerations for Sports Medicine

12

William E. Prentice

The use of medications prescribed for various medical conditions by qualified physicians may be of great value to the athlete, just as it may with any other individual in the population. Under normal circumstances, an athlete would be expected to respond to medication just as would anyone else. However, because of the nature of physical activity, the athlete is in a situation that is not normal, and it is true that with intense physical activity special consideration should be given to the effects of certain types of medication. For the sports therapist who often provides the primary health care to the athlete, some knowledge of the potential effects of certain types of drugs on performance during physical activity is essential.

The sports therapist, working under the direction of a team physician, is responsible for keeping the athlete healthy and ready to train and compete under physically, mentally, and emotionally demanding circumstances. The therapist should be concerned with prevention, acute management, evaluation, and rehabilitation of sport-related injuries. The sports therapist typically spends a considerable amount of time each day dealing with a particular group of athletes. Because of the competitive schedules that athletes follow, the sports therapist may also be asked to travel with a team to the site of competition. Consequently, many times a physician is not available for consultation should an athlete become ill or require some type of medication. On occasion, the sports therapist must make some decisions about the appropriate use of medications, based on knowledge of the indications for use and the possible side-effects in athletes who participate in intense physical activities. Although the sports therapist will likely be instructed to distribute only over-the-counter medications within the strict framework of preestablished guidelines and protocols, they must also be cognizant of the potential effects of prescription medications in the competitive athlete.

This chapter will concentrate on the special considerations that must be given for those medications most commonly used in a sports medicine environment.

DISPENSING OF MEDICATION

The methods by which drugs may be dispensed vary according to individual state laws. Sports medicine settings are subject to those laws. Usually, the team physician is the individual ultimately responsible for prescribing medications. These prescription medications are then dispensed by the physician or pharmacist or by a nurse. The sports therapist typically does not possess the background nor the expertise to make decisions about the appropriate use of medication and should use great caution when dispensing such.

Very often over-the-counter medications are simply placed on a counter top in the sports medicine clinic for use as the athlete sees fit. Although it is true that this method of dispensing medication is time-saving for the clinician, this somewhat indiscriminate use of even the over-the-counter drugs by an athlete should be discouraged. The sports therapist who is dispensing over-the-counter medication of any variety should be knowledgeable about the possible effects of various drugs during exercise. Likewise, they should be subject to strict protocols, which are established by the team physician for dispensing medication. Failure to follow these guidelines or protocols may make the sports therapist legally liable should something happen to the athlete that can be attributed to use or misuse of a particular drug.

RECORD KEEPING

Those involved in any health care-related profession are acutely aware of the necessity of maintaining complete up-to-date medical records. Again, the sports medicine setting is no exception. If medications are being dispensed by a sports therapist, it is just as important to maintain accurate records of the types of medications dispensed as it is to record progress notes, treatments given, and rehabilitation plans. The sports therapist, working in an athletic training room must function in an environment that is considerably different from that to which the normal therapist is accustomed. The sports therapist may be dealing with a number of different patients simultaneously while trying to get a team ready for practice or competition. At times, things become hectic, and it is difficult to stop and write down or to log each medication as it is administered. Nevertheless, the sports therapist should include the following information on a type of medication administration log:

- Name of the athlete
- Complaint or symptoms
- Type of medication given
- Quantity of medication given
- Time and date of administration

COMMON MEDICATIONS

The following section will provide the sports therapist with some special considerations for those medications most commonly prescribed and used by individuals
involved in some sport-related activity. The classifications of medication discussed
will include (1) analgesic, antipyretic, and anti-inflammatory agents, (2) drugs that
affect the respiratory tract, (3) drugs that affect the gastrointestinal tract, and (4)
use of antibiotic medications (Table 12-1).

Analgesic, Antipyretic, and Anti-Inflammatory Agents

Perhaps the medications most commonly used by the sports therapists are those
for the purpose of pain relief. Athletes continuously place themselves in situations
where injury is likely to occur. Fortunately, a large number of the injuries that do
occur are not serious and lend themselves to rapid rehabilitation. But there is no
question that there is pain associated with even minor injury.

The two nonnarcotic analgesics most often used are aspirin and acetaminophen.
Aspirin is the most commonly used drug in the world.[16] Because of its easy availability, it is also probably the most misused drug. Aspirin is a derivative of salicylic
acid and is used for its analgesic, anti-inflammatory, and antipyretic capabilities.

Analgesia may result from several mechanisms: aspirin may interfere with the
transmission of painful impulses in the thalamus; it may increase the sensitivity of
pain receptors by interference with synthesis of prostaglandins which cause redness, swelling, and pain; and it may facilitate fluid resorption from injured tissues
by blocking the release of lysosomal enzymes and by reducing capillary permeability and, thus, fluid loss which produces swelling.[11] Aspirin also has the capability of reducing fever by altering sympathetic outflow from the hypothalamus,
which produces increased vasodilation and heat loss through sweating.[11] Among
the side-effects of aspirin use are gastric distress, heartburn, some nausea, tinnitus, headache, and diarrhea. Other more serious consequences can develop with
prolonged use or high doses.[1]

An athlete should be very cautious about selecting aspirin as a pain reliever
for a number of reasons. Most importantly is that aspirin decreases aggregation
of platelets, thereby impairing the clotting mechanism should injury occur.[13] Prolonged bleeding at an injured site will increase the amount of swelling, which has
a direct effect on the time required for rehabilitation.

Use of aspirin as an anti-inflammantory should be recommended with caution
because other prescription anti-inflammatory medications are available that do not
produce many of the undesirable side-effects of aspirin. Generally, prescription
anti-inflammatory agents are considered to be a more effective therapy.

It is not uncommon for aspirin to produce gastric discomfort. In an athlete,
intense physical activity may exacerbate this side-effect. It is important to realize
that taking a buffered aspirin is no less irritating to the stomach than is regular
aspirin. Enteric-coated tablets do resist aspirin breakdown in the stomach and
may minimize gastric discomfort. Regardless of the form of aspirin ingested, it
is recommended that it be taken with meals or with large quantities of water (8 to
10 oz/tablet) to reduce the likelihood of gastric irritation.

(*Text continues on p. 266*)

TABLE 12-1
A Guide to Commonly Used Medications for the Sports Therapist

Generic Name	Trade Name	Primary Use of Drug	Sport Medicine Consideration
ANALGESICS, ANTIPYRETICS, ANTI-INFLAMMATORY			
Aspirin	Many trade names	Analgesic, antipyretic, anti-inflammatory	Gastric irritation, nausea tinnitus,
Acetaminophen	Tylenol, Datril, others	Analgesic, antipyretic	None
Nonsteroidal anti-inflammatory drugs (NSAID)		All are analgesic, antipyretic, Anti-inflammatory	Less common gastric irritation than with aspirin, except for indomethacin. These should be used on a long-term basis for reducing inflammation. Should not be substituted for aspirin or acetaminophen in cases of mild headache or low fever.
Indomethacin	Indocin		
Ibuprofen	Advil, Motrin, Nuprin		
Naproxen	Naprosyn, Anaprox		
Piroxicam	Feldene		
Zomepirac	Zomax		
Tolmetin	Tolectin		
Fenoprofen	Nalfon		
Meclofenamate	Meclomen		
DRUGS THAT AFFECT THE RESPIRATORY TRACT			
Chlorpheniramine	Chlor-Trimeton	Antihistamine for allergies	Used primarily for treatment of allergic reactions. Causes drowsiness and decreased coordination
Diphenhydramine	Benadryl	Antihistamine; sometimes used to treat cough caused by a cold	Produces marked drowsiness; found in OTC sleeping medications

Dimenhydrinate	Dramamine	Antihistamine; used for treatment of motion sickness, nausea, vomiting	Should be administered before travel begins; produces drowsiness
Oxymetazoline	Afrin, Dristan Long Lasting, Neo-Synephrine 12 Hour, Nostrilla, Sinex Long Lasting	Adrenergic decongestant; applied topically as spray	Do not exceed recommended dosage because of rebound congestion; may cause sneezing, dryness of nasal mucosa, and headache
Pseudoephedrin	Sudafed, Sudrin, Afrinol, Cenafed, Neofed, others	Adrenergic decongestion; used orally	Produces stimulation of the central nervous system; topically applied decongestants work faster but oral decongestants are preferred in long-term use
Diphenhydramine	Benylin Cough Syrup, Benydryl	Antihistamine; used primarily for its drying effect in reducing coughing; also used for motion sickness and preventing nausea and vomiting	Produces drowsiness and dry mouth
Dextromethorphan	Benylin DM, Romilar CF, Coughettes, Sucrets Lozange	Nonnarcotic antitussive; used for suppression of cough	Very effective for unproductive cough; does not produce drowsiness and other side effects as commonly
Benzonatate	Tessalon	Peripherally acting antitussive; acts as an anesthetic	May produce drowsiness and a chilled sensation

(Continued)

TABLE 12-1 (Continued)
A Guide to Commonly Used Medications for the Sports Therapist

Generic Name	Trade Name	Primary Use of Drug	Sport Medicine Consideration
Codeine or hydrocodone		Narcotic antitussives; depress the central cough mechanism	Used in combination with a decongestant, an antihistamine, or an expectorant; can produce sedation, dizziness, constipation, and nausea
Guaifenesin	Robitussin, Glycotuss, Anti-Tuss	Expectorant used for symptomatic relief of unproductive cough	Used for treating a dry or sore throat. May cause drowsiness & nausea.
DRUGS THAT AFFECT THE GASTROINTESTINAL TRACT			
Sodium bicarbonate	Soda Mint, Bell/ans	Antacid; used for quick relief of upset stomach	Produces gas, belching, and gastric distension; may cause systemic alkalinity
Aluminum hydroxide	Amphojel, Dialume AlternaGEL	Antacid; used for upset stomach	May produce constipation; moderate acidneutralizer
Calcium carbonate	Mallamint, Alka-2, Amitone, Chooz, Titralac	Antacid; used for stomach upset	May produce constipation and acid rebound. High acid neutrali-capability
Dihydroxaluminum sodium carbonate	Rolaids	Antiacid; used for upset stomach	May cause constipation; rapid neutralizing capabilities, but transient

Magnesium hydroxide (milk of magnesia), carbonate, oxide, or phosphate	Milk of Magnesia	Antacid; used for upset stomach	May cause diarrhea and last-neutralization of acid without rebound
Cimetidine	Tagamet	Antihistamine; used for relief of upset stomach	May produce drowsiness and either constipation or diarrhea
Common combination antacids and antiemetics	Alka-Seltzer, Di-Gel, Gaviscon, Gelusil, Maalox, Mylanta, Tempo, Titralac WinGel, others	OTC combination drugs; used for controlling nausea and vomiting	May produce either diarrhea or constipation
Promethazine hydrochloride	Phenergan	Antiemetic; used for preventing motion sickness, nausea, and vomiting	Causes sedation and drowsiness
Diphenoxylate HCl with	Lomotil, Enoxa, Colonil	Narcotic antidiarrheal	Causes dry mouth, nausea, drowsiness
Loperamide	Imodium	Systemic antidiarrhea	Abdominal discomfort and drowsiness
Common OTC antidiarrheals	Donnagel, Kaopectate, Pepto-Bismol Amogel, Devrom	Relief of diarrhea	Relatively safe with few side effects, although their effectiveness is questionable

Acetaminophen, like aspirin, has both analgesic and antipyretic effects, but it does not have significant anti-inflammatory capabilities. Acetaminophen is indicated for relief of mild somatic pain and for fever reduction through mechanisms similar to those of aspirin.[9]

The primary advantage of acetaminophen for the athlete is that it does not produce gastric irritation or gastrointestinal bleeding. Likewise, it does not affect platelet aggregation and, thus, does not increase clotting time after an injury.

For the athlete who is not in need of some anti-inflammatory medication, but who requires some pain-relieving medication, acetaminophen should be the drug of choice. If inflammation is a consideration, the team physician may elect to use either aspirin or a type of nonsteroidal anti-inflammatory drug (NSAID). Most NSAIDs are prescription medications which, like aspirin, have not only anti-inflammatory, but also analgesic and antipyretic effects. The NSAIDs are effective for patients who cannot tolerate aspirin and who tend to experience gastrointestinal distress associated with aspirin use. Their anti-inflammatory capabilities are thought to be equal to those of aspirin, the advantages being that NSAIDs have fewer side-effects and have relatively longer duration of action. Perhaps the biggest disadvantage of the NSAIDs is that they tend to be expensive.[10] Even though NSAIDs have analgesic and antipyretic capabilities, they should not be used in place of aspirin or acetaminophen for a mild headache or an increased body temperature. However, they can be used to relieve many other mild to moderately painful somatic conditions (i.e., menstrual cramps, soft-tissue injury).[10]

The NSAIDs are used primarily to reduce the pain, stiffness, swelling, redness, and fever associated with localized inflammation. This is probably accomplished by inhibiting the synthesis of prostaglandins. The sports therapist must be aware that inflammation is simply a response to some underlying trauma or condition and that the source of irritation must be corrected or eliminated for these anti-inflammatory medications to be effective.

FIGURE 12-1. Participation in sports activity involves some special consideration for the use of various medications.

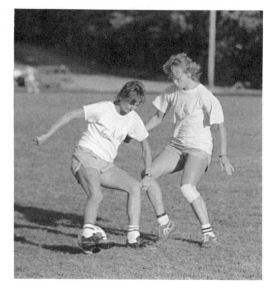

Drugs That Affect the Respiratory Tract

ANTIHISTAMINES

An antihistamine is a drug that reduces the effects of the chemical histamine on various tissues by selectively blocking receptor sites in the body to which histamines attach. Histamine is a chemical that is abundant in the mast cells of the skin and lungs and in the basophils of blood. It is also found in the gastrointestinal tract and in the brain, where it acts as a neurotransmitter.[5] Histamine is released in response to some toxin, physical or chemical agent, drug, or antigen that may be introduced into the system. Thus, it has a major function in many allergic or hypersensitivity reactions.[12]

Antihistamines are most typically used in the treatment of allergic reactions, but they may also be used as an antiemetic in the prevention of nausea and vomiting.[8] Histamine produces a number of systemic responses: (1) swelling and inflammation in the skin or mucous membranes (angioedema), (2) spasm of smooth bronchial muscle (asthma), (3) inflammation of nasal membranes (rhinitis), and (4) the possibility of anaphylaxis.[5] These responses in varying degrees are typical of allergic reactions to insect stings, food reactions, drug hypersensitivities, or anything else that may facilitate the release of histamine.

Histamine produces these reactions by binding with cells that compose the various tissues at specific receptor sites. An antihistamine medication has the capability of competitively blocking these receptor sites, thus preventing the typical histamine response. Antihistamines are classified as either H_1- or H_2-receptor blockers. The so-called true antihistamines affect the H_1-receptors only. The H_2-blockers affect cells in the stomach that secrete hydrochloric acid. It must be remembered that antihistamines do not reverse the effects of histamine, they simply block the receptor sites. An athlete would benefit from the use of different types of antihistamine medications for relief from various types of allergic reactions, prevention of motion sickness, and relief of coughing because of colds or throat irritations.

Athletes, particularly those involved with fall and spring sports, practice outdoors where they are exposed to a number of allergens (e.g., pollen, insects) that potentially can produce a histamine response. Usually, a mild allergic reaction will occur that may be treated by the sports therapist using an over-the-counter (OTC) antihistamine. These medications are most effective in reducing the effects of histamine on the vascular system which include uticaria, rhinitis, and angioedema. These medications are effective in approximately 70% of the patients treated.[5] Chlorpheniramine is the antihistamine that is most commonly used for the treatment of these mild allergic reactions.

A competitive schedule may require the athlete to do a great deal of traveling. It is not uncommon for people riding in a bus, car, or airplane to develop nausea and discomfort in response to motion. This motion sickness may be treated using a number of antihistamine medications. Dimenhydrinate and meclizine are the most commonly used drugs for the prevention of motion sickness. They are best used prophylactically before motion sickness occurs. Like the other antihistamines, the major side-effect produced is drowsiness and sedation.[3]

In the athlete, antihistamines should be administered with caution. The most common side-effects of an antihistamine are that they tend to cause drowsiness and, sometimes, decreased coordination. Both of these side-effects may adversely

affect athletic performance and may potentially predispose the athlete to unnecessary injury. Thus, use of antihistamine medication immediately before athletic
competition is not recommended. The athlete should also be reminded that use of
any antihistamine with consumption of alcohol will markedly increase drowsiness.

DECONGESTANTS

Nasal congestion may be associated with a number of causes including pollinosis
or hay fever; perennial rhinitis, a chronic inflammatory condition that occurs with
constant exposure to an allergen; and infectious rhinitis, which is symptomatic of
the common cold.[16] Antihistamines also have anticholinergic effects and can offer
help to "dry up" a "runny" nose. In addition, nasal congestion may be treated with
sympathomimetic or decongestant medications that may be used topically or orally.
Oxymetazoline is an adrenergic topical nasal decongestant that, when sprayed on
the nasal mucosa, produces prolonged vasoconstriction and reduces edema and
fluid exudation. Pseudoephedrine is also an adrenergic decongestant that is taken
orally. Athletes must use pseudoephedrine carefully if they are sensitive to sweating
or thermo regulatory disorders. Nose drops act more rapidly than do the oral
decongestants and the oral medications cause more side-effects, such as stimulation
of the CNS. However, the oral medications are preferred in long-term use.[10]

Some medications combine both antihistamines and nasal decongestants into
a single tablet, taken orally, that produces relatively lower degrees of drowsiness
and other side-effects.

ANTITUSSIVES AND EXPECTORANTS

Those drugs that suppress coughing are called antitussives. Coughing is a reflex
response to some irritation of the throat or airway. A cough may be termed
productive if some material is cleared, and it is beneficial in removing excessive
mucus or sputum. An unproductive cough may be caused by postnasal drip, dry
air, a sore throat, or anything else that may irritate the throat. An unproductive
cough is of no benefit and should be treated with medication. If the cause of the
cough is dry throat or a sore throat, an expectorant medication may be used to
increase production of fluid in the respiratory system to coat the dry and irritated
mucosal linings.[10]

Antitussive drugs are divided into those that depress the central cough center
in the medulla and may be either narcotic or nonnarcotic drugs, and those that act
peripherally to reduce irritation in the throat or trachea. Codeine and hydrocodone
are two of the more common narcotic antitussives that also have analgesic effects.
These are relatively weak narcotics, which are considered safe. Codeine is found
primarily in liquid form and is often combined with a decongestant, an analgesic,
an expectorant, or an antihistamine. Any liquid preparation that contains codeine
is a prescription medication. The side-effects of codeine include sedation, dizziness,
constipation, and nausea.[5]

The most common nonnarcotic antitussives are diphenhydramine, dextromethorphan, and benzonatate. Perhaps their biggest advantage is that they have
no analgesic effects and will not produce dependence. Diphenhydramine is an an-
tihistamine/antitussive that produces both drowsiness and a drying effect. Dextromethorphan is the most widely used antitussive. It has been shown to be equally

as effective as codeine in medicating an unproductive cough, but it does not cause side-effects that are as severe as those of codeine. Benzonatate causes a local anesthetic action on the stretch receptors in the throat and, thus, dampens the cough reflex. The side-effects include drowsiness and a chilled sensation.[5]

The peripherally acting antitussives are primarily expectorants. Although it is thought that the expectorants increase production of fluid in the throat, there is little experimental evidence to suggest that the use of an expectorant is any more effective than drinking water or sucking a piece of hard candy. Often, an expectorant is combined with some other medication, such as an antihistamine or a decongestant.[4]

The athlete who is in need of antitussive or expectorant medication may benefit greatly from their use. Physical activity only tends to exacerbate the problem of a dry or sore throat, which may be responsible for an unproductive cough. The biggest consideration for the sports therapist would be the effects of other medications (e.g., antihistamines or decongestants) that may also be contained in these fluids or lozenges. The drowsiness, gastric irritability, and lack of coordination that may occur will once again detract from athletic performance.

Drugs That Affect the Gastrointestinal Tract

The gastrointestinal tract is subject to numerous disturbances and disorders that are probably among the most common human ailments. The ailments may include indigestion, nausea, diarrhea, constipation, and the like, that virtually everyone has experienced at one time or another. Because of several factors, such as stress associated with competition, inconsistent travel schedules, eating patterns on road trips, and even motion sickness during travel, the athlete is even more likely to experience gastric upset.

ANTACIDS

The primary function of an antacid is to neutralize acidity in the upper gastrointestinal tract by raising the *p*H and inhibiting the activity of the digestive enzyme pepsin, thus reducing its action on the gastric mucosal nerve endings. Antacids are effective not only for relief of acid indigestion and heartburn but also in the treatment of peptic ulcer. A variety of antacids are available in the market that possess a wide range of acid-neutralizing capabilities and side-effects. It is important for the sports therapist to be aware of these side-effects when selecting one specific antacid preparation.

One of the most commonly used antacid preparations is sodium bicarbonate or baking soda. Sodium bicarbonate quickly neutralizes hydrochloric acid, yielding carbon dioxide gas and water. Sodium bicarbonate is rapidly absorbed by the blood, thereby producing systemic alkalinity. Belching is usually associated with sodium bicarbonate ingestion. It is important to realize that the ingestion of excess sodium bicarbonate will often produce a rebound effect in which the gastric acid secretion is increased in response to an alkaline environment.[18]

Other antacids include alkaline salts that again neutralize hyperacidity but are not easily absorbed in the blood. They also produce disturbances in the lower gastrointestinal tract. Many of these nonsystemic antacids will slow absorption of other medications from the gastrointestinal tract. Ingestion of antacids containing magnesium tend to have a laxative effect, whereas those containing aluminum or calcium seem to cause constipation. Consequently, many of the antacid liquids or tablets are combinations of magnesium and either aluminum or calcium hydroxides.[5] If the use of a specific antacid produces diarrhea, for example, it may be advantageous to select another antacid that is higher in aluminum or calcium content to counteract the effects of the magnesium. Conversely, an antacid high in magnesium content may reduce constipation. Simethicone is a silicone added to many of these preparations to reduce gas, trapped in the upper gastrointestinal tract, through its antifoaming action.[16]

Sodium bicarbonate is best used on a short-term basis for rapid relief of heartburn or acid indigestion because of the subsequent rebound effect, whereas the hydroxide salt preparations may be used on a more long-term basis.

Selection of specific antacids should be based on consideration of their potential side-effects, such as a tendency to produce diarrhea or constipation, and how well the patient tolerates their use in terms of taste, side-effects, and finally cost.[10]

Calcium supplementation for the purpose of increasing calcium uptake by bone and, hence, increasing bone density as a means of reducing the incidence at fractures is being recommended by some sports medicine specialists. Caution should be exercised in ingesting large amounts of calcium carbonate in an antacid because of the potential constipation that may accompany prolonged use.

Another medication used for relief of gastric discomfort is an antihistamine that is an H_2-receptor blocker. Cimetidine inhibits the action of histamine on cells in the stomach that secrete hydrochloric acid. Cimetidine is most typically used for treatment of ulcers. However, its use in the treatment of indigestion is thought to be no more effective than other antiacid preparations.[14]

ANTIEMETICS

The antiemetic drugs are used in the treatment of nausea and vomiting that may result from a variety of causes. Vomiting serves as a means of eliminating irritants from the stomach before they can be absorbed. Most of the time, however, it is not necessary to purge the stomach, and vomiting only serves to make the athlete uncomfortable. Frequently, nausea may be treated by giving the individual carbonated soda, tea, or ice to suck. If nausea and vomiting persist, some medications may be beneficial.

Antiemetics are classified as acting either locally or centrally. The locally acting drugs, such as most of the over-the-counter medications (e.g., Pepto-Bismol, Alka-Seltzer) are topical anesthetics that, reportedly, affect the mucosal lining of the stomach. However, the effects of soothing an upset stomach may be more of a placebo effect.[16] The centrally acting drugs affect the chemoreceptor trigger zone in the medulla by making it less sensitive to irritating nerve impulses from the inner ear or stomach.

A variety of prescription antiemetics can be used for controlling nausea and vomiting including phenothiazines, antihistamines and anticholinergic drugs for preventing motion sickness, and sedative drugs. The primary side-effect of these medications is, again, extreme drowsiness.

The sports therapist should deal with nausea and vomiting by first, using fluids that have a calming effect on the stomach, followed by the administration of one of the locally acting medications. If vomiting persists, the athlete will be drowsy and, thus, may be unable to perform at competitive levels. Also, dehydration and the problems that accompany it is an important consideration for an athlete who has been nauseated and vomiting. Antiemetics may also potentiate central nervous system depressants.

ANTIDIARRHEALS

Diarrhea may result from many causes, but it is generally considered to be a symptom rather than a disease in itself. Diarrhea can occur as a result of emotional stress, allergies to food or drugs, or many different types of intestinal problems. Diarrhea may be acute or chronic. Acute diarrhea is the most common. It comes on suddenly and may be accompanied by nausea, vomiting, chills, and intense abdominal pain. Acute diarrhea typically runs its course very rapidly and symptoms subside once the irritating agent is removed from the system. Chronic diarrhea may result from more serious disease states and may last for weeks.

The athlete suffering from acute diarrhea may be totally incapacitated in terms of being able to perform athletically. Potentially, the major problem of having diarrhea is dehydration. An athlete, particularly when exercising in a hot environment, depends on body fluids to maintain normal temperature. When an individual becomes dehydrated, there is difficulty with regulation of temperature, and the athlete may experience some heat-related problem. The sports therapist's primary concern should be replacing body fluids and electrolytes. Medication may be used on a short-term basis for relief of the symptoms. However, it is important to try and identify the cause of the problem and treat it as well.

Medications used for control of diarrhea are either locally acting or systemic. The locally acting medications most typically contain kaolin, which absorbs other chemicals, and pectin, which sooths irritated bowel. Others contain substances that add bulk to the stool. The effectiveness of the locally acting medications is questionable, although they are considered safe and inexpensive.[6]

The systemic agents, which are generally antiperistaltic or antispasmodic medications, are considered to be much more effective in relieving symptoms of diarrhea, although most of these are prescription drugs. The systemic medications are either opiate derivatives or anticholinergic agents, both of which, in effect, reduce peristalsis. Common side-effects of the systemic antidiarrheals include drowsiness, nausea, dry mouth, and constipation. Long-term use of the opiate drugs may lead to dependence.[2]

If the cause of diarrhea is a noninvasive bacteria, a physician may choose to administer multispectrum antibiotics along with an antiperistaltic agent.

CATHARTICS

Laxatives may be used to empty the gastrointestinal tract and eliminate constipation. Usually constipation may be relieved by proper diet, sufficient fluid intake, and exercise.[10] For the most part, the use of a cathartic medication is not necessary.

An athlete who complains of constipation should first be advised to consume those foods and juices that cause bulk in the feces and stimulate gastrointestinal peristalsis, such as bran cereals, fresh fruits, coffee, and chocolate. Increased fluid intake will also facilitate peristalsis in the bowel.

Generally, it seems as if fewer athletes tend to suffer from constipation than from diarrhea. This may be attributed as much to activity levels as to any other single factor.

If it is necessary to use a laxative medication the bulk-forming laxatives are among the safest, but they should be used only for short periods in addition to other previously indicated dietary modifications.

Use of Antibiotic Medications

Many of the medications discussed previously are over-the-counter medications that may be selected and administered by the sports therapist following the strict guidelines and protocols for adminstration that have been established by the team physician. With infectious diseases, the team physician must be directly involved in the selection of the specific antimicrobial agent. The sports therapist is often the individual who first recognizes the signs of developing infection in the athlete, such as fever, redness, swelling, tenderness, purulent drainage, swollen lymph nodes, and so on. It should be the responsibility of the sports therapist to refer the athlete with a suspected infection to the physician for a total assessment, including physical examination and laboratory tests. The team physician will prescribe an appropriate antibiotic medication for the athlete that is selectively capable of destroying the invading microorganism without affecting the patient.[15] The sports therapist may be asked to provide adjunctive therapy such as applying hot compresses or soaks in antiseptic solutions in the open infections.

For an athlete who is using an antibiotic medication, the sports therapist's role should be to monitor the patient for signs and symptoms of allergic response or drug-induced toxicity. Many individuals will exhibit hypersensitivity reactions to antimicrobial agents. Perhaps the most common reaction occurs with the use of penicillin. Antibiotics are also capable of damaging tissues with which they come into contact. They may damage the mucosa of the stomach and cause diarrhea, nausea, and vomiting. They can also affect kidney function and may interfere with nervous system function. Should these reactions occur, the athlete should be sent back to the physician, who may elect to change to another type of antibiotic medication.[20]

An athlete who has an infection, be it localized or systemic, that requires use of an antibiotic will usually be advised not to train or compete until the infection is under control. The sports therapist should be certain that the athlete adheres to this recommendation, both for the benefit of the infected athlete and to limit the possibility of the infection spreading or being transmitted to other athletes.

Suggested Protocol for Medication Administration

The protocols outlined in Table 12-2 should be viewed as guidelines to the disposition of the athlete/patient. The protocols are aimed at clarifying the use of over-the-counter drugs in the treatment of common problems encountered by the sports therapist with an athletic team. These guidelines do not cover every situation the sports therapist may encounter in assessing and managing the athlete/patient's physical problems. Therefore, physician consultation is recommended whenever there is uncertainty in making a decision about the appropriate care of the athlete.

The sports therapist is responsible for screening the athlete to identify the nature of the presenting illness. Subjective findings, such as onset, duration, medica-
(*Text continues on p. 279*)

TABLE 12-2
Guidelines for Use of OTC Medications*

Observations	Management of Problem	Requires Physician Attention
Headache		
Pain associated with elevated BP, temperature elevation, blurred vision, nausea, vomiting, or history of migraine		✓
Pain across forehead ("garden variety" headache)	Patient may be given acetaminophen. (*See* acetaminophen or aspirin administration protocol)	
Tension headache, occipital pain	Patient may be given acetaminophen. (*See* acetaminophen administration protocol)	
Pain in antrum or forehead associated sinus or nasal congestion.	Patient may be given pseudoephedrine tablets. (*See* protocol on pseudoephedrin administration)	
Head and facial injury		✓
Eye injury		✓
Extremity		
Deformity		✓
Localized pain and tenderness, impaired range-of-motion	First-aid to part as soon as possible. Ice Compression: Ace bandage Elevation Protection: crutches or sling and/or splint If this injury interferes with patient's normal activities, *consult physician within 24 hr*	
Pain with swelling, discoloration, no impaired movement or localized tenderness	Patient may be given acetaminophen. (*See* acetaminophen administration protocol)	✓

(Continued)

TABLE 12-2
Guidelines for Use of OTC Medications (*Continued*)

Observations	Management of Problem	Requires Physician Attention
Temperature		
Higher than or equal to 102°F, orally	Patient may be given acetaminophen. (See acetaminophen administration protocol)	✓
Lower than 102°F but more than 99.8°	Limit exercise of athlete. Do not allow participation in practice.	
	If fever decreases to less than 99.8° degrees, the athlete may participate in practice.	
	If athlete is to be involved in an intercollegiate event, *consult with one of the sports medicine physicians* concerning participation.	
Less than or equal to 99.6°F, orally	Follow management guidelines for fever less than 102° but allow athlete to practice or compete.	
Throat		
History of sore throat, no fever, no chills	Advise saline gargle (½-teaspoon salt in a glass of warm water)	
Sore throat	Patient may also be given throat lozenges. Before administering (a) determine whether patient is allergic to (phenol-containing lozenges. If yes, do not administer.	
	(b) Determine temperature. If fever, manage as outlined in temperature protocol. *Consult physician.*	
Sore throat and/or fever and/or swollen glands		✓
Nose		
Watery discharge	Patient may be given pseudoephedrine tablets. (See pseudoephedrine administration protocols)	

Nasal congestion

Patient may be given oxymetazoline HCl nasal spray. See oxymetazoline administration protocol.

Chest

Dry hacking cough

You may administer generic guaifenesin with dextromethorphan.

Cough with clear mucoid sputum

Before administering determine whether the patient is going to be involved in practice or game within 4 hr from administration of medication. If yes, do not give the above. You may administer one dose, 10 ml. (2 teaspoonfuls). Inform the patient that drowsiness may occur. Repeat doses may be administered every 6 hr. Push fluids, encourage patients to drink as much as possible.

Cough with green or rusty sputum

Severe, persistent cough

Athlete with known seasonal allergies who forgot to bring own medication on trip

Patient may be given chlorpheniramine 4-mg tablets. Before administering, determine:

(a) Is the patient sensitive to chlorphiramine?*

(b) Does the patient have asthma, urinary retention, or glaucoma?*

(c) Is patient going to be involved in training or a game within 4 hr from administration of medication?*

(d) Has the patient taken any other antihistamines, various cold medications, or other medications that cause drowsiness within the last 6 hr?*

*If yes, do not administer. *Consult physician.* You may administer one dose of chlorphanirmaine, 4 mg, one-half or one tablet. Repeat doses may be administered every 4 hr. Inform the patient that drowsiness may occur for 4–6 hr after taking this medication. Avoid alcoholic beverages. Avoid driving or operation of machinery for 6 hr after taking. *Contact physician* if allergic symptoms do not abate.

(Continued)

TABLE 12-2
Guidelines for Use of OTC Medications (*Continued*)

Observations	Management of Problem	Requires Physician Attention
Ears		
Discomfort caused by ears popping	Patient may be given pseudoephedrine tablets or oxymetazoline HCl nasal spray. (*See* pseudoephedrine administration protocol and/or oxymetazoline protocol)	
Earache (or external otitis)	Patient may be given acetaminophen. (*See* acetaminophen administration protocol)	
Recurrent earache		
(a) Associated with dietary indiscretion or tension	You may administer an antacid as a single dose, as defined by label of particular antacid	✓
(b) Associated with abdominal or chest pain		✓
Vomiting, nausea		
No severe distress	Monitor symptoms. Patient may be given dimenhydrinate orally. Same as under motion sickness.	
Vomiting		
Projectile, coffee ground, febrile		✓
Diarrhea		
Associated with abdominal pain or tenderness and/or dehydration, bloody stools, febrile, recurrent diarrhea		✓

✓

Frequent loose stools not associated with any of the above signs or symptoms

Encourage clear liquid diet

Patient may be given a kaolin and pectin solution. Before administering determine: (a) How long has patient had diarrhea? If longer than 48 hr, *see doctor.* (b) Is patient taking any digitalis medications, e.g., digoxin, Lanoxin, Lanoxicaps? If *yes, see doctor.*
You may administer one dose of Kaopectate 6–8 tablespoonfuls. Shake well. Repeat dose after each loose bowel movement until diarrhea is controlled. Should not be used for more than 2 days.
Discontinue use if fever develops, or if diarrhea is *not controlled within 24 hr of treatment, and consult physician.*

Motion Sickness
History of nausea, dizziness, and/or vomiting associated with travel

Patient may be given dimenhydrinate orally. Before administering, determine:
(a) Is the patient sensitive or allergic to any antihistamines?*
(b) Has the patient taken any other antihistamines various cold or other medications that cause sedation, within the last 6 hr?*
(c) Does the patient have asthma, glaucoma, or enlargement of the prostate gland?*
(d) Is the patient going to be involved in practice or game within 4 hr from administration of medication?

*If yes, do not administer.

Administer dose based on body weight, 30–60 min before departure time: Under 150 lb: one 50-mg tablet; over 150 lb: two 50-mg tablets

(Continued)

TABLE 12-2
Guidelines for Use of OTC Medications (Continued)

Observations	Management of Problem	Requires Physician Attention
	*Inform the patient that drowsiness may occur for 4–6 hr after taking this medication. Avoid driving or operation of machinery for 6 hr after taking. If traveling time is extended, another dose may be administered 6 hr after the first dose.	✓

Nausea, Vomiting: Prolonged, Severe

Acetaminophen Administration Protocol: Before administering; determine:
(a) Is the patient allergic to acetaminophen?*
   *If yes, do not give acetaminophen.

You may administer one dose of acetaminophen 325 mg #2. Repeat doses may be administered every 6 hr if needed.
Pseudoephedrin Administration Protocol: Before administering, determine:
(a) Is the patient allergic or sensitive to pseudoephedrine?*
(b) Does the patient have high blood pressure, heart disease, diabetes, urinary retention, glaucoma, or thyroid disease?*
(c) Does the patient have problems with sweating?*
   *If yes, do not give pseudoephedrine.
(d) Do not administer 4 hr before practice or game.

You may administer one dose of pseudoephedrine tablets. Repeat doses may be administered every 6 hr up to four times a day.
Oxymetazoline Administration Protocol: Before administering, determine:
(a) Is the patient allergic or sensitive to oxymetazoline?*
(b) Does the patient react unusually to nose sprays or drops?*
   *If yes, do not administer

You may administer 2–3 sprays of oxymetazoline 0.5% nasal spray into each nostril. Repeat doses may be administered every 12 hr. (The container should be marked with the patient's name and maintained by the trainer for repeat administration.)

*Compiled by Daniel N. Hooker, Ph.D., P.T., A.T.C., and Sandra Hak, Pharm.D., R.P.H., Student Health Service, University of North Carolina.

tions taken, and known allergies, should be included in the screening evaluation, along with the objective findings.

The athlete should always be advised by the sports therapist to seek further evaluation by a sports medicine physician if their symptoms persist or become worse.

DRUG TESTING

Perhaps no other topic related to pharmacology has received more attention from the media during recent years than the use and abuse of drugs by athletes. Much has been written and discussed about the use of performance-enhancing drugs among Olympic athletes, the widespread use of "street drugs" by professional athletes, and the use of pain-relieving drugs by athletes at all levels. Although much of the information being disseminated to the public by the media may be based on hearsay and innuendo, there is no question that the use and abuse of many different types of drugs can have a profound impact on athletic performance.

To say there is growing concern on the part of many experts in the field of sports medicine relative to drug abuse among athletes is a gross understatement. During testing of athletes at all levels to identify individuals who may have some problem with drug abuse is becoming commonplace. The International Olympic Committee has established a list of substances that are banned from use by Olympic athletes (Table 12-3). This list includes both performance-enhancing drugs as well as "street" or "recreational" drugs. The legality and ethics of drug-testing only those individuals involved with sport are still open to debate. The pattern of drug use among athletes may simply reflect that of our society in general.

In many sports medicine settings, the sports therapist is often the individual responsible for performing these drug tests. Detection of these drugs is usually done by urine analysis. Many substances can be detected in urine weeks or even months after use. Athletes will tend to have many questions about what the tests are looking for and what will be the consequences of a positive test. The sports therapist must be totally honest and open about the purpose of drug testing. Positive drug tests should result in drug education, rather than in some type of punitive action.

Familiarity with the banned substances is required by sports therapists working with athletes who will be undergoing drug testing. Many of the over-the-counter drugs used routinely contain substances that are banned. It would be most unfortunate to have an athlete disqualified because of the indiscriminate use of some over-the-counter drug.

Anabolic Steroids

The use of anabolic steroids to increase muscular strength and size appears to be widespread among athletes in many sports (e.g., football, track and field, body building).[17] These steroids have both *anabolic* (causing synthesis of protein) and *androgenic* (having to do with the effects of the male sex hormones) effects. The steroids most commonly used are synthetically produced male hormones that closely resemble testosterone.

TABLE 12-3
Categories of Substances Banned from the Olympic Games (with Examples of Each)

PSYCHOMOTOR STIMULANT DRUGS

Amphetamine
Benzphetamine
Chlorphentermine
Cocaine
Diethylpropion
Dimethylamphetamine
Ethylamphetamine
Fencamfamine
Meclofenoxate
Methylamphetamine
Methylphenidate
Norpseudoephedrine
Pemoline
Phendimetrazine
Phenmetrazine
Phentermine
Pipradrol
Prolintane
and related compounds

SYMPATHOMIMETIC AMINES

Clorprenaline
Ephedrine
Etafedrine
Isoetharine
Isoprenaline
Methoxyphenamine
Methylephedrine
and related compounds

**MISCELLANEOUS CENTRAL NERVOUS
SYSTEM STIMULANTS**

Amiphenazole
Bemegride
Doxapram
Ethamivan
Leptazol
Nikethamide
Picrotoxin
Strychnine
and related compounds

NARCOTIC ANALGESICS

Anileridine
Codeine
Dextromoramide
Dihydrocodeine
Dipipranone
Ethylmorphine
Heroin
Hydrocodone
Hydromorphone
Levorphanol
Methadone
Morphine
Oxocodone
Oxomorphone
Pentazocine
Pethidine
Phenazocine
Piminodine
Thebacon
Trimeperidine
and related compounds

ANABOLIC STEROIDS

Methandienone
Stanozolol
Oxymetholone
Nandrolone decanoate
Nandrolone phenpropionate
and related compounds

(Information from the International Olympic Committee: IOC Medical Controls, 1980).

Anabolic steroids are generally acknowledged to provide the intensively training athlete the potential for temporary increases in muscular strength and body weight. Physical and psychological problems are associated with their use. The improvement in athletic performance seems to be outweighed by potential risk of adverse side-effects.

The Appendix is a Position Statement issued by the American College of Sports Medicine.

CASE 1   **Assessment**

A 19-year-old female soccer player has traveled to an away game which is several hours from her university. During the morning approximately 4 hr before an afternoon game, she indicates to her sports therapist that she is having problems with her allergies. She is sneezing, complains of headache, and has nasal congestion that gives her a "stuffy" feeling. She indicates that she typically has problems with hay fever during this time of year and normally uses medication given to her by the team physician to control these symptoms. However, she has forgotten to bring her medication along with her on the trip.

Management

The sports therapist should administer an antihistamine, such as chlorpheniramine, along with a topical nasal decongestant. The purpose of using these medications is to alleviate the symptoms of perennial rhinitis, so that the young woman may be able to compete comfortably. Before administering the antihistamine, the sports therapist should determine (1) if the patient has any known sensitivity to chlorpheniramine, (2) if the patient has asthma, and (3) if any other antihistamines have been taken in the last 6-hr period. If not, the antihistamine should be effective if taken at least 4 hr before competition. A topical nasal decongestant will work rapidly to relieve her stuffy nose and will still be effective throughout the game. Recommendations for dosages should be closely followed.

CASE 2   **Assessment**

A 16-year-old high school football player has been seen by his family physician and a diagnoses of acute Achilles tendinitis was made. The physician elected to treat this tendinitis by prescribing two aspirin, taken every 6 hr to reduce inflammation. During a Friday evening game, while carrying the ball, the patient was tackled by an opponent. The initial contact occurred between the helmet of the tackler and the anterior right thigh of the ball carrier. The patient immediately complained of intense pain and loss of functional movement. The sports therapist determined that the patient had a deep contusion of the quadriceps muscle. During the next 24-hr period there was considerable swelling and ecchymosis associated with the development of a hematoma in the right anterior thigh.

Management

Although a certain amount of swelling could be expected with any contusion, the extent of bleeding may have been substantially reduced by selecting a different type of anti-inflammatory medication for treating the Achilles tendinitis. Aspirin decreases platelet aggregation and, thus, increases the time required for clotting. Had a non-steroidal anti-inflammatory drug (NSAID) been selected, the likelihood of increased swelling and clotting time after injury would have been greatly reduced. Because the time required for rehabilitation is, to some extent, related to the amount of swelling that occurs, controlling initial bleeding is critical. The sports therapist must rely on ice, compression, and elevation as a means of controlling swelling.

The use of aspirin as an anti-inflammatory drug should be avoided for an athlete who is involved in a contact sport.

REFERENCES

1. Beaver W, Kantor T, Levy G: On guard for aspirin's harmful side effects. Patient Care 13:48, 1975
2. Bertholf C: Protocol, acute diarrhea. Nurs Pract 3:8, 1980
3. Black F, Correia M, Stucker F: Easing proneness to motion sickness. Patient Care 14(6):114, 1980
4. Boyd E: A review of expectorants and inhalants. Int J Clin Pharmacol Ther Toxicol 3:55, 1970
5. Clark J, Queener S, Karb V: Pharmacology Basis of Nursing Practice. St Louis, CV Mosby, 1982
6. Dahr G, Soergel K: Principles of diarrhea therapy. Am Fam Physician 19(1):165, 1979
7. Dretchen K, Hollander D, Kirsner J: Roundup on antacids and anticholinergics. Patient Care 9(6):94, 1975
8. Krausen A: Antihistamines: Guidelines and implications. Annu Rev Otol Rhinol Laryngol 85:686, 1976
9. Koch-Weser J: Acetaminophen. N Eng J Med 255:1297, 1976
10. Malseed R: Pharmacology: Drug Therapy and Nursing Considerations. Philadelphia, JB Lippincott, 1985
11. Moncada S, Vane J: Mode of action of aspirin like drugs. Adv Intern Med 24:1, 1979
12. Pearlman D: Antihistamines: Pharmacology and clinical use. Drugs 12:258, 1976
13. Quick AJ: Salicylates and bleeding: The Aspirin tolerance test. Am J Med Sci 252:265, 1966
14. Rodman M: A fresh look at OTC drug interactions: Antacid preparations. RN 46:84, 1981
15. Rodman M: Antiinfectives you administer choosing the right drug for every job. RN 40:73, 1977
16. Rodman M, Smith D: Clinical Pharmacology in Nursing. Philadelphia, JB Lippincott, 1984
17. Strauss R: Sports Medicine, pp 482–485. Philadelphia, WB Saunders, 1984
18. Texter E, Smart D, Butler R: Antiacids. Am Fam Physician 11(4):111, 1975
19. Vane JR: Inhibition of prostaglandin synthesis as a mechanism of action for aspirin like drugs. Nature 231:232, 1971
20. Weinstein L: Some principles of antibiotic therapy. Ration Drug Ther 11(3):1, 1977

Appendix.
The Use and Abuse of Anabolic-Androgenic Steroids in Sports*

Based on a comprehensive survey of the world literature and a careful analysis of the claims made for and against the efficacy of anabolic–androgenic steroids in improving human physical performance, it is the position of the American College of Sports Medicine that:

1. The administration of anabolic–androgenic steroids to healthy humans below age 50 in medically approved therapeutic doses often does not of itself bring about any significant improvements in strength, aerobic endurance, lean body mass, or body weight.
2. There is no conclusive scientific evidence that extremely large doses of anabolic–androgenic steroids either aid or hinder athletic performance.
3. The prolonged use of oral anabolic–androgenic steroids (C_{17}-alkylated derivatives of testosterone) has resulted in liver disorders in some persons. Some of these disorders are apparently reversible with the cessation of drug usage, but others are not.
4. The administration of anabolic–androgenic steroids to male humans may result in a decrease in testicular size and function and a decrease in sperm production. Although these effects appear to be reversible when small doses of steroids are used for short periods of time, the reversibility of the effects of large doses over extended periods of time is unclear.
5. Serious and continuing efforts should be made to educate male and female athletes, coaches, physical educators, physicians, trainers, and the general public regarding the inconsistent effects of anabolic–androgenic steroids on improvement of human physical performance and the potential dangers of taking certain forms of these substances, especially in large doses, for prolonged periods.

RESEARCH BACKGROUND FOR THE POSITION STATEMENT

This position stand has been developed from an extensive survey and analysis of the world literature in the fields of medicine, physiology, endocrinology, and physical education. Although the reactions of humans to the use of drugs, including hormones or drugs which simulate the actions of natural hormones, are individual and not entirely predictable, some conclusions can nevertheless be drawn with regard to what desirable and what undesirable effects may be achieved. Accordingly, whereas positive effects of drugs may sometimes arise because persons have been led to expect such changes ("placebo" effect) (8), repeated experiments of a similar nature often fail to support the initial positive effects and lead to the conclusion that any positive effect that does exist may not be substantial.

*Position statement issued by the American College of Sports Medicine. Reproduced with permission.

283

1. Administration of testosterone-like synthetic drugs which have anabolic (tissue building) and androgenic (development of male secondary sex characteristics) properties in amounts up to twice those normally prescribed for medical use have been associated with increased strength, lean body mass and/or body weight in some studies (6,19,20,26,27,33,34,36) but not in others (9,10,12,13,21,35,36). One study (13) reported an increase in the amount of weight the steroid group could lift compared with controls but found no difference in isometric strength, which suggests a placebo effect in the drug group, a learning effect or possibly a differential drug effect on isotonic compared with isometric strength. An initial report of enhanced aerobic endurance after administration of an anabolic–androgenic steroid (20) has not been confirmed (6,9,19,21,27). Because of the lack of adequate control groups in many studies it seems likely that some of the positive effects on strength that have been reported are due to "placebo" effects (3,8), but a few apparently well-designed studies have also shown beneficial effects of steroid administration on muscular strength and lean body mass. Some of the discrepancies in results may also be due to differences in the type of drug administered, the method of drug administration, the nature of the exercise programs involved, the duration of the experiment, and individual differences in sensitivity to the administered drug. High protein dietary supplements do not insure the effectiveness of the steroids (13,21,36). Because of the many failures to show improved muscular strength, lean body mass, or body weight after therapeutic doses of anabolic–androgenic steroids it is obvious that for many individuals any benefits are likely to be small and not worth the health risks involved.

2. Testimonial evidence by individual athletes suggests that athletes often use much larger doses of steroids than those ordinarily prescribed by physicians and those evaluated in published research. Because of the health risks involved with the long-term use of high doses and requirements for informed consent, it is unlikely that scientifically acceptable evidence will be forthcoming to evaluate the effectiveness of such large doses of drugs on athletic performance.

3. Alterations of normal liver function have been found in as many as 80% of one series of 69 patients treated with C_{17}-alkylated testosterone derivatives (oral anabolic–androgenic steroids) (29). Cholestasis has been observed histologically in the livers of persons taking these substances (31). These changes appear to be benign and reversible (30). Five reports (4,7,23,31,39) document the occurrence of peliosis hepatitis in 17 patients without evidence of significant liver disease who were treated with C_{17}-alkylated androgenic steroids. Seven of these patients died of liver failure. The first case of hepatocellular carcinoma associated with taking an androgenic–anabolic steroid was reported in 1965 (28). Since then at least 13 other patients taking C_{17}-alkylated androgenic steroids have developed hepatocellular carcinoma (5,11,14,15,16,17,18,25). In some cases dosages as low as 10–15 mg/day taken for only 3 or 4 months have caused liver complications (13,25).

4. Administration of therapeutic doses of androgenic–anabolic steroids in men often (15,22), but not always (1,10,19), reduces the output of testosterone and gonadotropins and reduces spermatogenesis. Some steroids are less potent than others in causing these effects (1). Although these effects on the reproductive system appear to be reversible in animals, the long-term results of taking large doses by humans is unknown.

5. Precise information concerning the abuse of anabolic steroids by female athletes is unavailable. Nevertheless, there is no reason to believe females will not be tempted to adopt the use of these medicines. The use of anabolic steroids by females, particularly those who are either prepubertal or have not attained full growth, is especially dangerous. The undesired side effects include masculinization (2,29,30), disruption of normal growth pattern (30), voice changes (2,30,32), acne (2,29,30,32), hirsutism (29,30,32), and enlargement of the clitoris (29). The long-term effects on reproductive function are unknown, but anabolic steroids may be harmful in this area. Their ability to interfere with the menstrual cycle has been well documented (29).

For these reasons, all concerned with advising, training, coaching, and providing medical care for female athletes should exercise all persuasions available to prevent the use of anabolic steroids by female athletes.

APPENDIX REFERENCES

1. Aakvaag, A. and S.B. Stromme. The effect of mesterolone administration to normal men on the pituitary–testicular function. *Acta Endocrinol.* 77:380–386, 1974.
2. Allen, D.M., M.H. Fine, T.F. Necheles, and W. Dameshek. Oxymetholone therapy in aplastic anemia. *Blood* 32:83–89, July 1968.
3. Ariel, G. and W. Saville. Anabolic steroids: the physiological effects of placebos. *Med. Sci. Sports* 4:124–126, 1972.
4. Bagheri, S.A. and J.L. Boyer. Peliosis hepatitis associated with androgenic–anabolic steroid therapy. *Ann. Intern. Med.* 81:610–618, 1974.
5. Bernstein, M.S., R.L. Hunter and S. Yachrin. Hepatoma and peliosis hepatitis developing in a patient with Fanconi's anemia. *N. Engl. J. Med.* 284:1135–1136, 1971.
6. Bowers, R. and J. Reardon. Effects of methandro-stenolone (Dianabol) on strength development and aerobic capacity. *Med. Sci. Sports* 4:54, 1972.
7. Burger, R.A. and P.M. Marcuse. Peliosis hepatitis, report of a case. *Am. J. Clin. Pathol.* 22:569–573, 1952.
8. Byerly, H. Explaining and exploiting placebo effects. *Prosp. Biol. Med.* 19:423–436, 1976.
9. Casner, S., R. Early, and B.R. Carlson. Anabolic steroid effects on body composition in normal young men. *J. Sports Med. Phys. Fitness* 11:98–103, 1971.
10. Fahey, T.D. and C.H. Brown. The effects of an anabolic steroid on the strength, body composition and endurance of college males when accompanied by a weight training program. *Med. Sci. Sports* 5:272–276, 1973.
11. Farrell, G.C., D.E. Joshua, R.F. Uren, P.J. Baird, K.W. Perkins, and H. Kraienberg. Androgen-induced hepatoma. *Lancet* 1:430–431, 1975.
12. Fowler, Jr., W.M., G.W. Gardner, and G.H. Egstrom. Effect of an anabolic steroid on physical performance of young men. *J. Appl. Physiol.* 20:1038–1040, 1965.
13. Golding, L.A., J.E. Freydinger, and S.S. Fishel. Weight, size and strength–unchanged by steroids. *Physican Sports Med.* 2:39–45, 1974.
14. Guy, J.T. and M.O. Auxlander. Androgenic steroids and hepato-cellular carcinoma. *Lancet* 1:48, 1973.
15. Harkness, R.A., B.H. Kilshaw, and B.M. Hobson. Effects of large doses of anabolic steroids. *Br. J. Sports Med.* 9:70–73, 1975.
16. Henderson, J.T., J. Richmond, and M.D. Sumerling. Androgenic–anabolic steroid therapy and hepato-cellular carcinoma. *Lancet* 1:934, 1972.
17. Johnson, F.L. The association of oral androgenic–anabolic steroids and life threatening disease. *Med. Sci. Sports* 7:284–286, 1975.

18. Johnson, F.L., J.R. Feagler, K.G. Lerner, P.W. Majems, M. Siegel, J.R. Hartman, and E.D. Thomas. Association of androgenic–anabolic steroid therapy with development of hepato-cellular carcinoma. *Lancet* 2:1273–1276, 1972.
19. Johnson, L.C., G. Fisher, L.J. Sylvester, and C.C. Hofheins. Anabolic steroid: Effects on strength, body weight. O_2 uptake and spermatogenesis in mature males. *Med. Sci. Sports* 4:43–45, 1972.
20. Johnson, L.C. and J.P. O'Shea. Anabolic steroid: Effects on strength development. *Science* 164:957–959, 1969.
21. Johnson, L.C., E.S. Roundy, P. Allsen, A.G. Fisher, and L.J. Sylvester. Effect of anabolic steroid treatment on endurance. *Med. Sci. Sports* 7:287–289, 1975.
22. Kilshaw, B.H., R.A. Harkness, B.M. Hobson, and A.W.M. Smith. The effects of large doses of the anabolic steroid, methandrostenolone, on an athlete. *Clin. Endocrinol.* 4:537–541, 1975.
23. Kintzen, W. and J. Silny. Peliosis hepatitis after administration of fluoxymesterone. *Can. Med. Assoc. J.* 83:860–862, 1960.
24. McCredie, K.B. Oxymetholone in refractory anaemia. *Br. J. of Haemtol.* 17:265–273, 1969.
25. Meadows, A.T., J.L. Naiman, and M.V. Valdes-Dapena. Hepatoma associated with andro-gen therapy for aplastic anemia. *J. Pediatr.* 84:109–110, 1974.
26. O'Shea, J.P. The effects of an anabolic steroid on dynamic strength levels of weight lifters. *Nutr. Rep. Int.* 4:363–370, 1971.
27. O'Shea, J.P. and W. Winkler. Biochemical and physical effects of an anabolic steroid in competitive swimmers and weight lifters. *Nutr. Rep. Int.* 2:351–362, 1970.
28. Recant, L. and P. Lacy (eds.). Fanconi's anemia and hepatic cirrhosis. Clinicopathologic Conference. *Am. J. Med.* 39:464–475, 1965.
29. Sanchez-Medal, L., A. Gomez-Leal, L. Duarte, and M. Guadalupe-Rico. Anabolic-androgenic steroids in the treatment of acquired aplastic anemia. *Blood* 34:283–300, 1969.
30. Shahidi, N.T. Androgens and erythropoiesis. *N. Engl. J. Med.* 289:72–79, 1973.
31. Sherlock, S. *Disease of the Liver and Biliary System.* 4th Edition, Philadelphia: F.A. Davis, p. 371, 1968.
32. Silink, J. and B.G. Firkin. An analysis of hypoplastic anaemia with special reference to the use of oxymetholone ("Adroyd") in its therapy. *Aust. Ann. Med.* 17:224–235, 1968.

Index

Page numbers in italic indicate figures; page numbers followed by *t* indicate tables.

A

Absorption, of drugs, in the elderly, physiologic and pharmacokinetic changes in, 148–149
Acetaminophen, 262t, 265
  for pain management, 39, 40t
Acetylcholine, role of, in parasympathetic nervous system, 13
ACTH, for treatment of dermatomyositis, adverse effects of, 199
Acute renal failure, 248
Affective disorders, 210–223
Aging, changes in, effect on drug-taking behavior, 146–147
Agonists
  definition of, 6
  partial, definition of, 6
Albuterol, for management of pulmonary disease, 102t, 103
Alcohol, effect on pregnancy, 92
Allergic disorders, in the elderly, drug therapy for, 162–163
Allergies, in the elderly, drug therapy for, 163
Allopurinol, for treatment of gout, 133
Alpha-adrenergic agents, uses of, 14
Amantadine
  for treatment of influenza type A, 23
  for treatment of parkinsonism, 49
Aminocaproic acid, uses of, 16
Aminoglycosides
  for management of pulmonary disease, 108t, 109
  types of, 11t
Amiodarone hydrochloride, for treatment of dysrhythmias, 68
Amoxicillin, for treatment of acute otitis media in children, 193

Amphetamines, for treatment of depression, 219
Ampicillin
  for treatment of acute otitis media in children, 192–193
  for treatment of bacterial meningitis in children, 190–191
  for treatment of urinary tract infections in children, 194
  uses of, 11t, 12
Analgesics
  for back pain, 232–233, 234t
  for CNS disorders, 19t, 19–20
  narcotic, 19t
    for back pain, 233–234, 235t
    for pain management, 42–43, 43t, 44t
  nonnarcotic, for pain management, 39, 40t
  in sports medicine, 261–265, 262t-264t
Anesthetics
  effect on pregnancy, 93
  local
    for back pain, 240–244
    for pain management, 42
Angina, 69–71
  in the elderly, drug therapy for, 152–153
  treatment of, medications for, 70–71
  types of, 69
Angiotensin-converting enzyme (ACE) inhibitors, for treatment of hypertension, 18, 18t, 62–63
Angiotensin II, for treatment of hypertension, 18, 18t
Ankylosing spondylitis (AS)
  in the elderly, drug therapy for, 163–166
  overview of, 128

viral meningoencephalitis in, 191–192

Chloramphenicol, for treatment of bacterial meningitis in children, 190–191

Chorea
   dopamine agonist-induced, management of, 52
   management of, 50

Chronic renal failure, 248–249

Cimetidine
   for treatment of gastroesophageal reflux in children, 186
   for treatment of gastrointestinal disorders in the elderly, 158
   for treatment of renal dysfunction, adverse effects of, 252

Clindamycin, uses of, 11t, 12

Clofibrate, for lowering cholesterol, 77

Clonidine, for treatment of hypertension, 17, 18t

CNS. *See* Central nervous system

Colchicine, for treatment of gout, 133

Cold, for pain management, 42

Collagen diseases, in children, 196–198

Confusion
   drug-induced, in the elderly, 169–170
   in the elderly, drug therapy for, 162

Congestive heart failure, in the elderly, drug therapy for, 153–155

Constipation, laxatives for treatment of, 29, 30t

Corticosteroids
   for back pain, 238t
   classification of, 41t
   for management of pulmonary disease, 106–107, 107t
   for pain management, 40–41
   for treatment of dermatomyositis, adverse effects of, 199
   for treatment of juvenile rheumatoid arthritis, 197
   adverse effects of, 198

Coumarin drugs, uses of, 15

Cromolyn sodium, for management of pulmonary disease, 106

Cyclophosphamide, for treatment of rheumatoid diseases, 138

Cystic fibrosis, definition of, 98

D

Dantrolene, for treatment of spasticity in children, 55, 200–201

Decongestants, effect on respiratory tract, in sports medicine, 267

Delusions, in schizophrenic disorders, 223

Dementia
   drug-induced, in the elderly, 171
   in the elderly, drug therapy for, 162

Depolarizing agents, description of, 27, 28t

Depression
   antidepressants for treatment of, 217–223, 218t
   case study, 222
   cognitive levels of, 220
   course of the disease, 221
   drug-induced, in the elderly, 169
   in the elderly, drug therapy for, 161–162
   rehabilitation in, 221
   treatment of, drugs for, 23, 24t

Dermatomyositis
   in children, 199
   overview of, 125–126

Desiccated thyroid, for treatment of hypothyroidism in children, 185

Dextrothyroxine, for lowering cholesterol, 77

Diabetes, effect on pregnancy, 92–93

Diabetes mellitus
   insulin for, 33, 33t
   in the elderly, drug therapy for, 158

Dialysis, for treatment of renal dysfunction, 250–251

Diarrhea
   antidiarrheal agents for treatment of, 29–31, 30t
   effect on gastrointestinal tract in sports medicine, 270

Diazepam, for treatment of spasticity in children, 200–201